Evidence-Based Dentistry

Evidence-Based Dentistry

Edited by Preston Bailey

hayle
medical

New York

Hayle Medical,
750 Third Avenue, 9th Floor,
New York, NY 10017, USA

Visit us on the World Wide Web at:
www.haylemedical.com

ISBN: 978-1-63241-567-7

Cataloging-in-Publication Data

Evidence-based dentistry / edited by Preston Bailey.
    p. cm.
Includes bibliographical references and index.
ISBN 978-1-63241-567-7
1. Dentistry. 2. Oral medicine. 3. Teeth. I. Bailey, Preston.
RK51 .E95 2019
617.6--dc23

Table of Contents

Preface

The purpose of the book is to provide a glimpse into the dynamics and to present opinions and studies of some of the scientists engaged in the development of new ideas in the field from very different standpoints. This book will prove useful to students and researchers owing to its high content quality.

The field of dentistry is concerned with the diagnosis, prevention and treatment of disorders, diseases and conditions of the dentition, oral mucosa and oral cavity. Evidence-based dentistry (EBD) is an approach to oral health, which makes use of current scientific data and evidence for guiding decision-making related to a patient's medical and oral health. It allows practitioners to stay abreast of the latest researches and procedures in dentistry in order to provide the best possible care for patients. Modern dentistry applies restorative procedures to treat diseases of the teeth like cavities and dental trauma. For dental caries, the condition may be reversed if caught in its early stages but in its later stages, restorative methods of intervention become vital. The incorporation of dental technologies incorporating digitally-controlled components is an upcoming aspect of dentistry. Some of these technologies are dental lasers, computer-aided implant dentistry, CAD/CAM and intraoral imaging, photogrammetry-based intraoral scanning, etc. This integration makes dental procedures more efficient both for restorative or diagnostic purposes. This book is a valuable compilation of topics, ranging from the basic to the most complex advancements in the field of evidence-based dentistry. It presents this upcoming discipline in the most comprehensible language. The extensive content of this book provides the readers with a thorough understanding of the subject.

At the end, I would like to appreciate all the efforts made by the authors in completing their chapters professionally. I express my deepest gratitude to all of them for contributing to this book by sharing their valuable works. A special thanks to my family and friends for their constant support in this journey.

Editor

Multiple, Multiloculated, and Recurrent Keratocysts of the Mandible and Maxilla in Association with Gorlin-Goltz (Nevoid Basal-Cell Carcinoma) Syndrome: A Pediatric Case Report and Follow-up over 5 Years

P. Santander ⓘ,[1] E. M. C. Schwaibold,[2] F. Bremmer,[3] S. Batschkus,[1] and P. Kauffmann[4]

[1]Department of Orthodontics, University Medical Center, Göttingen, Germany
[2]Institute of Human Genetics, University Medical Center, Göttingen, Germany
[3]Institute of Pathology, University Medical Center, Göttingen, Germany
[4]Department of Maxillofacial Surgery, University Medical Center, Göttingen, Germany

Correspondence should be addressed to P. Santander; petra.santander@med.uni-goettingen.de

Academic Editor: Rui Amaral Mendes

Background. We report a case of multiple keratocysts first diagnosed in an 8-year-old boy. *Case report*. The incidental radiographic finding of a cystic lesion in an 8-year-old boy led to the surgical enucleation and further diagnosis of a keratocyst associated with a tooth crown. In the course of dental maturation from deciduous to permanent teeth, the boy presented new lesions, always associated with the crowns of teeth. Gorlin-Goltz (nevoid basal-cell carcinoma) syndrome was suspected, and the genetic analysis detected a previously undescribed germline variant in the *PTCH1* gene. *Treatment*. This included a surgical removal of the cystic lesions, as well as the affected teeth. *Follow-up*. Due to the high recurrence rate of the keratocysts, frequent radiological checks were performed over a 5-year period.

1. Introduction

Keratocysts are comparatively rare benign neoplasms. In 2005, this formerly designated odontogenic cyst was reclassified by the World Health Organization as a tumor [1] due to its local aggressive and recurrent behavior. This term "tumor," however, has been somewhat controversial due to a lack of clearly described neoplastic etiology. In the new revision by the WHO in 2017 [2], the name of "odontogenic keratocyst" (OKC) was reinstituted [3]. OKCs are mostly solitary lesions that can radiologically present a single chamber or septations. Despite their heterogeneous features, OKCs appear most frequently in the 3rd molar area of the mandible, in the 2–4th decade of life, with a slight predominance in males [4, 5]. The nature and mainly the high recurrence of OKCs is still a matter of discussion. It has been proposed that difficult operative access, leaving affected teeth in place after treatment, cystic satellite formation, and the association with

Gorlin-Goltz syndrome are correlated with a higher recurrence of OKCs [6, 7].

The "Gorlin-Goltz syndrome" has also been called "nevoid basal-cell carcinoma syndrome" or more descriptively "multiple basal epithelioma, jaw cysts, and bifid rib syndrome" [8, 9]. This syndrome is an autosomal dominant condition characterized by the presence of recurrent basal cell carcinoma and skeletal anomalies such as bifid ribs, OKCs, palmar and plantar pits, and other heterogeneous symptoms which often make diagnosis difficult [10–12]. Pathogenic heterozygous variants in the genes *PTCH1*, *PTCH2*, and *SUFU* are associated with Gorlin-Goltz syndrome. Apart from Gorlin-Goltz syndrome, the presence of multiple keratocystic lesions is exceptionally rare. According to the first international colloquium on nevoid basal-cell nevus syndrome [13] and to Evans et al. [14], the diagnosis of a Gorlin-Goltz syndrome should be suspected when (a) one major criteria and molecular confirmation, (b) two

TABLE 1: Diagnostic criteria for nevoid basal-cell carcinoma syndrome. A diagnosis can be made when two major or one major and two minor criteria are fulfilled. Extracted from Evans et al. [14].

Major criteria	Minor criteria
More than two basal cell carcinomas, or BCCs; one BCC at younger than 30 years of age; or more than 10 basal cell nevi	Congenital skeletal anomaly: bifid, fused, splayed or missing rib or bifid, wedged or fused vertebra
Any odontogenic keratocyst (proven on histology) or polyostotic bone cyst	Occipital-frontal circumference, more than 97 percentile, with frontal bossing
Three or more palmar or plantar pits	Cardiac or ovarian fibroma
Ectopic calcification: lamellar or early—at younger than 20 years of age—falx calcification	Medulloblastoma
	Lymphomesenteric cysts
Positive family history of nevoid basal-cell carcinoma syndrome	Congenital malformation such as cleft lip or palate, polydactylism, or eye anomaly (cataract, coloboma, microphthalmos)

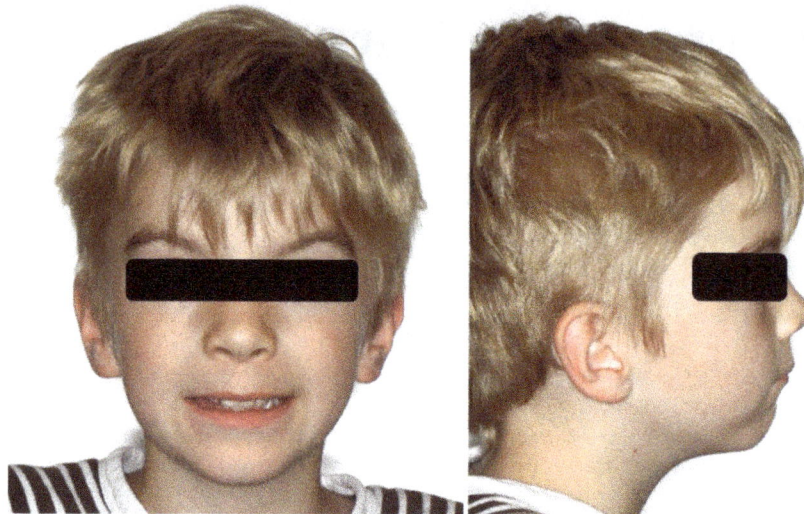

FIGURE 1: Extraoral photographs of the patient at first presentation in 2012.

major criteria, or (c) one major and two minor criteria are found as listed in Table 1.

Due to the high recurrence rate of the OKCs and the consequences of the mostly extensive lesions, different therapeutic approaches and control schemes have been discussed [7]. In the following report, we present a pediatric male patient diagnosed with Gorlin-Goltz syndrome with heterogeneous, recurrent, and multiple OKCs. We describe the surgical management and the development over 5 years after the initial presentation.

2. Case Presentation

The 8-year-old boy first presented in January 2012, having been referred by the family dentist, to the Department of Orthodontics at the Medical Center of the University of Göttingen for a routine orthodontic control and evaluation of treatment need (Figure 1). The clinical examination of the asymptomatic patient showed no extra- or intraoral pathological findings. The medical history of the boy included a mild pulmonary valve stenosis and a secundum atrial septal defect with a left-right shunt. He showed a good physical

and cardiac fitness and a normal nutritional status. The family history was positive for maxillofacial anomalies: the boy's older sister had been previously diagnosed with a dysplastic fibroma, a rare benign fibrovascular defect in the mandible, and a resection of the affected area in the mandible had been performed. His father and paternal grandmother had a positive history of odontogenic cysts as well as basal cell carcinomas, although the family history of OKCs was negative. The radiological examination showed three suspicious hypomineralisations visible as radiolucencies in the panoramic radiograph associated with the retained teeth 13 and 23 and the ectopic tooth 27 (Figure 2). The young patient was referred to the Department of Maxillofacial Surgery for a surgical examination of the radiologic anomalies.

2.1. Treatment. The operation was performed under general anesthesia. The suspected pathological area around teeth 23 and 13 showed no visible intraoperative pathological signs. A bone and soft tissue biopsy for histological examination was taken. In the area of tooth 27, a well-marked membrane was revealed, filled with a viscid fluid and fully enclosing the dental crown. The clinical aspect was consistent with

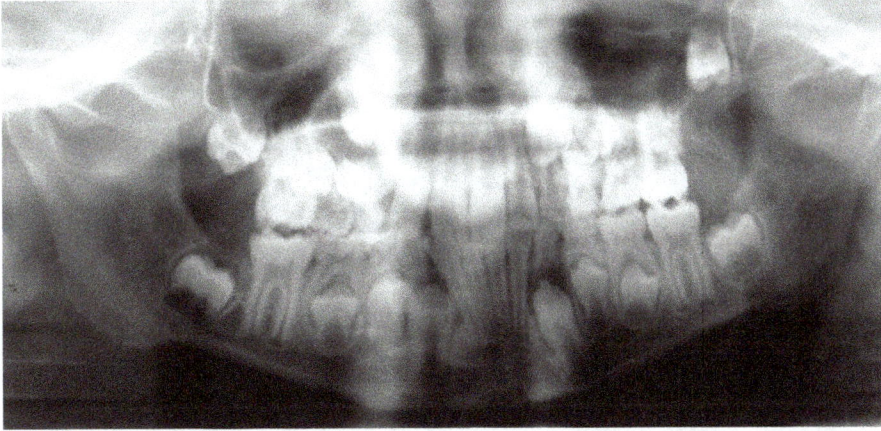

FIGURE 2: Panoramic radiograph (January 2012). Unclear radiolucency at teeth 13 and 23. Ectopic tooth 27.

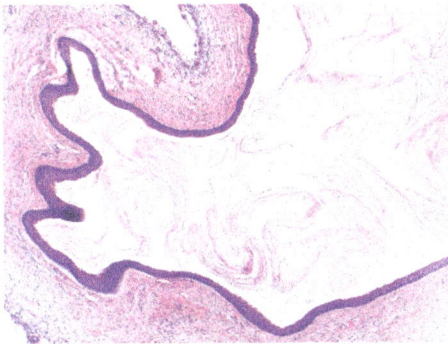

FIGURE 3: Histopathologic specimen (HE stain, 5x magnification).

a follicular cyst. During the radical cystectomy, tooth 27 was removed due to massive attachment loss. The histopathological biopsy showed a fibroosseous lesion in the area of teeth 13 and 23. The biopsy from region 27 showed an odontogenic connective tissue cyst wall with intramural odontogenic cell islands. On request of the surgeon, samples were sent for further diagnosis to the Bone Tumor Reference Center of the Swiss Society of Pathology at the University Hospital in Basel, Switzerland. The initial histological diagnosis was corrected to an OKC of the parakeratin variant. Microscopically, the cyst shows a squamous epithelium. The basal cells are palisading, with hyperchromatic nuclei (HE staining, 5x magnification) (Figure 3). Due to the high recurrence of OKCs, a radiological control interval of 6 months was indicated (Figure 4). Furthermore, orthodontic treatment was initiated.

In August 2014, during a regular radiological control, a new radiolucency was detected, associated with the retained and displaced teeth 47 and 48 (Figure 5). The surgical removal of the cystic lesion and tooth 47 was performed under general anesthesia. The pathological finding was consistent with an OKC.

The regular control examinations were interrupted by missed appointments, so the next evaluation took place one year later, in October 2015 (Figure 6). New radiolucencies

were detected in the panoramic radiograph associated with the retained teeth 18, 17, 37, 38, and 48 as well as an evident enlargement of the radiolucency around the crown of tooth 13. A cone beam computer tomography scan was performed and showed well-defined radiolucent areas, associated with the retained teeth. Details of the surgical enucleation of the cysts with the extraction of teeth 18, 17, 13, 37, 38, and 48 are shown below. The postoperative radiological examination is depicted in Figure 7. Clinical and radiological examinations were then performed every 6 months.

2.2. Surgery. We describe the surgical enucleation of the cystic lesions using the example of the third operation (2015). This was performed under general anesthesia; the affected regions were exposed after lifting a mucoperiosteal flap. After a careful removal of a thin bone cortex, the cystic capsule was found (Figure 8(a)) and separated from the bone with an obtuse instrument. The aim was to leave no epithelial remnants on the trabecular bone. All four lesions were associated with a retained tooth, which was only loosely anchored in the alveolar bone. Due to the high recurrence rate of the cystic lesions in this particular case, all affected teeth were extracted. In the area of the mandible, the use of Carnoy's solution was not indicated because of the exposure of the lower alveolar nerve (Figure 8(e)). Due to their large size, the cystic cavities were filled with a collagen graft, which stabilized the formation of a coagulum. No reconstruction with iliac crest bone or allogenic bone grafts was attempted. Subsequently, the mucoperiosteal flap was reverted back to its original position and fixed by sutures.

By October 2016 and August 2017, bone remodeling of the affected area had been detected and no new lesions were observed (Figures 9 and 10).

Due to the recurrence and the appearance of new lesions, Gorlin-Goltz syndrome was suspected in the patient. After genetic counselling at the Institute of Human Genetics of the University Medical Center of Göttingen, molecular genetic analysis of the genes *PTCH1* and *PTCH2* was performed in 2015. Sanger sequencing revealed the heterozygous germline variant c.2779_2793del (p.Ser927_Val931del)

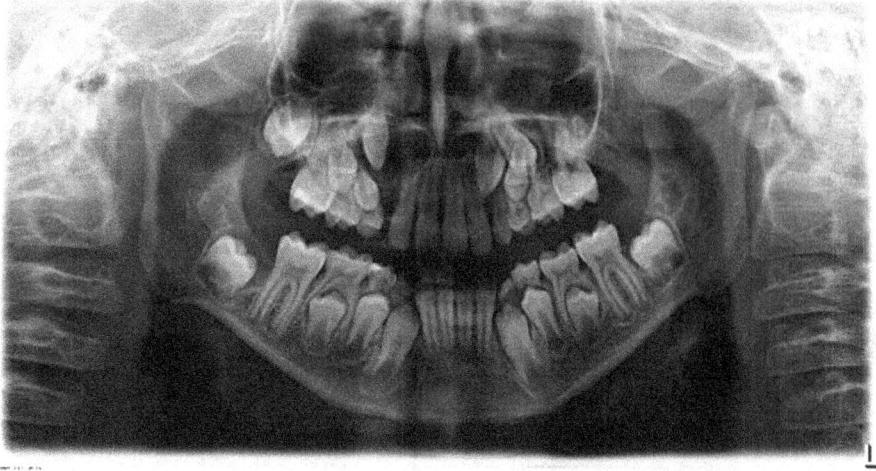

FIGURE 4: Panoramic radiograph (August 2012). 6 months after therapy, the radiolucent area in the region of tooth 23 was controlled. On the basis of the previous pathological findings, no further surgery was indicated.

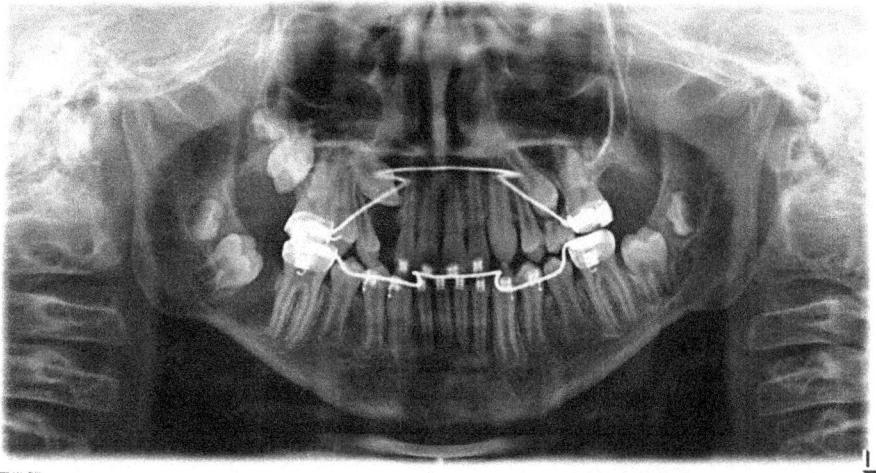

FIGURE 5: Panoramic radiograph (August 2014). Evaluation of the region of tooth 13. No manifest change and therefore no indication for further therapy. Radiolucency around the crown of the retained tooth 47, with indication for cystectomy.

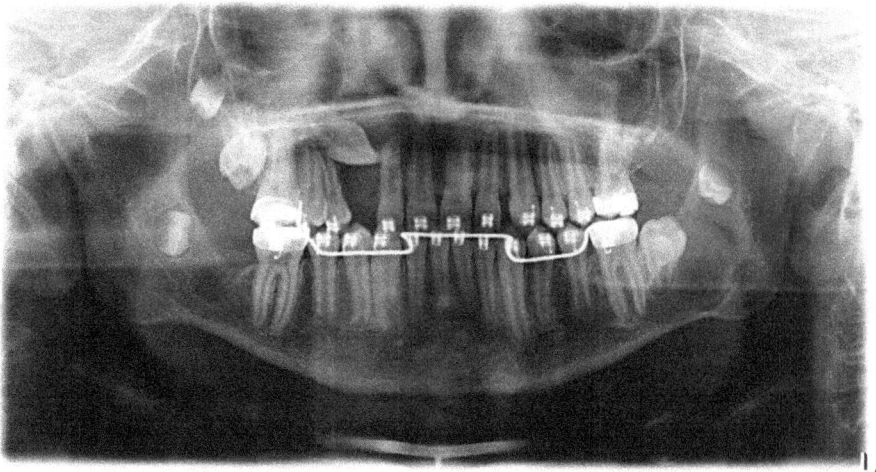

FIGURE 6: Follow-up panoramic radiograph (October 2015) shows a clear enlargement of the translucent area at tooth 13, as well as new changes associated to the crowns of teeth 18, 17, 37, 38, and 48.

Multiple, Multiloculated, and Recurrent Keratocysts of the Mandible and Maxilla...

5

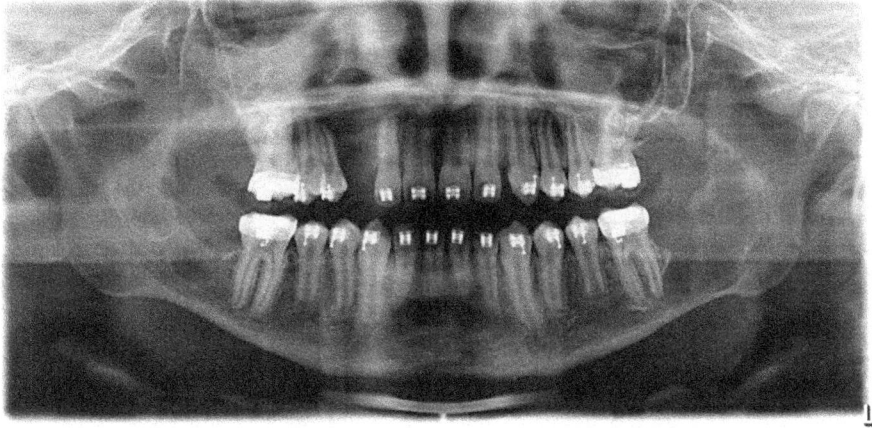

FIGURE 7: Postoperative control panoramic radiograph (October 2015).

in the *PTCH1* gene. This variant leads to an "in-frame" deletion of 5 amino acids between amino acid positions 927 and 931 of the protein. This variant is listed neither in the Human Gene Mutation Database (HGMD) nor in the Leiden Open Variation Database (LOVD). However, a pathogenic effect of the variant seemed likely as many pathogenic variants have already been described in this region of the *PTCH1* gene, even several in-frame deletions [15, 16]. Since the boy's father had shown similar symptoms (odontogenic cysts, basal cell carcinomas) that could be in line with a Gorlin-Goltz syndrome, he, too, was tested for the *PTCH1* variant and resulted to be carrier of the variant.

In summary, clinical and molecular data together with the positive segregation analysis led to the classification of the variant as "probably pathogenic" and being responsible for Gorlin-Goltz syndrome in the patient and his father. The importance of talking precautions (e.g., sun protection due to the high risk of basal cell carcinomas) and regular medical surveillance (e.g., regular orthodontic care and annual dermatologic examinations) was emphasized.

3. Discussion

Gorlin-Goltz syndrome is an autosomal dominant inherited disorder resulting from pathogenic heterozygous germline variants in either of the genes *PTCH1*, *PTCH2*, and *SUFU*. It is relatively rare, and its phenotype can vary with more than 100 anomalies being associated with this syndrome. This diversity in clinical manifestations can lead to misdiagnoses and often to late diagnoses, associated with major bone defects. Hence, the experience of the practitioner, who correctly interprets the signs and draws a connection to a possibly underlying syndrome, and the experience of the pathologist, who is able to identify subtle histological differences, are essential [13].

According to the recommendations of Evans et al. [14] and Lo Muzio et al. [11], initially, no direct link to Gorlin-Goltz syndrome had been established in our patient since only one of the major criteria was fulfilled. The conspicuous repetitive appearance of the cystic lesions, which were all pathologically confirmed as OKCs, led to the

recommendation of performing a genetic evaluation of the patient and his direct relatives. A positive family history of "odontogenic cysts" as well as basal cell carcinoma additionally pointed towards Gorlin-Goltz syndrome. As reported by Kulkarni et al. [17], only a few patients with multiple OKCs have other characteristic symptoms of Gorlin-Goltz syndrome. However, it has been suggested that multiple keratocysts alone may be confirmatory of this syndrome.

According to Casaroto et al. [18], OKCs are often the first manifestation of Gorlin-Goltz syndrome in children. Nevertheless, and as mentioned by Lo Muzio et al. [11], Gorlin-Goltz syndrome should be suspected in pediatric patients under 10 years of age presenting with OKCs at this early age. Reinforcing this recommendation, the study group of Ahn et al. [19] pointed out that 90% of the Gorlin-Goltz syndrome patients presented with OKCs.

The boy's presentation with bilateral or more than three lesions at the same time, which were mainly localized in the posterior region of the mandible and associated with retained teeth, even causing tooth or germ displacement, is also highly associated with Gorlin-Goltz syndrome [20]. This conclusion of Gupta et al. [20] is consistent with the manifestations in the boy. A substantial difference was observed regarding the occurrence of new lesions, since Gupta et al. [20] described that there were no recurrences or new manifestations after an observation period of 11–20 months. This should not be confused with a reoccurrence of the initial lesion. Reoccurrence of OKCs is frequent, ranging from 2.5% to 62%, as reported by Bell and Dierks [21]. As presented in our patient, reoccurrence as well as new lesions can be observed, especially as a manifestation for Gorlin-Goltz syndrome.

Despite not being characteristic of Gorlin-Goltz syndrome, 40% of the OKCs are associated with retained teeth, as mentioned by Díaz-Belenguer et al. [22]. This is a property that makes a differential diagnosis to follicular cysts difficult. Our patient was remarkable for the relation of the cystic lesions and the tooth crown, as all lesions were associated with retained teeth and involved the tooth crown.

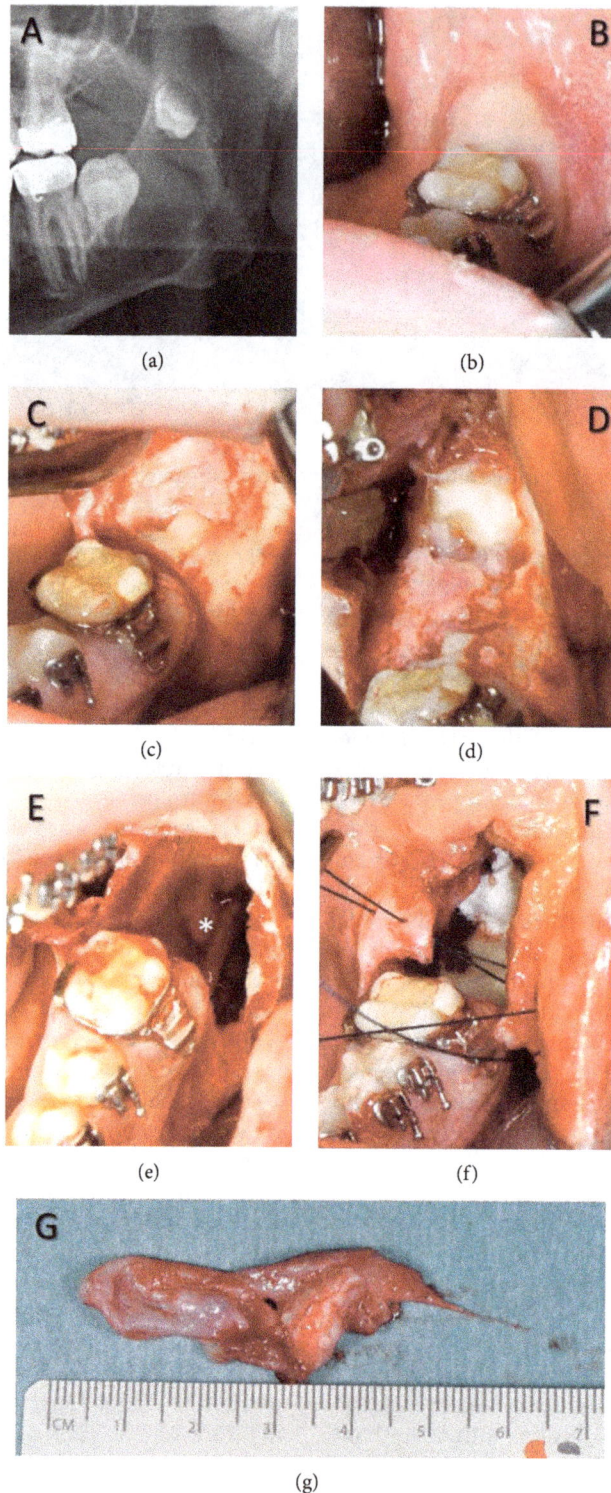

FIGURE 8: Enucleation of the cystic lesion. (a) Radiological finding of the affected area on the left side of the mandible. (b) Clinical situation, tooth 37 is not erupted. (c) Lifting of the mucoperiosteal flap, a perforation of the cortical bone is visible, as well as tooth 37. (d) Exposition of the displaced tooth 38. (e) Clinical situation after radical cystectomy. The lower alveolar nerve is intact and marked with an asterisk (*). (f) Insertion of a collagen graft and suture. (g) Cystic lesion *in toto*.

4. Conclusions

The suspected diagnosis of an OKC is possible with radiological images and should be confirmed histopathologically. Due to the high recurrence risk, regular radiological follow-ups are important for treatment success. A possible presence of Gorlin-Goltz syndrome should be suspected in case of multilocular cysts in pediatric patients, even if further signs of the

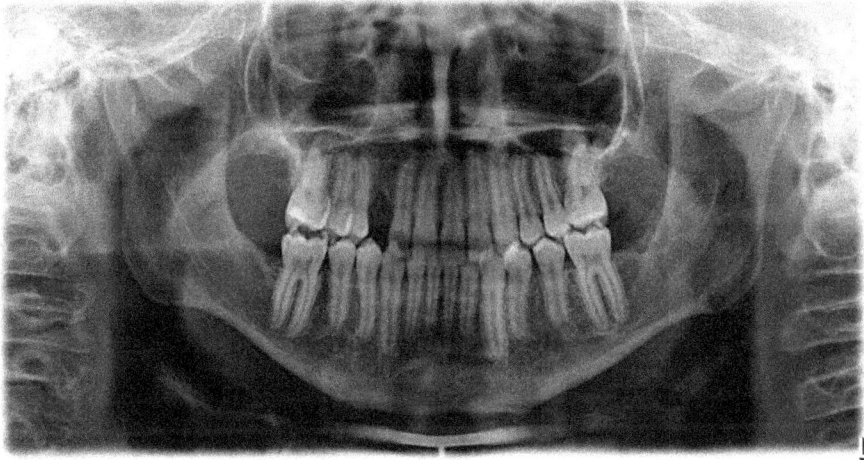

FIGURE 9: Panoramic radiograph (October 2016) 12 months after the third surgery.

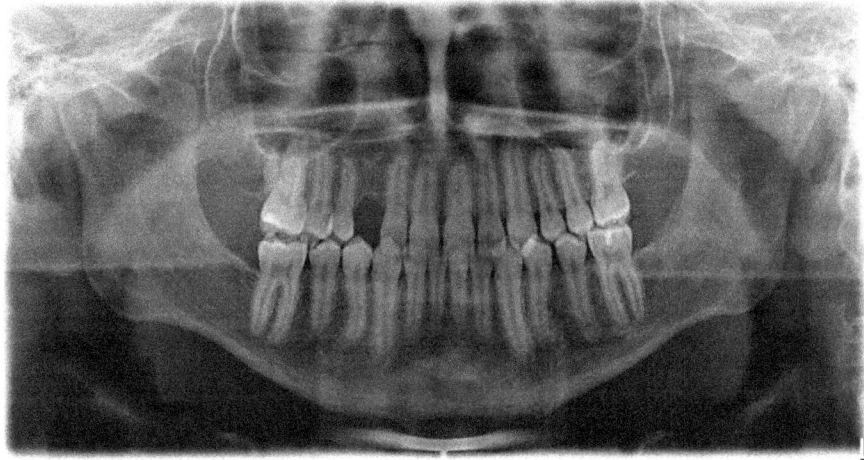

FIGURE 10: Follow-up panoramic radiograph (August 2017). Bone apposition in the former cystic cavities. No new lesions or recurrence is visible.

syndrome are not discernible at first sight and all pediatric patients with OKC diagnosis should be followed into adulthood. A genetic analysis confirms the diagnosis. In our patient, it led to the detection of a new, probably pathogenic germline variant in the *PTCH1* gene.

Consent

Informed consent was obtained from patient and parents.

Disclosure

For author name Schwaibold EMC, the current affiliation is Institute of Human Genetics, Heidelberg University, Heidelberg, Germany.

Acknowledgments

We would like to thank Professor G. Jundt and Professor D. Baumhoer from the Bone Tumor Reference Center and the DÖSAK Reference Registry at the University Hospital in Basel for their support in the histopathological assessment. We would also like to express our gratitude to Professor B. Zoll, Dr. U. Engel, and Dr. F. Schnabel from the Institute for Human Genetics at the University of Göttingen and Dr. H. Skladny from the SYNLAB-MVZ Humangenetik Mannheim GmbH. Without their valuable support, this work would not have been possible.

References

[1] L. Barnes, J. W. Eveson, and P. Reichart, Eds.D. Sidransky, *Pathology and Genetics of Head and Neck Tumours*, L. Barnes, J. W. Eveson, and P. Reichart, Eds., IARC (International Agency for Research on Cancer), Lyon, 2005.

[2] A. K. El-Naggar, J. K. C. Chan, and J. R. Grandis, Eds.T. Takata and P. J. Slootweg, *WHO Classification of Head and Neck Tumours*, A. K. El-Naggar, J. K. C. Chan, and J. R. Grandis, Eds., IARC (International Agency for Research on Cancer), Lyon, 2017.

[3] P. M. Speight and T. Takata, "New tumour entities in the 4th edition of the World Health Organization classification of head and neck tumours: odontogenic and maxillofacial bone tumours," *Virchows Archiv*, vol. 472, no. 3, pp. 331–339, 2017.

[4] P. J. Stoelinga, "Long-term follow-up on keratocysts treated according to a defined protocol," *International Journal of Oral and Maxillofacial Surgery*, vol. 30, no. 1, pp. 14–25, 2001.

[5] J. A. Regezi, "Odontogenic cysts, odontogenic tumors, fibroosseous, and giant cell lesions of the jaws," *Modern pathology*, vol. 15, no. 3, pp. 331–341, 2002.

[6] E. Ahlfors, A. Larsson, and S. Sjögren, "The odontogenic keratocyst: a benign cystic tumor?," *Journal of oral and maxillofacial surgery*, vol. 42, no. 1, pp. 10–19, 1984.

[7] R. A. Mendes, J. F. C. Carvalho, and I. van der Waal, "Characterization and management of the keratocystic odontogenic tumor in relation to its histopathological and biological features," *Oral Oncology*, vol. 46, no. 4, pp. 219–225, 2010.

[8] R. J. Gorlin and R. W. Goltz, "Multiple nevoid basal-cell epithelioma, jaw cysts and bifid rib—a syndrome," *The New England Journal of Medicine*, vol. 262, no. 18, pp. 908–912, 1960.

[9] L. Lo Muzio, "Nevoid basal cell carcinoma syndrome (Gorlin syndrome)," *Orphanet Journal of Rare Diseases*, vol. 3, no. 1, p. 32, 2008.

[10] A. Spiker and M. Ramsey, *Gorlin Syndrome (Basal Cell Nevus)*, StatPearls, Treasure Island, FL, USA, 2017.

[11] L. Lo Muzio, P. Nocini, P. Bucci, G. Pannone, U. Consolo, and M. Procaccini, "Early diagnosis of nevoid basal cell carcinoma syndrome," *JADA*, vol. 130, no. 5, pp. 669–674, 1999.

[12] L. Lo Muzio, P. Nocini, A. Savoia et al., "Nevoid basal cell carcinoma syndrome. Clinical findings in 37 Italian affected individuals," *Clinical Genetics*, vol. 55, no. 1, pp. 34–40, 1999.

[13] A. F. Bree and M. R. Shah, "Consensus statement from the first international colloquium on basal cell nevus syndrome (BCNS)," *American Journal of Medical Genetics Part A*, vol. 155, no. 9, pp. 2091–2097, 2011.

[14] D. G. Evans, E. J. Ladusans, S. Rimmer, L. D. Burnell, N. Thakker, and P. A. Farndon, "Complications of the naevoid basal cell carcinoma syndrome: results of a population based study," *Journal of Medical Genetics*, vol. 30, no. 6, pp. 460–464, 1993.

[15] A. B. Unden, E. Holmberg, B. Lundh-Rozell et al., "Mutations in the human homologue of Drosophila patched (PTCH) in basal cell carcinomas and the Gorlin syndrome: different in vivo mechanisms of PTCH inactivation," *Cancer Research*, vol. 56, no. 20, pp. 4562–4565, 1996.

[16] N. Soufir, B. Gerard, M. Portela et al., "PTCH mutations and deletions in patients with typical nevoid basal cell carcinoma syndrome and in patients with a suspected genetic predisposition to basal cell carcinoma: a French study," *British Journal of Cancer*, vol. 95, no. 4, pp. 548–553, 2006.

[17] G. H. Kulkarni, S. I. Khaji, S. Metkari, H. S. Kulkarni, and R. Kulkarni, "Multiple keratocysts of the mandible in association with Gorlin-Goltz syndrome: a rare case report," *Contemporary clinical dentistry*, vol. 5, no. 3, pp. 419–421, 2014.

[18] A. R. Casaroto, D. C. N. R. Loures, E. Moreschi et al., "Early diagnosis of Gorlin-Goltz syndrome: case report," *Head & Face Medicine*, vol. 7, no. 1, p. 2, 2011.

[19] S.-G. Ahn, Y.-S. Lim, D.-K. Kim, S. G. Kim, S. H. Lee, and J. H. Yoon, "Nevoid basal cell carcinoma syndrome: a retrospective analysis of 33 affected Korean individuals," *International Journal of Oral and Maxillofacial Surgery*, vol. 33, no. 5, pp. 458–462, 2004.

[20] S. R. Gupta, V. Jaetli, S. Mohanty, R. Sharma, and A. Gupta, "Nevoid basal cell carcinoma syndrome in Indian patients: a clinical and radiological study of 6 cases and review of literature," *Oral surgery, oral medicine, oral pathology and oral radiology*, vol. 113, no. 1, pp. 99–110, 2012.

[21] R. B. Bell and E. J. Dierks, "Treatment options for the recurrent odontogenic keratocyst," *Oral and Maxillofacial Surgery Clinics of North America*, vol. 15, no. 3, pp. 429–446, 2003.

[22] Á. Díaz-Belenguer, A. Sánchez-Torres, and C. Gay-Escoda, "Role of Carnoy's solution in the treatment of keratocystic odontogenic tumor: a systematic review," *Medicina oral, patologia oral y cirugia bucal*, vol. 21, no. 6, pp. e689–e695, 2016.

2

A Predictable Aesthetic Rehabilitation of Deciduous Anterior Teeth in Early Childhood Caries

Priyanka Agarwal, Rashmi Nayak⊙, and Ghayathri Elangovan

Department of Pedodontics and Preventive Dentistry, Manipal College of Dental Sciences, Manipal 576104, Karnataka, India

Correspondence should be addressed to Rashmi Nayak; rashmi.nayak@manipal.edu

Academic Editor: Andrea Scribante

Aesthetic dentistry plays a significant role not only in adults but also in pediatric patients. However, a pediatric dentist is faced with the dual problem of satisfying the aesthetic expectations of the patient and parents as well as managing the pediatric patient. In the present era, there are numerous restorative techniques that can be applied to different clinical scenarios. However, we have to choose the technique that best suits our patient, not only biologically but also aesthetically, psychologically, functionally, and financially. The following paper presents the clinical sequence of rehabilitation of severely carious maxillary anterior teeth from left to right lateral incisors in a child with early childhood caries. Severely carious anterior teeth were endodontically treated. The central incisors were restored with gamma loop posts which is mainly used for pediatric patients in endodontically treated teeth. Lateral incisors were treated with Ribbond polyethylene fibre posts. Following this, all the teeth were restored aesthetically with free-hand composite buildup after proper shade selection. The occlusion was restored, and the restorations were finished and polished.

1. Introduction

Early childhood caries is an infectious disease of the primary teeth in children which if not intervened at an early stage can lead to severe destruction of the teeth not only in the primary dentition but can also affect their successors [1]. Inspite of the increasing awareness among parents about dental caries and its ill effects, we are frequently faced with situations when we need to extract the teeth with its imminent consequences. The concept of parents insisting for extraction of an extensively decayed tooth of their child has become obsolete. There has been a paradigm shift in the attitude of parents wherein a good portion of the society is more determined to maintain the primary teeth in the oral cavity of their children for as long as they should naturally last. This expectation of the parents cannot be denied, and the final outcome is that more teeth are being restored than used to be during the last century. Not surprisingly, there are diverse techniques and materials [2] that are being used to maintain the primary teeth in the oral cavity of children in a healthy condition. It is the responsibility of the pediatric dentist to

choose the technique and the material that best suit the patient's condition. Pediatric dentists have to face the dual challenge of restoring severely decayed teeth at the same time managing the behaviour of the child because children are among the youngest and the least adaptable groups of patients. In addition to management problems, there are a number of procedural problems that need to be addressed while restoring primary incisors. Their crowns are short and narrow, while the pulp chamber is large with respect to the size of the crown [3]. In pulpectomised primary anterior teeth where the entire crown is destroyed by the carious process, only a small amount of the tooth structure is available for bonding. Enamel, if and when present, is also less amenable to acid etching than the permanent teeth because of more aprismatic enamel [4]. In many cases, the entire coronal structure is destroyed, sparing only the root and hence only dentine to bond to the restorative materials. Not surprisingly, in the past, and often even now, many of these teeth are extracted [5]. The following paper elaborates the clinical sequence of rehabilitation of severely mutilated maxillary anterior teeth from left to right lateral incisors in a child with early childhood caries.

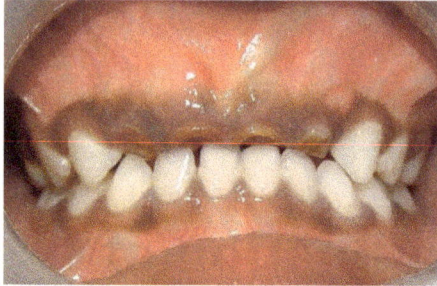

FIGURE 1: Preoperative frontal view.

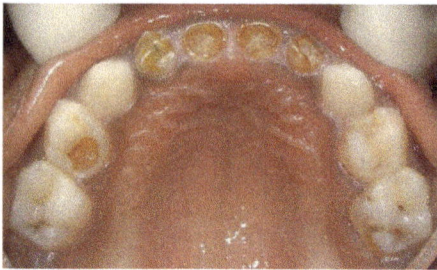

FIGURE 2: Preoperative maxillary occlusal view.

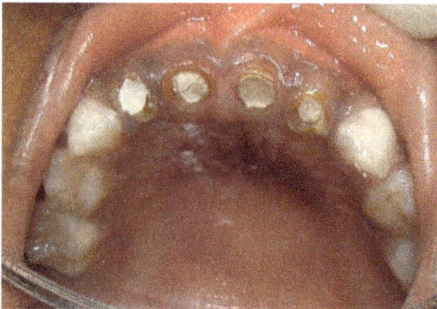

FIGURE 3: Obturated 51, 52, 61, and 62.

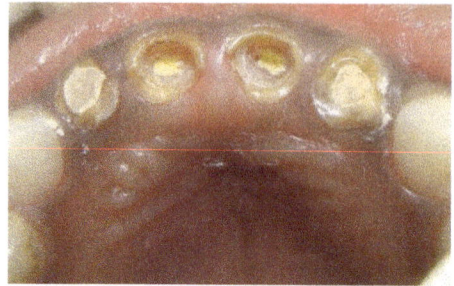

FIGURE 4: Post space preparation 51 and 61.

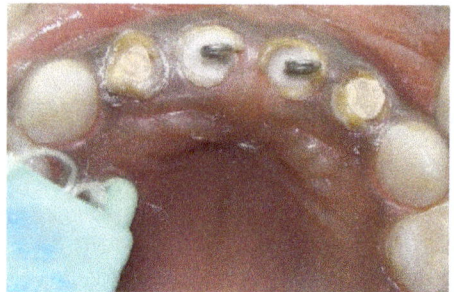

FIGURE 5: Gamma post cemented.

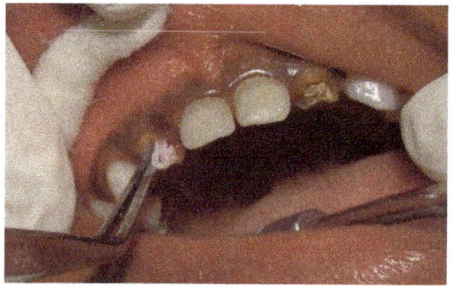

FIGURE 6: Placement of the Ribbond post.

2. Case Report

A four-and-a-half-year-old boy reported along with his parents to the Department of Pedodontics and Preventive Dentistry with the chief complaint of decayed teeth in the upper front region since many months. His medical history was not significant. On intraoral examination, he was found to have several carious lesions with grossly decayed 52, 51, 61, and 62 (Figures 1 and 2) and deep dental caries in 85. However, the radiographs of the maxillary anterior teeth revealed good root length of these teeth (Figure 3). Hence, it was planned to restore the maxillary anterior teeth by performing pulpectomy followed by the post and core for these teeth. The parents were informed, and a written consent was obtained.

3. Clinical Procedure

(i) The maxillary central incisors and lateral incisors were pulpectomised and obturated with Vitapex (Neo Dental Chemical Products Co. Ltd.) (Figure 4).

(ii) Space was created for the intracanal post by removing Vitapex from the canals (coronal 3-4 mm) (Figure 5) with a small spoon excavator, and a thin layer of luting GIC (Luting and Lining Cement, GC Corporation, Tokyo, Japan) was placed over the root canal filling.

(iii) Gamma loop posts (made of a 0.6 mm stainless steel wire) were placed in 51 and 61. Care was taken to secure the posts with a floss for the fear of accidental aspiration until they were cemented in the canal with the help of luting GIC (Figures 6 and 7). Following this, the GIC and the coronal tooth structure were cleaned with saline, dried, etched (Eco-Etch, Ivoclar Vivadent), washed, dried, and cured after application of the bonding agent (Adper™ Single Bond 2, 3M, ESPE).

(iv) The core and crown buildup was done using free-hand buildup with composite resin (Filtek™ Z350 XT, 3M, ESPE) (Figure 8).

(v) 52 and 62 were planned for the Ribbond post (Ribbond Inc., Seattle, Washington, USA).

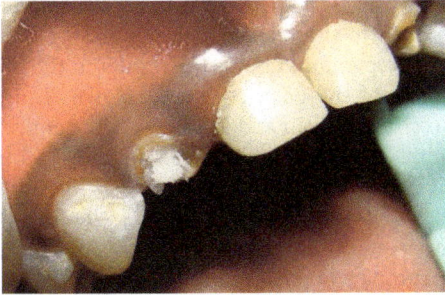

FIGURE 7: Ribbond post cured.

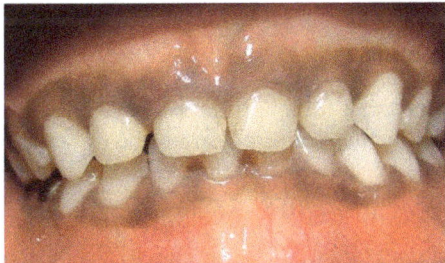

FIGURE 8: Postoperative frontal view.

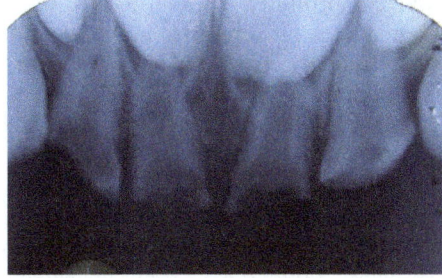

FIGURE 9: Preoperative IOPAR 52, 51, 61, and 62.

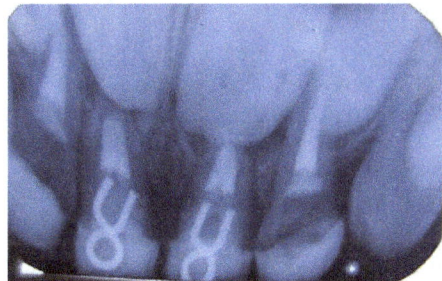

FIGURE 10: IOPA of 51, 61 showing intraradicular gamma post.

(vi) For this, Vitapex was removed from the coronal portion (3 mm) of the root canal. This length of the root canal was measured using a Williams probe.

(vii) The width of Ribbond was decided based on the root canal space available. A 3 mm wide Ribbond fibre was cut to a length double of this measurement plus an excess of 2-3 mm. Care was taken not to contaminate the Ribbond fibre.

(viii) The root canal was prepared to receive the Ribbond post by etching for 15 seconds (Eco-Etch, Ivoclar Vivadent), washing for 30 seconds, and gently air-drying [6], after which the bonding agent was applied (Adper Single Bond 2, 3M, ESPE) and cured.

(ix) The Ribbond fibre was placed on a paper pad and was coated with a layer of unfilled resin (Clinpro™ Sealant, 3M, ESPE). The excess resin was removed by pressing the Ribbond between the prongs of a pair of tweezers.

(x) Following this, the length of the fibre was folded over itself and then inserted in the canal so as to maximise the reinforcement of the canal with the fibre (Figure 8).

(xi) Ribbond was stabilised with flowable composite (G-ænial Universal Flo, GC Corporation, Tokyo, Japan), which was then cured. Care was taken to keep 2-3 mm of the fibre above the cementoenamel junction (Figure 9). The protruding ends of the Ribbond strip aided in reinforcing the core buildup that was done to substitute the missing coronal tooth structure. Utmost caution was exercised to make sure that the resin filled the space between the extended Ribbond strips so as not to leave any voids.

(xii) Free-hand composite build up was done to restore the coronal structure.

(xiii) Occlusal interferences were checked with an articulating paper, and occlusion was restored. Restorations were finished and polished (Figure 10).

(xiv) 54, 55, 64, 65, 74, and 75 were restored with glass ionomer cement (high-strength posterior restorative, GC Corporation, Tokyo, Japan).

(xv) 85 was pulpectomised and restored with a stainless steel crown (Hu-Friedy Pedo Crowns).

4. Discussion

In the past, the only treatment option for severely decayed teeth was to extract them and replace them with a prosthesis till the permanent successors erupted. However, with the numerous techniques and materials [2] available now, we are duty-bound to encourage the parents to succumb to extraction only as a last resort while making every effort to salvage these teeth till their natural exfoliation time. The importance of preserving the primary teeth, the role of primary teeth in preventing future malocclusions, and the consequences of premature loss of primary teeth, if explained to the parents well, will lead to more number of primary teeth being restored rather than being extracted. In the present case also, the parents were convinced to save the primary teeth, although they were so critically broken down.

In order to improvise on retention and stress distribution, the post and core were needed as the coronal tooth structure was compromised [7, 8]. The post interconnects the two fragments and minimises stresses on the tooth structure that is being reinforced [9]. The reconstructed crown will be more stable and will be able to endure masticatory forces in function [10]. A diversity of techniques have been used for intracanal reinforcement of anterior teeth, such as metal screw posts, Ni-Cr coil spring posts, short composite posts, biologic posts which are procured from a tooth bank, short wire posts (omega or gamma loop), ready-made glass fibre posts, and polyethylene fibre posts/Ribbond. The coronal tooth structure may be reestablished by direct incremental composite buildup, composite buildup using celluloid strip crowns, indirect composite buildup, and biological shell crowns [2]. In this patient, gamma loop posts were used for the central incisors and Ribbond posts for the lateral incisors, and the coronal structures were replaced with free-hand direct composite buildup.

Prefabricated posts do not follow the discrete contour of the root canal, although they are quick, inexpensive, and easy to use. Even though metal posts can be used for primary teeth, there is an aesthetic concern owing to their colour. Furthermore, these may affect the resorption of the root during the natural exfoliation. Composite posts offer reasonable esthetics; however, the associated and inherent polymerization shrinkage could result in a compromised retention. The accessibility of a tooth bank is a prerequisite for biological posts which are also still a subject to new studies for future conclusions. Wire loops curved in altered shapes, that is, alpha, gamma, and delta, have long been used by many clinicians as posts for primary teeth. Wire curved in the form of alpha is pressure-bonded within the root canals, and this may cause stresses in the dentine. Although with wire curved in the form of gamma, a success rate of 93% has been reported [2].

Composite materials have been reinforced with different fibre types such as carbon fibres, Kevlar fibres, Vectran fibres, glass fibres, and polyethylene fibres. Carbon fibres avert fatigue fracture and fortify composite materials; however, their colour is dark, which makes them objectionable esthetically. Kevlar fibres made of an aromatic polyamide upsurge the impact strength of composites but are unaesthetic and hence have limited use. Vectran fibres are synthetic fibres made of aromatic polyesters. They possess good abrasion resistance and impact strength, but they are expensive and difficult to manipulate [11]. The adhesion of the polyethylene fibre post to the composite resin matrix is better when compared to the adhesion of the glass fibre post to composite resin. Ribbond fibre posts offer good impact strength to composite resin used for coronal reconstruction. This is because of their modulus of elasticity and flexural strength being close to dentine [2]. In Ribbond, the fibres are not arranged longitudinally and are instead woven in alternating patterns. This arrangement results in improved distribution of the internal tension lines and thus provides fracture resistance [12].

The advantage of using the reinforced composite material as an intracanal post includes resin composite crown reinforcement, translucency, and relative ease of manipulation [11]. The resin adapts to the intimate shape of the canal space ensuring that there would be negligible, if any, voids. It bonds to the resin which is used for building the core and the crown, and hence, it results in the creation of a single block of the post, core, and crown. Thus, there is excellent resistance against debonding of the entire unit and also favourable occlusal force transmission. Another advantage of using Ribbond as a post is that there is no metal which needs to be masked while building the core and crown with composite. After the Ribbond (although opaque in nature) is completely enclosed in the composite, it does not adversely affect the colour of the core or the crown [13]. According to Memarpour et al. [14], polyethylene posts associated with extensive composite restoration show excellent clinical performance.

5. Conclusion

The importance of retaining the primary anterior teeth till their natural exfoliation time cannot be overemphasized. It plays a pivotal role in maintaining esthetics, development of speech, and building up of a confident individual.

Disclosure

This paper has been presented in the IAACD 2017 annual conference (http://conf2017.iaacd.org/freepaperlist.php).

References

[1] Y. Kawashita, M. Kitamura, and T. Saito, "Early childhood caries," *International Journal of Dentistry*, vol. 2011, Article ID 725320, 7 pages, 2011.

[2] N. Mittal, H. P. Bhatia, and K. Haider, "Methods of intracanal reinforcement in primary anterior teeth—assessing the outcomes through a systematic literature review," *International Journal of Clinical Pediatric Dentistry*, vol. 8, no. 1, pp. 48–54, 2015.

[3] W. F. Waggoner, "Restorative dentistry for the primary dentition in pediatric dentistry," in *Infancy through Adolescence*, pp. 341–374, Elsevier Saunders, Philadelphia, PA, USA, 4th edition, 2005.

[4] F. R. Tay and D. H. Pashley, "Etched enamel structure and topography: interface with materials in dental hard tissues and bonding interfacial phenomena and related properties," in *Dental Hard Tissues and Bonding*, pp. 3–33, Springer, Berlin, Germany, 2005.

[5] A. Mortada and N. M. King, "A simplified technique for the restoration of severely mutilated primary anterior teeth," *Journal of Clinical Pediatric Dentistry*, vol. 28, no. 3, pp. 187–192, 2004.

[6] S. Acharya and S. Tandon, "Fiber-reinforced composite: post and core material in a pediatric patient: an alternative to usual," *SRM Journal of Research in Dental Sciences*, vol. 6, no. 3, pp. 206–210, 2015.

[7] R. S. Schwartz and J. W. Robbins, "Post placement and restoration of endodontically treated teeth: a literature review," *Journal of Endodontics*, vol. 30, no. 5, pp. 289–301, 2004.

[8] A. Kumar, S. Tekriwal, B. Rajkumar, V. Gupta, and R. Rastogi, "A review on fibre reinforced composite resins," *Annals of Prosthodontics and Restorative Dentistry*, vol. 2, no. 4, pp. 11–16, 2016.

[9] R. Saha and P. Malik, "Paediatric aesthetic dentistry: a review," *European Journal of Paediatric Dentistry*, vol. 13, no. 1, pp. 6–12, 2012.

[10] V. Khokhar, S. Kawatra, and K. Datta, "Use of glass fiber post for esthetic rehabilitation of severely mutilated primary incisors: case report of 2 cases," *International Journal of Recent Scientific Research*, vol. 7, no. 7, pp. 12359–12362, 2016.

[11] L. Verma and S. Passi, "Glass fibre-reinforced composite post and core used in decayed primary anterior teeth: a case report," *Case Reports in Dentistry*, vol. 2011, Article ID 864254, 4 pages, 2011.

[12] N. Arhun and A. Arman, "Fiber-reinforced technology in multidisciplinary chairside approaches," *Indian Journal of Dental Research*, vol. 19, no. 3, pp. 272–277, 2008.

[13] S. Acharya and S. Tandon, "Fibre-reinforced composite as post and core," *Journal of Clinical and Diagnostic Research*, vol. 8, no. 11, pp. 29–31, 2014.

[14] M. Memarpour and F. Shafiei, "Restoration of primary anterior teeth using intracanal polyethylene fibers and composite: an in vivo study," *Journal of Adhesive Dentistry*, vol. 15, no. 1, pp. 85–91, 2013.

3

Comprehensive Treatment of Severe Periodontal and Periimplant Bone Destruction Caused by Iatrogenic Factors

Gregor-Georg Zafiropoulos (ID),[1] Andreas Parashis (ID),[2] Taha Abdullah,[3] Evangelos Sotiropoulos,[3] and Gordon John[4]

[1]College of Dental Medicine, University of Sharjah, Sharjah, UAE
[2]College of Dentistry, Ohio State University, Columbus, OH, USA
[3]College of Dental Medicine, Mohammed Bin Rashid University of Medicine and Health Sciences, Dubai, UAE
[4]School of Dentistry, University of Duesseldorf, Duesseldorf, Germany

Correspondence should be addressed to Gregor-Georg Zafiropoulos; ggzafi@gmx.de

Academic Editor: Sukumaran Anil

Dental implant success requires placement after periodontal therapy, with adequate bone volume, plaque control, primary stability, control of risk factors, and use of well-designed prostheses. This report describes the surgical and prosthetic management of a patient with severe iatrogenic periodontal/periimplant bone destruction. *Methods.* A 55-year-old female smoker with fixed partial dentures (FPDs) supported on teeth and implants presented with oral pain, swelling, bleeding, and a 10-year history of multiple implant placements and implants/prosthesis failures/replacements. Radiographs showed severe bone loss, subgingival caries, and periapical lesions. All implants and teeth were removed except implants #4 and #10 which served to retain an interim maxillary restoration. Bone defects were covered with nonresorbable dPTFE membranes. In the mandible, three new implants were placed and loaded immediately with a bar-retained temporary denture. *Results.* Seven months postoperatively, the bone defects were regenerated, and three additional mandibular implants were placed. All mandibular implants were splinted and loaded with a removable overdenture. *Conclusions.* In this case, periimplant infection and tissue destruction resulted from the lack of periodontal treatment/maintenance and failure to use evidence-based surgical and loading protocols. Combination therapy resolved the disease and the patient's severe discomfort while providing immediate function and an aesthetic solution.

1. Background

Nowadays, implant-supported restorations are generally accepted as a state-of-the-art treatment option. Many advances in materials and techniques, in surgical and loading protocols, in restorative design as well as a better understanding of the biological/mechanical concepts of osseointegration and of the importance of infection resolution before placement and maintenance, made implants more acceptable by the dental community. Furthermore, appropriate implant treatments are becoming increasingly important also for the general dentists as the number of implants placed per year continues to increase. Gaviria et al. [1] analyzing data of the American Association of Oral and Maxillofacial Surgeons reported that approximately 100,000 to 300,000 dental implants are being placed every year. Also in Germany, the published data showed 200,000 placed implants in the year 2000, and according to statements of scientific societies, the recent number of placed implants is 1.2 million [2].

Periimplantitis, one of the main factors of implant failure, is an inflammatory condition involving the soft and hard tissue surrounding the implant. The 6th European Workshop on Periodontology considered bacterial plaque as the main etiological factor for periimplant tissue damage

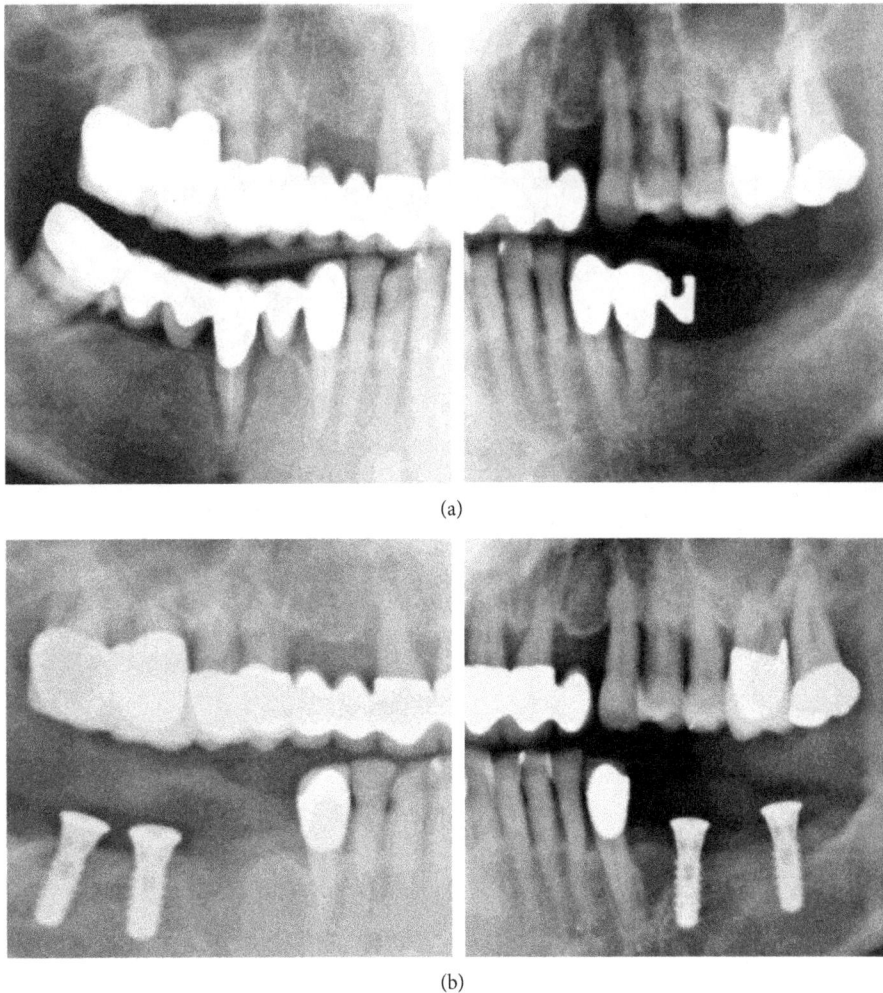

(a)

(b)

FIGURE 1: OPGs (original OPG of previous treatment modified for presentation reasons). (a) Before the initiation of previous treatment (January 2004). (b) After mandibular tooth extraction and implant placement (April 2004).

and also included poor oral hygiene and history of periodontitis as risk indicators [3]. Despite technological, surgical, and material advancements that contribute to enhanced implant survival and/or success, placing dental implants still requires thorough education, training, and continuous professional development in order to acquire the knowledge of which materials, which surgical techniques, which type of loading, and which type of restorations are indicated in every clinical scenario. In other words, implants should be placed by well-trained, qualified clinicians [4].

This report describes the surgical and prosthetic management of a patient with severe iatrogenic periodontal and periimplant bone destruction.

2. Case Presentation

A 55-year-old female, smoker (4–6 cigarettes/day), in good general health presented in our clinic in May 2015 with the chief complaint of strong and acute pain in both arches as well as generalized spontaneous bleeding and suppuration (see Case Management). The patient did not

consent to intraoral photography at the initial visit. She reported that the same dentist had performed all prior treatments.

2.1. Treatment History. In January 2004, generalized severe periodontal disease with deep pockets and severe mobility was diagnosed (Figure 1(a)). The patient was not informed about the presence of or need to treat severe periodontitis. In April 2004, teeth #21, #29, and #32 were extracted, and implants were placed in positions #18, #20, #30, and #31/32 (Figure 1(b)). The bone defect at position #21 was not augmented, and no periodontal treatment was performed. In July 2004, the implants were loaded with fixed partial dentures (FPDs) connecting to teeth #22 and #27 (Figure 2(a)). The bone defect at position #21, periimplant bone loss at position #20, and progressing periodontal disease were not treated.

In January 2006, partial healing of extraction socket #21, a bone defect with periapical involvement (#23), and two periimplant defects (#20 and #31; >50% and <50% implant length, resp.) were diagnosed (Figure 2(b)). Tooth #15 was

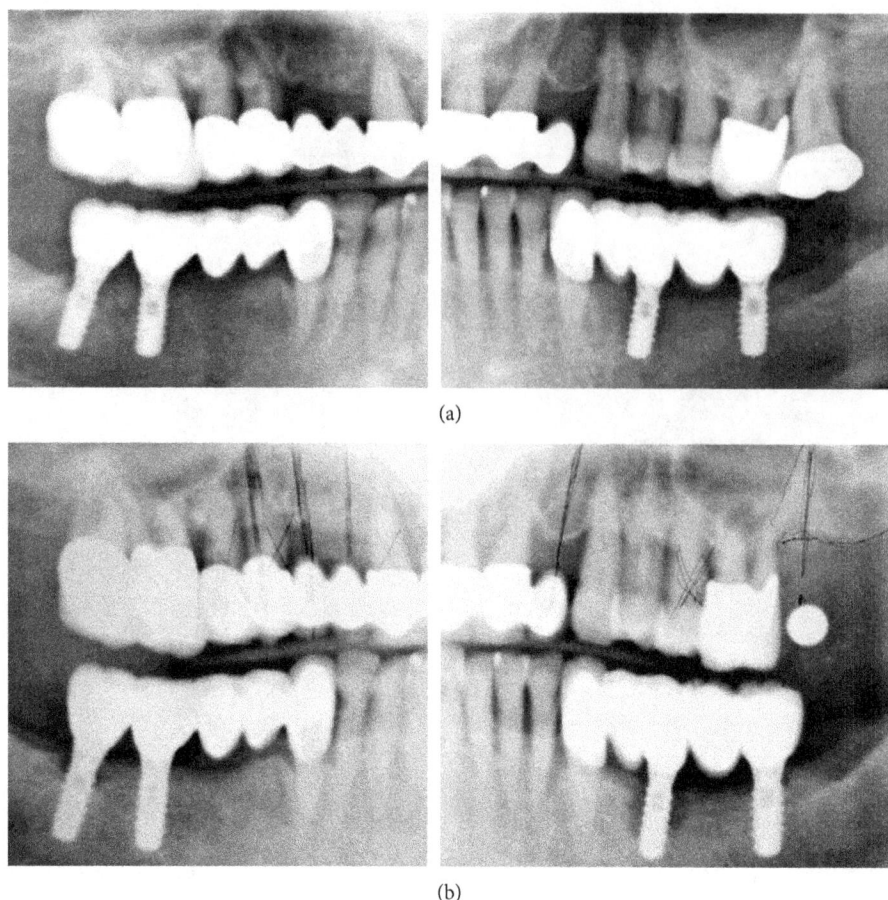

FIGURE 2: OPGs (original OPG of previous treatment modified for presentation reasons). (a) After mandibular implant loading (July 2004). (b) After extraction of tooth #15 (January 2006).

extracted, an implant plan was made (as shown in the orthopantomograph (OPG)), and no further periodontal/periimplant treatment was performed. Between the end of January and October 2006, teeth #5–8, #10, #12, and #15 were extracted; a composite veneered FPD was inserted with teeth #4, #9, and #11 as abutments; and an implant in position #15/16 was placed, but appeared to have only 50% bone contact (Figure 3(a)). No further periodontal/periimplant treatment was performed.

The patient reported visiting the dental office often due to pain, resulting in the fitting of a new maxillary restoration with immediate implant placement and loading in November 2006. The mandibular periimplant defects showed further progression (Figure 3(b)). A new implant in position #15 was placed (compare with implant geometry on Figure 3(a)), tooth #12 was replaced with an implant, and additional implants were placed in positions #1, #4–6, and #8. The new implants had insufficient bone contact; the implant in position #1 had only apical contact with bone. In the subsequent 2 years, the patient complained often about pain and visited the dental office regularly. However, other than superficial cleaning, no periodontal/periimplant treatment was performed.

An OPG taken in November 2009 demonstrated further progression of bone loss (Figure 4(a)). The patient reported

that the dentist in 2010 removed the mandibular FPDs, implants, and the majority of teeth and inserted another fixed restoration with immediate placement and loading, connecting the three implants with teeth #22 and #27. No OPG showing this treatment or follow-up were available. The patient visited the dental office regularly for cleaning and complained of new pain. In 2015, she was referred for periodontal consultation. Comparison of Figures 4(a) and 4(b) shows that the mandibular implants were explanted, and three new implants were placed and loaded.

2.2. Case Management. Comprehensive dental and periodontal examinations were performed, and an OPG was made (Figure 4(b)). All maxillary and mandibular implants and teeth showed radiographic severe bone loss, and teeth #9, #11, and #27 additionally showed subgingival caries and periapical lesions. Periimplant pockets were 6–10 mm deep with spontaneous bleeding, soft-tissue swelling, and pain on palpation.

After receiving oral and written descriptions of the proposed treatment, including surgical procedures, the patient provided written informed consent. To address the acute condition, mandibular periimplant abscesses were drained through the pockets, and clindamycin (800 mg/day) was prescribed, due to the patient's reported allergy to penicillin.

(a)

(b)

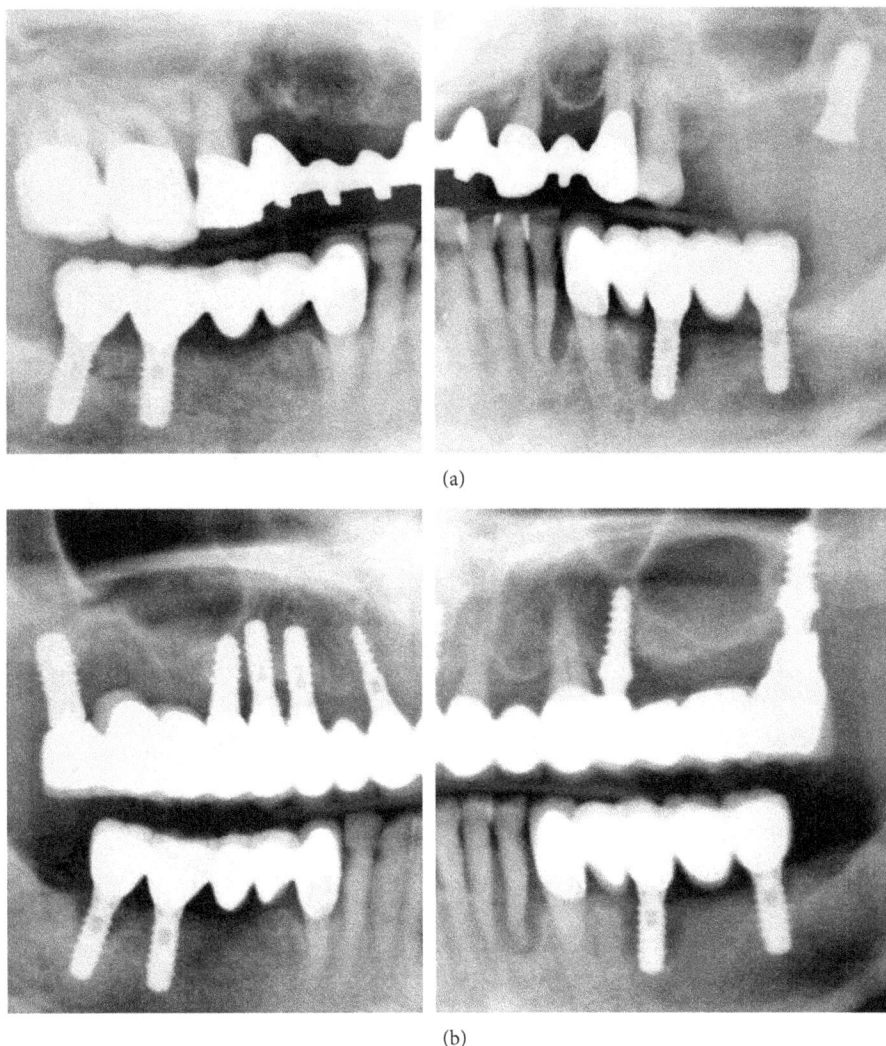

FIGURE 3: OPGs (original OPG of previous treatment modified for presentation reasons). (a) After extraction of tooth #14 and implant placement in position #15/16 (November 2006). (b) After maxillary restoration (November 2007).

The patient's file and radiographs were retrieved from her former dentist.

All mandibular and maxillary implants and teeth were removed, except implants #4 and #10 which served to temporarily retain an interim maxillary restoration. During surgery and after removal of the mandibular teeth and implants and cleaning of the bone defects, a cone beam computed tomograph (CBCT) was made (Figures 5(a) and 5(b)). The extraction sockets and periimplant bone defects were cleaned, and gentamicin-loaded collagen fleeces (Jason; Botiss Biomaterials, Zossen, Germany) were placed in the defects [5]. Subsequently, the defects were covered with nonresorbable dense polytetrafluoroethylene membranes (dPTFE; Cytoplast Ti-250; Osteogenics Biomedical, Lubbock, TX, USA) without additional bone grafting, as previously described [6]. Implants (K3Pro rapid; 3.5 mm diameter, 11 mm length: Argon Dental, Bingen/R, Germany) were placed in positions #24, #26, and #30 and loaded the same day with a bar-retained removable temporary denture. The membranes were removed 4 weeks postoperatively (Figures 5(c), 6(a), and b6(b)). The bar was milled of type 3 CrCo alloy (ZENOTEC NP; Wieland, Pforzheim, Germany), a metal base was constructed, and elastic plastic clips (Preci Matrice, CEKA, Waregem, Belgium) were used to retain the base over the bar.

On the same day, all remaining maxillary teeth and implants, except #4 and #10, were extracted, periimplant lesions on #4 and #10 were treated (Figures 6(c) and 6(d)), and the maxilla was temporarily restored with a milled FPD fixed on the implants #4 and 10 using provisional cement (Implant Provisional; Alvelogro Inc., Snoqualmie, WA, USA) and a removable partial denture for the molar areas (Figure 7).

Seven months postoperatively, the bone defects were regenerated, and three additional mandibular implants were placed in positions #22, #28, and #31/32 (K3Pro rapid; 4.5 mm diameter, 9 and 11 mm lengths, Argon Dental) (Figure 8(a)). All six mandibular implants were splinted with a milled bar and loaded as described previously (Figures 8(b) and 9).

(a)

(b)

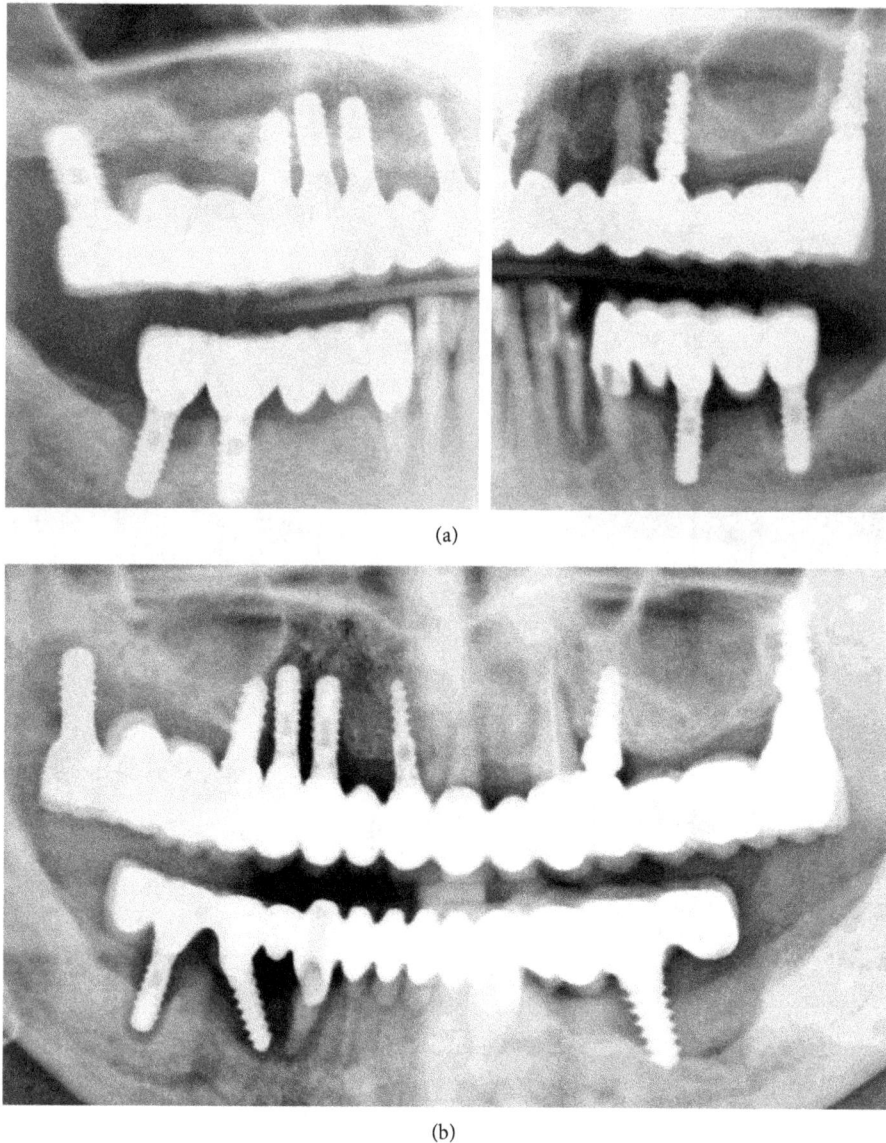

FIGURE 4: OPGs. (a) Further progression of bone loss on November 2009 (not modified radiograph taken during current treatment). (b) At initial examination in June 2015 (not modified radiograph taken during current treatment).

3. Discussion and Conclusions

In the present case report, the surgical and prosthetic management of a patient with multiple teeth and implants with severe bone loss and a hopeless prognosis due to iatrogenic factors, with extractions, bone regeneration, immediate implant placement, and insertion of prosthesis, is discussed. The patient was treated by the same dentist in the period between January 2004 and April 2015.

Dental implant success and survival requires placement after periodontal therapy, adequate bone volume/quality, nontraumatic surgery, primary stability, control of risk factors, and use of well-designed prostheses. In addition, adequate plaque control and regular maintenance (infection control) and early detection and treatment of periimplant inflammation are also important for long-term success [7–14].

Implants in patients treated for periodontal disease are associated with higher incidence of biologic complications and lower survival rates than those in periodontally healthy patients, and severe forms of periodontal disease are associated with higher rates of implant loss [7]. Several studies and systematic reviews have concluded that, before implant placement, any existing periodontal disease must be treated, periodontally susceptible patients have a higher risk of developing periimplantitis, and in cases with periodontally compromised teeth with probing depths >5 mm, the colonization of implants by periodontal pathogens is possible and could be considered as a risk factor. Furthermore, there is evidence that bone loss in periodontitis patients will progress in the absence of periodontal treatment [7–11].

The importance of an accurate diagnosis and an appropriate treatment plan are essential in management of periodontal disease [7]. Based on the radiographs and the

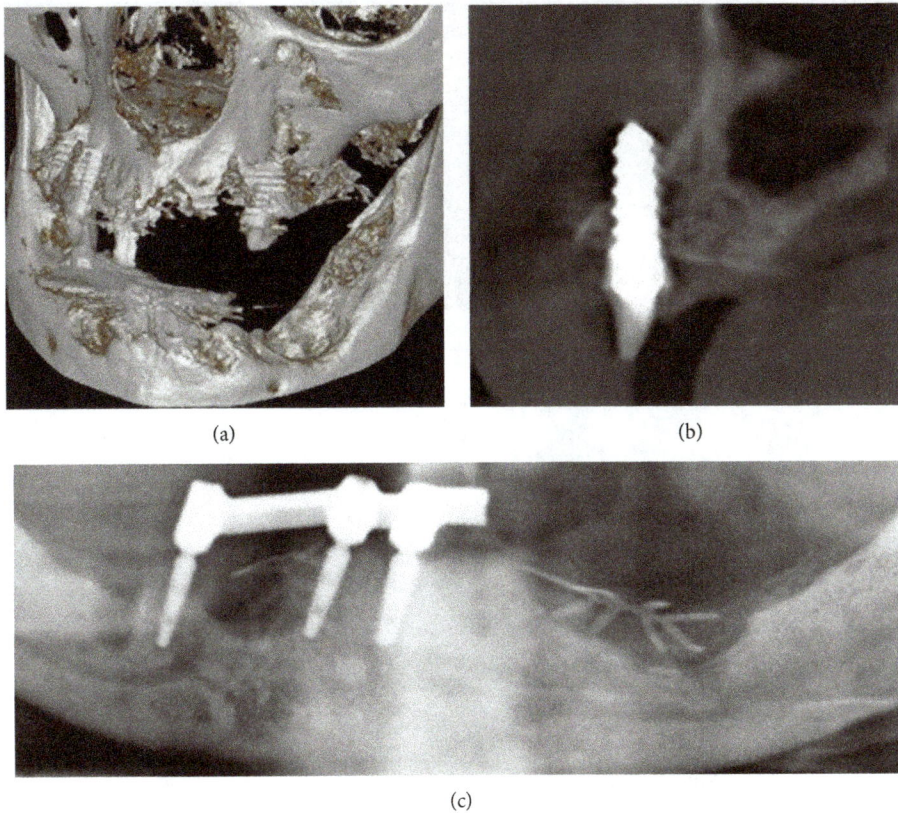

(a)

(b)

(c)

Figure 5: (a) Volumetric 3D representation of hard tissue and maxillary implants, taken during mandibular surgery, demonstrating large bone defects and loss of buccal bone plate in the maxilla. (b) Axial CBCT section of the maxilla showing misplaced implant #4. (c) OPG section showing bar retained on the remaining three mandibular implants (not modified radiograph taken during current treatment).

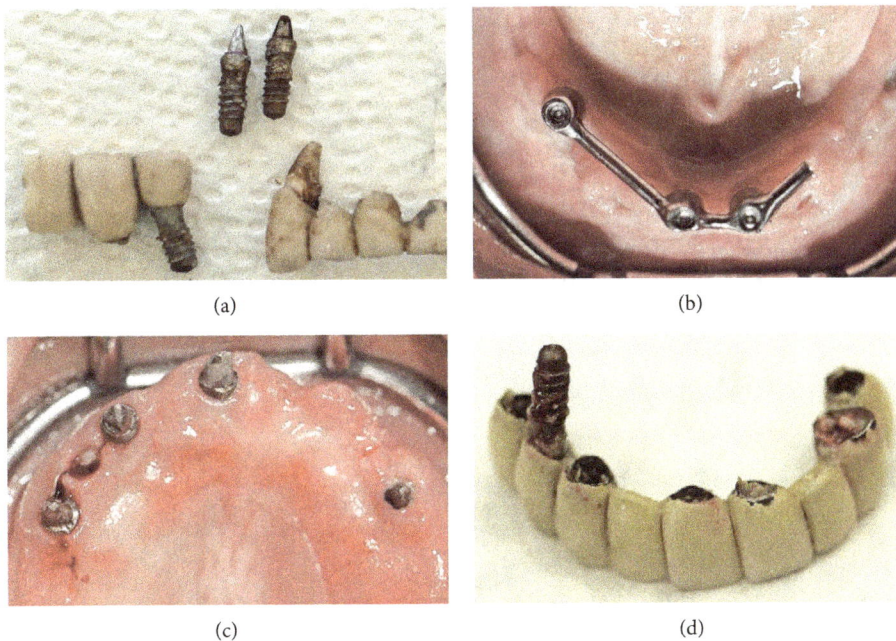

(a)

(b)

(c)

(d)

Figure 6: (a) Explanted mandibular implants and tooth #27. (b) Clinical view of the mandible 4 weeks postoperatively, before membrane removal. (c) The maxilla after FPD removal. (d) Explanted maxillary implant during FPD removal.

information obtained by the patient's file submitted by the previous dentist, one can conclude that she was suffering from severe chronic periodontal disease which was left untreated. In addition, the progression of periimplant inflammation was ignored and not treated although periimplant bone destruction was visible on the regularly taken

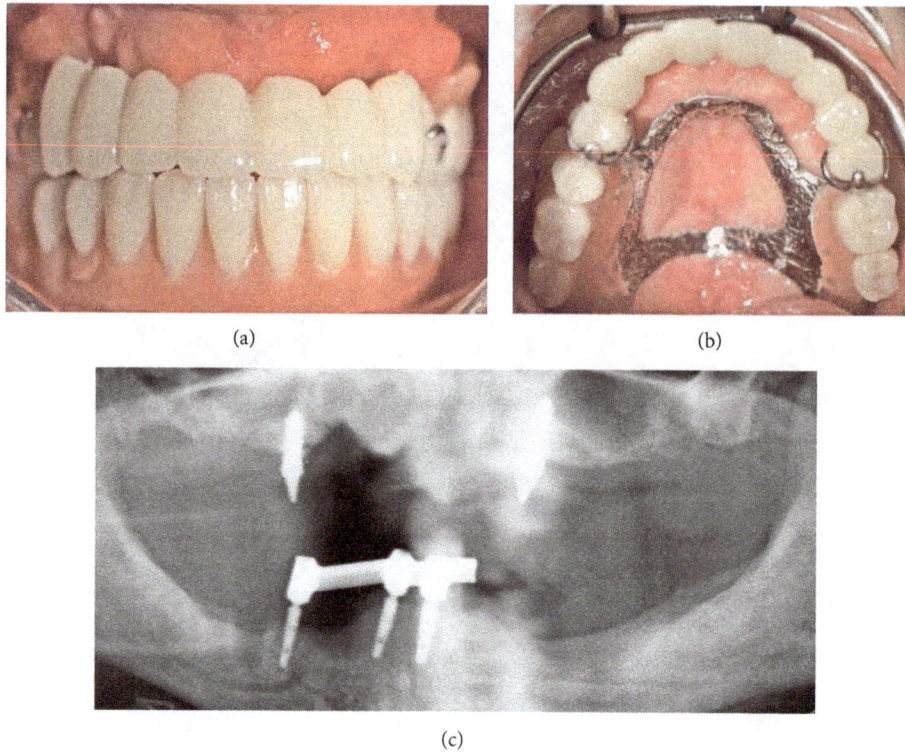

(a)

(b)

(c)

FIGURE 7: (a, b) Maxillary temporary rehabilitation with FPD retained on implants #4 and #10 and removable denture for the molar areas. (c) OPG 4 weeks after surgery with the mandibular overdenture (not modified radiograph taken during current treatment).

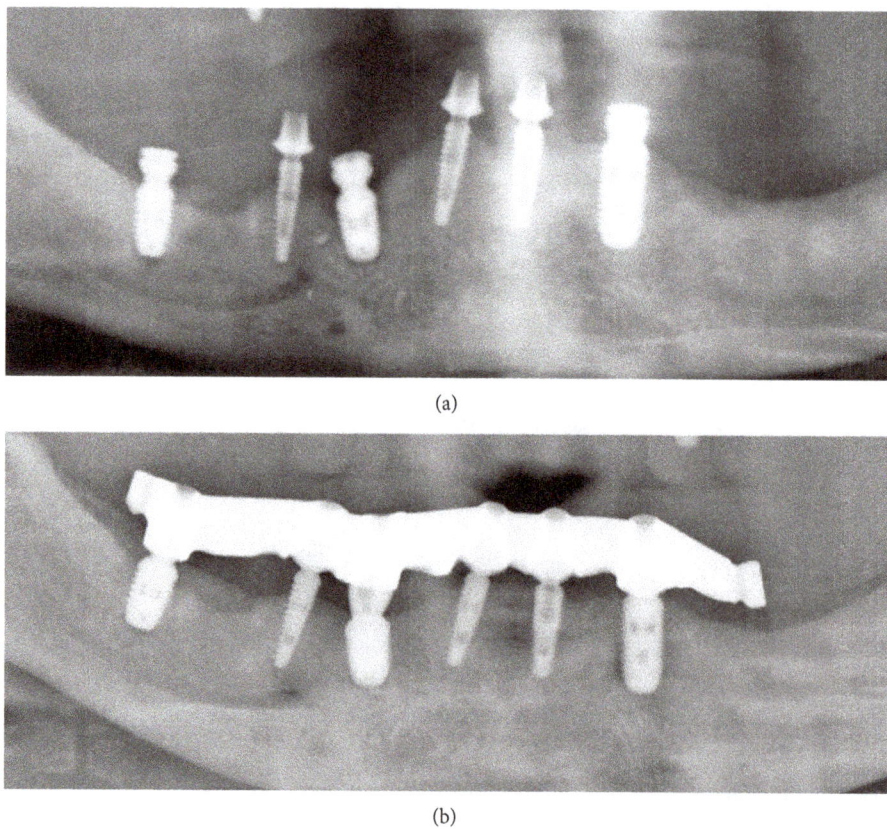

(a)

(b)

FIGURE 8: Mandibular OPG sections eight months postoperatively (not modified radiograph taken during current treatment). (a) After placement of three additional implants. (b) After bar mounting.

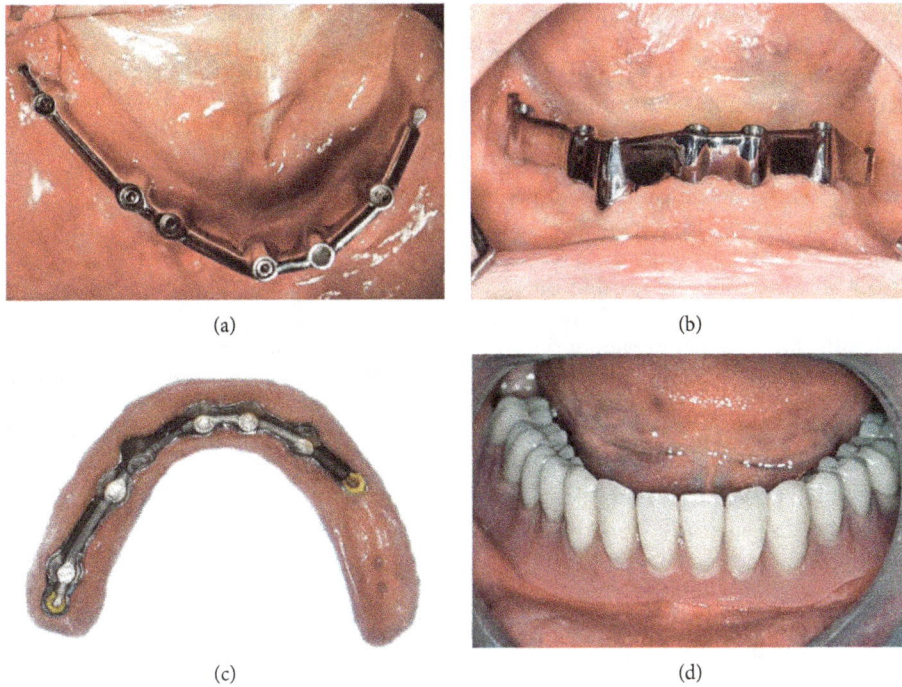

Figure 9: Clinical view of the final mandibular bar restoration after bar mounting. (a) Occlusal view after one week. (b) 30 days after loading. (c) Denture's base. (d) Mandibular denture in situ.

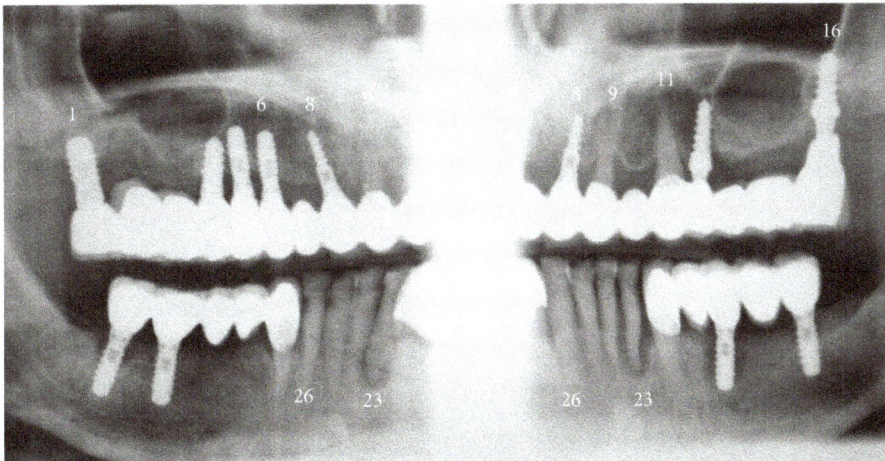

Figure 10: Original not modified OPG of previous treatment with significant distortion. Please compare with Figure 3(b). Double representation of teeth and implants is indicated.

radiographs. The patient reported regular oral hygiene appointments in the dental office but only supragingival debridement was performed.

Currently, there is not enough focus on the prevention of periimplant diseases, as compared to periodontal maintenance [7, 13]. It is well known that, in periodontitis susceptible patients treated with dental implants, residual pockets represent a significant risk for the development of periimplantitis and implant loss. Moreover, patients in supportive periodontal treatment developing reinfections are at greater risk for periimplantitis and implant loss than periodontally stable patients [14].

An additional finding, after examining the patient's file, was the absence of accurate radiographs of diagnostic quality

or the use of surgical guidance for implant placement. The used OPGs were of extremely poor quality, with a double representation of teeth and implants and significant distortion (Figures 1–3, 4(a), and 10). Thus, they had to be processed with a raster graphics editor (Photoshop Elements 15, Adobe Systems, Munich, Germany) for presentation reasons (Figures 1–3 and 4(a)). An accurate diagnosis was not possible on these OPGs, and they should not have been used for surgical planning. Although the use of two- or three-dimensional radiography in all or selected implant cases [15] and the routine use of different types of surgical guides or navigated implantology [16] is still a debate, the use of minimal appropriate diagnostic tools and procedures as well as medical and dental standards is mandatory for a successful result after implant placement.

Another treatment modality, which was repeatedly applied in the presented case, was immediate implant placement and loading in infected and compromized periodontal tissues as well as the connection of teeth and implants. Furthermore, the restorations did not fit on the abutments (Figure 4(b)). These could be additional factors for teeth and implants loss. In the present case, an immediate implant placement and eventually loading could be possible, only by following established rules and clinical protocols as well as guidelines from the scientific literature. However, the lack of knowledge has led to a disaster [4, 17, 18].

Combination therapy resolved the disease and the patient's severe discomfort while providing immediate function and an aesthetic solution. Patient's rehabilitation was achieved by elimination of the infection, bone regeneration, and implant placement. In the mandible, three implants were placed during the first surgery, splinted and loaded with an overdenture, restoring function, and aesthetics. In addition, the bar-retained mandibular overdenture protected the augmented areas from pressure during the healing period. In the maxilla, implants were removed, periimplant lesions in the remaining two implants were treated, and an aesthetic and functionally acceptable long-term provisional restoration was fabricated.

The long-term periodontal and periimplant infection and tissue destruction presented in this case resulted from lack of periodontal and periimplant treatment as well as maintenance and failure to use evidence-based diagnostic, surgical, and restorative procedures. Combination therapy resolved the disease and the patient's severe discomfort while providing immediate function and an aesthetic solution.

References

[1] L. Gaviria, J. P. Salcido, T. Guda, and J. L. Ong, "Current trends in dental implants," *Journal of the Korean Association of Oral and Maxillofacial Surgeons*, vol. 40, no. 2, pp. 50–60, 2014.

[2] S. Paleczek, *Bruchfestigkeit provisorischer Bruecken gelagert auf Implantaten bzw. Implantaten und Zaehne*, Doctoral Thesis, University of Regensburg, Regensburg, Germany, 2010.

[3] J. Lindhe, J. Meyle, and Group D of European Workshop on Periodontology, "Peri-implant diseases: Consensus Report of the Sixth European Workshop on Periodontology," *Journal of Clinical Periodontology*, vol. 35, no. 8, pp. 282–285, 2008.

[4] N. Harel, Z. Ormianer, E. Zecharia, and A. Meirowitz, "Consequences of experience and specialist training on the fabrication of implant-supported prostheses: a survey," *Journal of Prosthetic Dentistry*, vol. 117, no. 6, pp. 743–748, 2016.

[5] O. Kilian, H. Hossain, I. Flesch et al., "Elution kinetics, antimicrobial efficacy, and degradation and microvasculature of a new gentamicin-loaded collagen fleece," *Journal of Biomedical Materials Research Part B: Applied Biomaterials*, vol. 90B, no. 1, pp. 210–222, 2009.

[6] O. Hoffmann, B. K. Bartee, C. Beaumont, A. Kasaj, G. Deli, and G. G. Zafiropoulos, "Alveolar bone preservation in extraction sockets using non-resorbable dPTFE membranes: a retrospective non-randomized study," *Journal of Periodontology*, vol. 79, no. 8, pp. 1355–1369, 2008.

[7] N. Donos, L. Laurell, and N. Mardas, "Hierarchical decisions on teeth vs. implants in the periodontitis-susceptible patient: the modern dilemma," *Periodontology 2000*, vol. 59, no. 1, pp. 89–110, 2012.

[8] M. A. Stokman, A. J. van Winkelhoff, A. Vissink, F. K. Spijkervet, and G. M. Raghoebar, "Bacterial colonization of the peri-implant sulcus in dentate patients: a prospective observational study," *Clinical Oral Investigations*, vol. 21, no. 2, pp. 717–724, 2017.

[9] S. Eick, C. A. Ramseier, K. Rothenberger, U Brägger, D. Buser, and G. E. Salvi, "Microbiota at teeth and implants in partially edentulous patients. A 10-year retrospective study," *Clinical Oral Implants Research*, vol. 27, no. 2, pp. 218–225, 2016.

[10] G. Kalykakis, G.-G. Zafiropoulos, M. Yildirim, H. Spiekermann, and R. J. Nisengard, "Clinical and microbiological status of osseointegrated implants," *Journal of Periodontology*, vol. 65, no. 8, pp. 766–770, 1994.

[11] H. Wennström and N. P. Lang, "Treatment planning for implant therapy in the periodontally compromised patient," in *Textbook of Clinical Periodontology and Implant Dentistry*, J. Lindhe, N. P. Lang, and T. Karring, Eds., pp. 675–686, Blackwell Munksgaard, Oxford, UK, 5th edition, 2008.

[12] A. Ramanauskaite and T. Tervonen, "The efficacy of supportive peri-implant therapies in preventing peri-implantitis and implant loss: a systematic review of the literature," *Journal of Oral and Maxillofacial Research*, vol. 7, no. 3, p. e12, 2016.

[13] B. E. Pjetursson, C. Helbling, H. P. Weber et al., "Peri-implantitis susceptibility as it relates to periodontal therapy and supportive care," *Clinical Oral Implants Research*, vol. 23, no. 7, pp. 888–894, 2012.

[14] G. C. Armitage and P. Xenoudi, "Post-treatment supportive care for the natural dentition and dental implants," *Periodontology 2000*, vol. 71, no. 1, pp. 164–184, 2016.

[15] M. M. Bornstein, K. Horner, and R. Jacobs, "Use of cone beam computed tomography in implant dentistry: current concepts, indications and limitations for clinical practice and research," *Periodontology 2000*, vol. 73, no. 1, pp. 51–72, 2017.

[16] M. Vercruyssen, T. Fortin, G. Widmann, R. Jacobs, and M. Quirynen, "Different techniques of static/dynamic guided implant surgery: modalities and indications," *Periodontology 2000*, vol. 66, no. 1, pp. 214–227, 2014.

[17] O. Hoffmann and G. G. Zafiropoulos, "Tooth-implant connection: a review," *Journal of Oral Implantology*, vol. 38, no. 2, pp. 194–200, 2012.

[18] D. P. Tarnow, S. J. Chu, and P. D. Fletcher, "Clinical decisions: determining when to save or remove an ailing implant," *Compendium of Continuing Education in Dentistry*, vol. 37, pp. 233–243, 2016.

4

Soft-Tissue Chondroma of Anterior Gingiva: A Rare Entity

Dhana Lakshmi Jeyasivanesan ⓘ**, Shameena Pazhaningal Mohamed** ⓘ**, and Deepak Pandiar**

Department of Oral Pathology and Microbiology, Government Dental College, Kozhikode, India

Correspondence should be addressed to Dhana Lakshmi Jeyasivanesan; dhanikamds@gmail.com

Academic Editor: Giuseppe Colella

Soft-tissue chondroma is a rare, benign, slow-growing tumor made up of heterotopic cartilaginous tissue. It occurs most commonly in the third and fourth decades in the hands and feet. Oral soft-tissue chondromas are uncommon and soft-tissue chondroma of gingiva is extremely uncommon. Here, we report an unusual case of soft-tissue chondroma of gingiva in a 50-year-old woman.

1. Introduction

Soft-tissue chondroma is a rare soft-tissue tumor. It is also called extraskeletal chondroma or chondroma of soft-tissue parts. Soft-tissue chondromas constitute only 1.5% of benign soft-tissue tumors [1]. They arise principally in extremities (96%) with 72% in the upper limb, 24% in the lower limb, 2% in the head and neck, and 2% in the trunk [2].

Oral soft-tissue chondromas are uncommon. If it occurs intraorally, then the most common intraoral site is tongue. In the oral cavity, only few cases of soft-tissue chondroma have been reported in the English literature till date, with very few cases in the gingiva [2–6]. This report describes an unusual case of soft-tissue chondroma occurring in the gingiva.

2. Case Report

A 50-year-old female patient reported to the Department of Oral Pathology and Microbiology, Government Dental College, Kozhikode, with a chief complaint of swelling on gums in the upper front tooth region for 4 years. The patient recalled an initial small swelling in the upper front tooth region. Now, the swelling has grown slowly to a size of 3 × 2.5 cm. She has neither consulted any physician nor did she have any discomfort due to the lesion. There was no relevant past medical history. Presently, the lesion has caused an obvious bulge of the upper lip.

2.1. Clinical Findings. On examination, a firm ovoid swelling of size 3 × 2.5 cm was found on the attached gingiva with respect to 11 and 12 extending from free marginal groove inferiorly to the buccal sulcus superiorly (Figure 1). The marginal gingiva was uninvolved. No ulceration of the skin or the oral mucosa was observed. Silness and Loe plaque index was used to assess the plaque status of the patient which was 1.2 (fair). Since the lesion presented as a firm painless well-circumscribed swelling in the anterior gingiva and additionally the patient had a fair Silness and Loe plaque index, reactive lesions due to chronic low-grade irritation (dental plaque and food impaction) like peripheral ossifying fibroma, healing pyogenic granuloma, peripheral giant cell granuloma, and giant cell fibroma were considered as differential diagnoses. Also, fibroma and peripheral odontogenic tumors were considered. Considering the indolent painless nature of the swelling, malignancies were not included in the differential diagnoses. The commonest reactive lesion found more commonly in females, exclusively in gingiva and not in any other oral mucosal location, is peripheral ossifying fibroma. Hence, it was topmost in our list of differential diagnoses. Next, other reactive lesions like healing pyogenic granuloma, peripheral giant cell granuloma, and giant cell fibroma were considered. A fibroma is most common in buccal mucosa, and peripheral odontogenic tumors are extremely rare in occurrence. Hence, they both were considered last in the list of differential diagnoses.

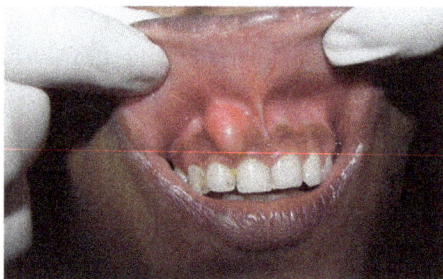

FIGURE 1: Intraoral view of lesion in anterior maxillary region.

2.2. Radiological Findings. IOPA showed mild alteration in the trabecular pattern in relation to 11 and 12 (Figure 2).

2.3. Pathological Findings. With all the above differential diagnoses in mind, the tumor was excised under local anesthesia. The diagnostic clue of the lesion is "histological examination showed well-circumscribed lobulated mass (Figure 3) of cartilaginous tissue with no cellular atypia, necrosis, or vascular invasion. Chondrocytes showed no nuclear pleomorphism or size variation. There was no binucleation or multinucleation (Figure 4)". Immunohistochemically, most of the tumor cells were positive for vimentin and S100 protein (Figures 5 and 6). For academic interest, toluidine blue staining was done, which showed typical metachromatism (Figure 7). The lesion was diagnosed as a chondroma of the gingiva.

3. Discussion

Chondroma is a benign tumor composed of mature hyaline cartilage. Most commonly, chondromas are centrally located in bone and such tumors are called enchondromas. Less often they are distinctly eccentric and cause the overlying periosteum to bulge. This type has been called periosteal chondroma [7]. Extraskeletal chondromas occur in three variants: articular, paraarticular, and soft-tissue chondromas [8]. When chondroma arises from soft tissue without attachment to the underlying bone, it is known as soft-tissue chondroma or chondroma of soft parts. Soft-tissue chondroma was first described by Baumuller in 1883, and since then, around 200 cases have been reported in the world literature. They commonly arise as painless slow-growing swelling in the extremities, especially in the hands and feet. It can also be seen in the dura, larynx, pharynx, oral cavity, skin, parotid gland, and fallopian tube [9].

Soft-tissue chondroma of the oral cavity is uncommon; very few [2–6] cases have been reported in the English literature. The tongue is the most common site for soft-tissue chondroma followed by the buccal mucosa, hard palate, gingiva, soft palate, and lips. Patients' age ranged from 3 to 79 years old (average 36.4 years old) [3]. There is a female preponderance. The lesion has a slow and indolent course and occasionally is present for many years [10]. The mean disease duration was 6.86 years [3]. Lesions range from 1.5 mm to 45 mm (average 14.7 mm) in size. Clinically, the lesion appears as a solitary, firm, slow-growing, and painless mass [11].

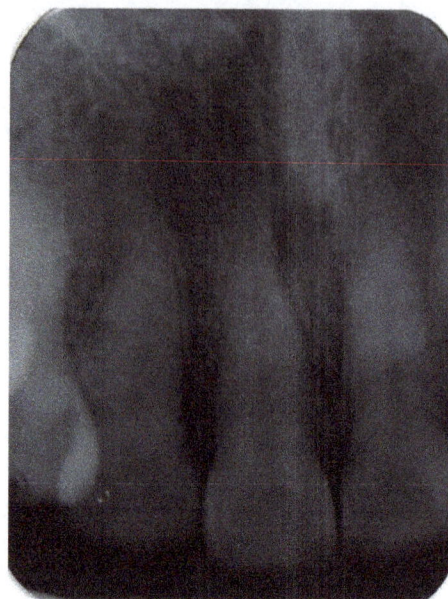

FIGURE 2: Intraoral periapical radiograph showing mild alteration in the trabecular pattern in relation to 11 and 12.

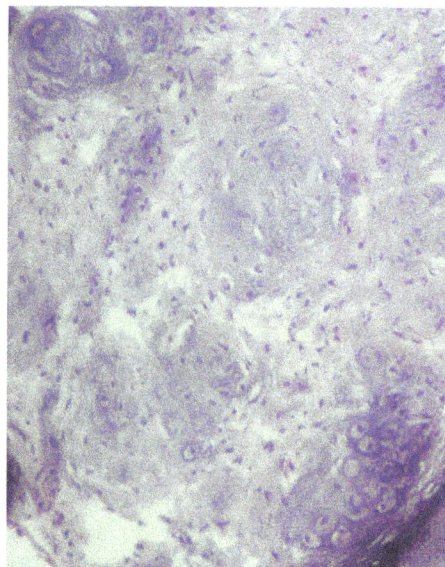

FIGURE 3: Photomicrograph showing lobulated mass of cartilaginous tissue (H&E, 10x).

Radiograph of soft-tissue chondroma in general may show an unmineralised soft-tissue mass or a soft-tissue mass with calcification typical of cartilage tumors [7]. Calcifications are seen in 33% to 70% of soft-tissue chondromas. Often, the densest calcification is in the center of the tumor mass [1]. The bones around the lesion are rarely affected. The best radiologic modality is MRI, as it can define the extent, the contour, the shape, and the intensity of the tumor in addition to its relation to the surrounding structures and calcifications, if any [12]. Although Chung and Enzinger reported that the tumor never involved the underlying bones, compression deformity, bone remodeling, bone

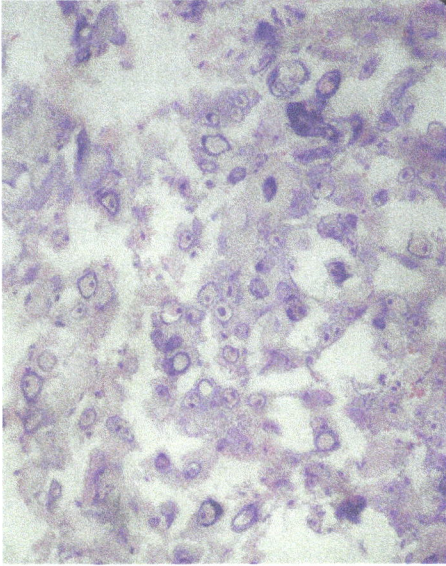

FIGURE 4: Photomicrograph showing no cellular atypia (H&E, 40x).

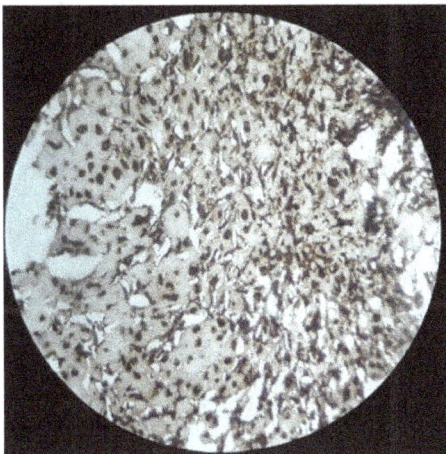

FIGURE 6: Immunostaining showing positivity for S100 (H&E, 10x).

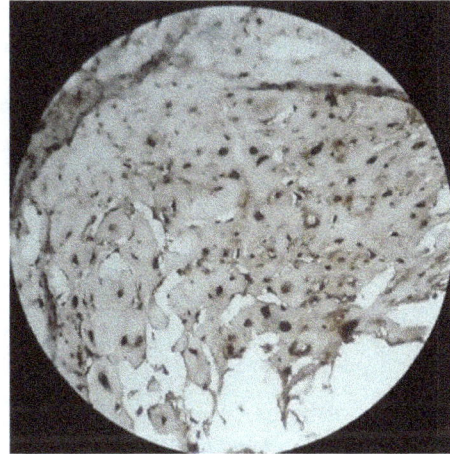

FIGURE 5: Immunostaining showing positivity for vimentin (H&E, 10x).

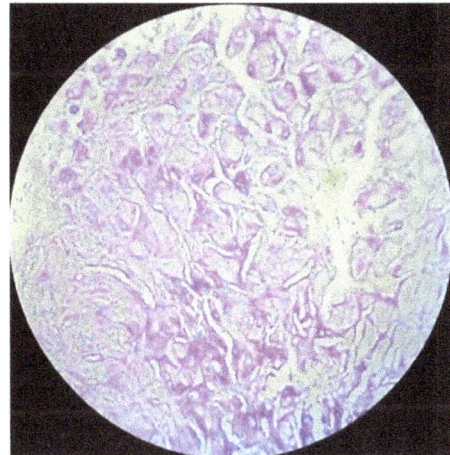

FIGURE 7: Toluidine blue staining showing typical metachromasia of cartilage.

erosion, or bone sclerosis due to the soft-tissue tumor have also been reported [1].

Grossly, chondromas of soft tissues are well encapsulated with lobular architecture. Biopsy frequently reveals a benign lobulated cartilaginous tumor composed of mature hyaline cartilage, with remarkable cellularity and prominent calcification [13]. Within the chondroid lobules, chondrocytes are in lacunae and have a tendency to cluster with large amounts of intervening chondroid matrix. This clustering arrangement is typical of soft-tissue chondromas and synovial chondromatosis but is not unique to them [7]. The external border of the tumor is usually well delineated from the adjacent tissues. The chondrocytes are located in rounded spaces and have usually single nucleus. The tumor can demonstrate marked cellularity, binucleated cells, and mitoses [14]. These findings may lead to the misdiagnosis of chondrosarcoma; however, the location and characteristic clustering arrangement should lead to a correct diagnosis. Chunky or powdery

calcification is typical of soft-tissue chondroma. It may be focal or involve the lesion diffusely [7]. It is necessary to differentiate other soft-tissue tumors from chondroma, especially in the presence of calcification. It is also important to make a differential diagnosis that considers malignancies. Fibrosis, myxoid content, and occasionally, hemorrhage are also seen in soft-tissue chondromas. Less frequently, there are granulomatous reactions and giant cells. Necrosis is rather rare [1].

Immunohistochemically, the tumor cells are positive for vimentin and S100 and negative for epithelial and myoepithelial markers [9]. The present case showed positivity for S100 and vimentin (Figures 5 and 6).

3.1. Toluidine Blue Stain. Majority of the dyes stain tissues in differing degrees of intensity of the same color; however, certain tissue components, which in the presence of certain basic dyes, will stain a color other than that of the original color of the dye. Such staining reaction is known as metachromasia, and the dyes exhibiting metachromatic properties are known as metachromatic dyes. Toluidine blue stains tissues based on the principle of metachromasia. It is a basic, metachromatic dye with high affinity for acidic tissue components, thereby staining tissues rich in DNA and RNA. It is used to highlight the principal tissue components that exhibit metachromasia like mucin, cartilage, and mast cell granules. Attached to DNA or RNA, in chromatin or Nissl substance, this dye appears blue (the original color of the dye). Attached to glycosaminoglycans, in mast cell granules or cartilage matrix, the dye displays a purple metachromatic color [15]. In our case also, the nucleus has taken blue color and the matrix of the cartilage has taken purple color demonstrating the principle of metachromasia which is the characteristic of a cartilage (Figure 7).

3.2. Theories of Soft-Tissue Chondroma. There are several theories explaining the origin of soft-tissue chondromas of head and neck. Sood et al. concluded that they arise due to metaplastic change from the adipose tissue. Dahlin and Salvador suggested a synovial origin. While Uehara, Rosenfeld, Kurzer, and Becker postulated that they arise due to the activation of heterotopic cartilaginous tissue [2]. Several authors have proposed various histogenetic theories to explain the origin of cartilage in the soft tissues of the oral cavity, but the exact cause of such cartilaginous masses is unknown [3, 16].

(1) Embryonal theory: according to this theory, cartilage is developed from the heterotopic fetal cartilaginous remnants.

(2) Metaplastic theory: According to this theory of histogenesis, development from the pluripotent mesenchymal cells is presumed either de novo or stimulated by some type of trauma, irritation, or chronic inflammation. In the present case, the probable cause of origin of the tumor could be due to metaplasia arising out of chronic irritation and inflammation triggered by plaque. Hence, it is in accordance with metaplastic theory.

According to Kho and Chen, there are reports of multiple soft-tissue chondromas as a result of an autosomal-dominant inheritance. Recently, nonrandom clonal changes of chromosomes 6, 11, and 12 have been implicated in the etiology of soft-tissue chondroma [13].

4. Conclusion

Soft-tissue chondromas are characterized by benign clinical behaviour. Surgical excision is the treatment of choice [3]. Once excised adequately, would rarely recur. Thus, recurrence is not exceptional [11]. They can show worrying radiologic and histological pictures simulating chondrosarcoma. Positive diagnosis can only be provided by the histopathological examination. Surgical treatment is the only successful solution, but recurrence is not uncommon. The present lesion was removed completely. After a 12-month follow-up, there were no signs of recurrence and there was no evidence of complications.

Disclosure

Dr. Dhana Lakshmi Jeyasivanesan is currently at the Department of Oral Pathology, Tamilnadu Government Dental College and Hospital, Chennai, India. Dr. Shameena Pazhaningal Mohamed is currently at the Department of Oral Pathology, Government Dental College, Thrissur, India. Dr. Deepak Pandiar is currently at the Faculty of Dental Sciences, Institute of Medical Sciences, Banaras Hindu University, Varanasi, India.

References

[1] H. T. Hondar Wu, W. Chen, O. Lee, and C. Y. Chang, "Imaging and pathological correlation of soft-tissue chondroma: a serial five-case study and literature review," *Clinical Imaging*, vol. 30, no. 1, pp. 32–36, 2006.

[2] M. T. Khadim, M. Asif, and Z. Ali, "Extraskeletal soft tissue chondromas of head and neck region," *Annals of Pakistan Institute of Medical Sciences*, vol. 7, pp. 42–44, 2011.

[3] T. Kawanoa, S. Yanamoto, G. Kawasaki, A. Mizuno, S. Fujita, and T. Ikeda, "Soft tissue chondroma of the hard palate: a case report," *Asian Journal of Oral and Maxillofacial Surgery*, vol. 23, no. 2, pp. 92–95, 2011.

[4] P. Vescovi, M. Meleti, E. Merigo et al., "Soft tissue chondroma of the oral cavity: an extremely rare tumour localized on the hard palate," *Case Reports in Medicine*, vol. 2014, Article ID 414861, 5 pages, 2014.

[5] A. Attakkil, V. Thorawade, M. Jagade et al., "Chondroma of tongue: a rare case report & review of literature," *International Journal of Otolaryngology and Head & Neck Surgery*, vol. 3, no. 6, pp. 359–363, 2014.

[6] R. Nehete, A. Nehete, S. Singla, and S. Sankalecha, "Soft tissue chondroma of hard palate associated with cleft palate," *Indian Journal of Plastic Surgery*, vol. 45, no. 3, pp. 550–552, 2012.

[7] K. K. Unni and C. Y. Inwards, "Chondroma," in *Dahlins Bone tumors*, K. K. Unni, Ed., pp. 22–39, Lippincott Williams and Wilkins Publishers, Philadelphia, PA, USA, 6th edition, 2009.

[8] R. A. Marcial-Seoane, M. A. Marcial-Seoane, E. Ramos, and R. A. Marcial-Rojas, "Extraskeletal chondromas," *Boletín de la Asociación Médica de Puerto Rico*, vol. 82, no. 9, pp. 394–402, 1990.

[9] D. Podder, V. Monappa, and P. Shetty, "Soft tissue chondroma: a rare tumor presenting as a cutaneous nodule," *Our Dermatology Online*, vol. 6, no. 2, pp. 173–175, 2015.

[10] J. Falleti, R. De Cecio, A. Mentone et al., "Extraskeletal chondroma of the masseter muscle: a case report with review of the literature," *International Journal of Oral and Maxillofacial Surgery*, vol. 38, no. 8, pp. 895–899, 2009.

[11] O. Norris and P. Mehra, "Chondroma (cartilaginous choristoma) of the tongue: report of a case," *Journal of Oral and Maxillofacial Surgery*, vol. 70, no. 3, pp. 643–646, 2012.

[12] M. Bahnassy and H. Abdul-Khalik, "Soft tissue chondroma: a case report and literature review," *Oman Medical Journal*, vol. 24, pp. 296–298, 2009.

[13] E. A. Gomes, J. J. Saliba, E. P. Junior, G. A. M. Saliba, C. M. D. S. Coelho, and A. C. D. M. Almeida, "Soft tissue chondroma case report and review of the literature," *Revista Brasileira de Cirurgia Plástica (RBCP)–Brazilian Journal of Plastic Surgery*, vol. 30, no. 3, pp. 477–481, 2015.

[14] M. Smida, W. Abdenaji, W. Douira-Khomsi, N. Nessib, I. Bellagha, and M. B. Ghachem, "Childhood soft tissue chondroma. Two cases report," *La tunisie Medicale*, vol. 89, no. 4, pp. 379–382, 2011.

[15] G. Sridharan and A. A. Shankar, "Toluidine blue: a review of its chemistry and clinical utility," *Journal of Oral and Maxillofacial Pathology*, vol. 16, no. 2, pp. 251–255, 2012.

5

Dental Management of a Young Child Affected by Galactosialidosis and a Gigantic Abdominal Growth

Yoselín Méndez-Salado, Paola De Ávila-Rojas, Amaury Pozos-Guillén ⓘ, Raúl Márquez-Preciado, Miguel Ángel Noyola-Frías, Socorro Ruiz-Rodríguez, and Arturo Garrocho-Rangel ⓘ

Pediatric Dentistry Postgraduate Program, Faculty of Dentistry, San Luis Potosi University, San Luis Potosi, SLP, Mexico

Correspondence should be addressed to Arturo Garrocho-Rangel; agarrocho@hotmail.com

Academic Editor: Maria Beatriz Duarte Gavião

Galactosialidosis (GS) is a rare form of lysosomal storage disease that involves a broad spectrum of skeletal and soft tissue abnormalities. We report here on a 4-year 7-month-old boy with mild mental retardation, exhibiting multiple caries cavities and associated infectious foci and macroglossia. A huge abdominal enlargement due to peritoneal ascites was evident. Behavioral management and patient positioning on the dental chair represented a true challenge. The patient was treated under general anesthesia. However, life-threatening postoperative complications occurred because of the impossibility of extubating the patient. A very careful preanesthetic assessment is crucial in children affected by general conditions associated with airway anomalies, such as GS.

1. Introduction

Lysosomal storage diseases (LSDs) are uncommon metabolic disorders produced by an accumulation of glycoconjugates (glycosaminoglycans, glycoproteins, or glycosphingolipids) within lysosomes, which affects normal tissue architecture in diverse areas of the human body. LSDs can be very rare individually; however, as a group, these anomalies comprise around 70 pathologic conditions with an incidence of 1 : 5000 live births [1, 2]. *Galactosialidosis* (GS) is an uncommon lysosomal storage condition, which belongs to the glyco-proteinosis subgroup of LSDs, inherited as an autosomal recessive trait [3]. The prevalence of the disease is, to our knowledge, unknown. It is caused by genetic mutations in the CTSA gene, which causes a deficiency or reduced activity of the protective protein cathepsin A (PCCA) [4, 5]; PCCA forms a complex with other two glycosidases: beta-galactosidase (beta-GAL) and neuraminidase 1 (NEU1). Thus, loss of PPCA function results in a severe secondary deficiency of NEU1 and partial deficiency of beta-GAL [6]. As a consequence of this, there is poor formation of elastic fibers, which are essential components of the connective tissues that form the body's supportive framework [7]. The diagnosis of GS is therefore made by measuring the activity of PCCA and by confirming the secondary deficiency of beta-GAL and NEU1 [8].

Children with GS present with a broad spectrum of clinical manifestations. Based on the age of onset of the disease during childhood and disease severity, GS is classified into three subtypes [3]. The *early infantile* type initiates between 0 and 3 months of age. It is the most severe form of GS and is associated with premature mortality [9, 10]. This form includes fetal hydrous (or *hydrops fetalis*, a severe life-threatening edema in the fetus or newborn), abdominal hernias, ascites, coarse face, proteinuria, telangiectasia (abnormal dilation of the superficial capillaries, arterioles, or venules, typically localized immediately below the skin surface), skeletal dysplasia (dysostosis multiplex, stippled epiphyses, and osteoporosis), nephrotic syndrome, cardiac failure, neurological deficit, and ocular defects. The most affected patients die early, within the first year of life, due to renal and cardiac involvement. The second subtype,

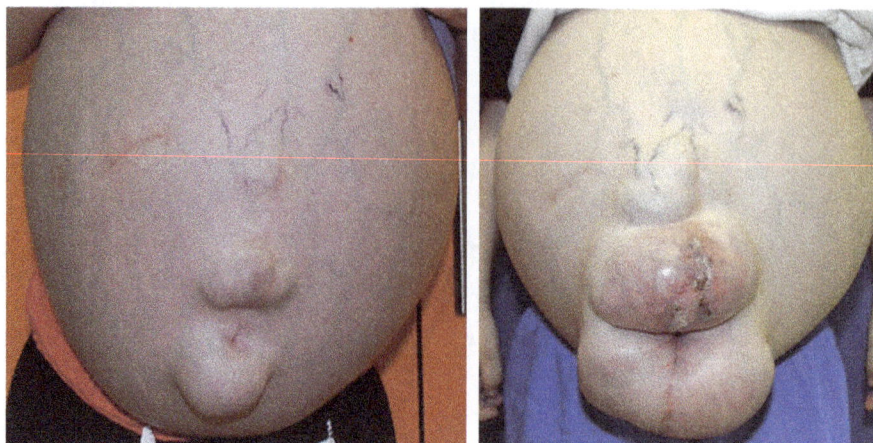

FIGURE 1: Abdominal enlargement: at the initial visit (June 2016) and at the last control appointment (November 2017).

late infantile, begins during the first 2 years of life, slowly progressing into adulthood. It is characterized primarily by absent or mild neurological/cognitive disability and mental deterioration. This condition consists of dysostosis multiplex, especially of the spine, growth retardation-associated muscular atrophy, hepatosplenomegaly, cardiac involvement (thickening of the heart valves), macroglossia, and hearing loss [1, 3, 9]. Additionally, there is a third subtype of GS, the *juvenile/adult* type. It represents the most common form of the disorder (approximately 60%), and it is more prevalent in the Japanese population. This subtype is characterized by the presence of myoclonus (a sudden and involuntary jerking of a muscle or group of muscles), ataxia, angiokeratoma (a skin condition manifested by clusters of dilated blood vessels, thickened skin, and warty growths), mental retardation, and long survival [8].

We describe the specific clinical body and oral characteristics of a 4-year 7-month-old male patient affected by early infantile GS and mild mental retardation, who presented an enormous abdominal enlargement. Due to this anatomical condition, there were diverse difficulties regarding the oral approach and body positioning of the patient on the dental chair.

2. Case Report

A 4-year 7-month-old boy and his parents were referred to the Pediatric Dentistry Postgraduate Program Clinic in June 2016, requesting dental treatment due to multiple dental caries cavities, local infectious processes, and associated pain. Two years previously, the patient had been diagnosed with early infantile GS, confirmed on the analysis of the beta-GAL both in peripheral blood leucocytes and in cultured skin fibroblasts (sequencing of the CTSA gene was not carried out). Previously, the child was insufficiently treated by a pediatric dentist, due to the child's very poor level of cooperation. Only the upper right anterior segment was treated: a pulpectomy procedure on the lateral incisor and extraction of the root remnant of the central incisor. However, the patient did not continue the treatment.

Medical and dental history revealed that when the child was 1 year of age, his parents noticed the existence of a mild soft outpouching swelling in his lower abdomen, which progressively increased in size. The patient was evaluated at a local public hospital, and the condition was diagnosed as peritoneal ascites, together with three abdominal hernias, due to enlarged liver and spleen.

At the moment of the patient's first dental visit, the presence was evident of a huge abdominal growth due to ascites (Figure 1). According to the treating medical team, this anomaly was unable to be surgically repaired. Because of the significant swelling, the patient had difficulty in maintaining a straightened body posture, and he could not be adequately positioned on the dental chair. In addition, the patient manifested mild mental retardation, language delay, severe bilateral hypoacusia, hepatic damage, and bilateral hydrocele (swelling in the scrotum).

The patient's head exhibited a squared form, coarse face, and short neck. The facial profile was markedly convex with an increased lower third, retrusive chin, protruding maxilla, closed nasolabial angle, and manifested lip incompetence (mouth permanently open) (Figure 2). Intraorally, the examination showed both arches with interdental spacing, carious cavities in all primary molars, a root remnant of the upper left lateral incisor with related abscess fistula and gingival swelling, and macroglossia associated with an evident anterior open bite (Figure 3). Oral hygiene was very poor, and halitosis was significant.

The programmed treatment plan consisted of the placement of composite restorations, pulpotomies and preformed metallic crowns, and extraction of the root remnant. Due to the greatly reduced level of cooperation exhibited by the patient (rated as Frankl's scale level I, definitely negative), it was not possible to obtain X-rays. The patient was very fearful, with clear evidence of treatment refusal, forceful crying, and extreme negativism. Therefore, it was decided to start the treatment with an oral examination, dental prophylaxis, topical fluoride-varnish applications, and the teaching of tooth brushing. Traditional behavioral management techniques, such as conditioning, desensitization, "tell-show-do," and positive reinforcement,

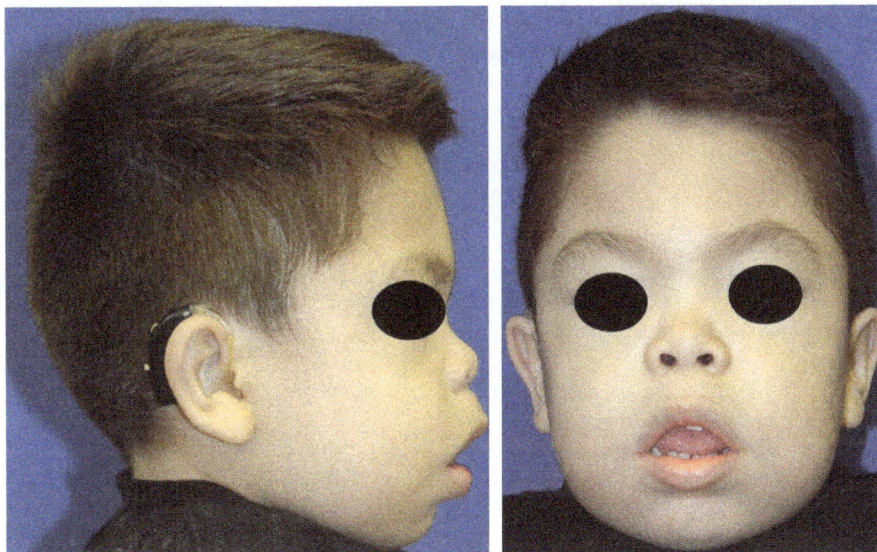

FIGURE 2: Extraoral views. Note the audition appliances.

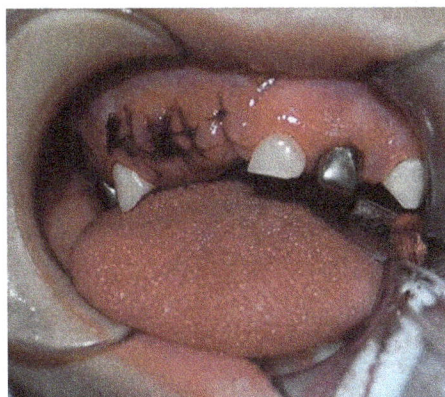

FIGURE 3: View of the macroglossia.

were persistently employed. On the other hand, the patient was unable to maintain a supine or horizontal position on the dental chair due to pain caused by the abdominal hernia. Thus, the patient was approached when he was in a 90-degree seated position, with the aid of his mother. However, all these efforts were unsuccessful. Then, it was decided to treat the patient under general anesthesia, in agreement with the parents, who signed a special informed consent document.

The patient was managed according to the American Academy of Pediatric Dentistry (AAPD) guidelines on sedation and general anesthesia. First, the child was sent to the pediatric anesthesiologist for a physical examination and a presurgical health and risk evaluation; respiratory, cardiovascular, and gastrointestinal systems were exhaustively assessed, and blood and urine laboratory tests were indicated; only coagulation times appeared slightly increased. The patient was classified as American Society of Anesthesiologists (ASA) physical status classification III, with lower pulmonary capacity, limited open aperture, macroglossia, and

challenging airway access due to decreased diameter. The parents were instructed, through printed guidance, regarding their child's eating and drinking on the day prior to the intervention.

The surgical intervention was carried out in August 2016 at the university hospital. After placing routine monitors, according to the American Society of Anesthesiologists standards, general anesthesia was induced via facemask with inhaled fentanyl, lidocaine, propofol, rocuronium bromide, and sevoflurane. Supplemental local anesthesia was also provided at the site of the root-remnant extraction. The extraction site was fully sutured with fine absorbable 6-0 Dexon in order to prevent a potential hemorrhagic episode. The whole surgical procedure lasted approximately 2 hours and ensued without complications. However, the extubation procedure was not possible due to respiratory restriction, and the patient was subsequently transferred to the pediatric intensive care unit (PICU). After 4 days under pharmacological management (dexamethasone, metamizole, ephedrine, clindamycin, and midazolam), together with assisted mechanical ventilation, the extubation could finally be performed. The patient was remitted to the pediatric area, where he was maintained with oxygen nebulization; the case proceeded uneventfully thereafter. He was discharged from the hospital 2 days later.

The patient was evaluated at our clinic 15 days after the intervention conducted under general anesthesia. Restorations were found to be in place adequately, and the cicatrization process at the extraction site was uneventful. Then, an individualized oral preventive program was initiated, including dental hygiene practice with a fluoridated paste (1,450 ppm), topical fluoride varnish, MI Paste Plus® applications, and diet counseling. Since then, the patient has been reviewed closely, every month; at each of the visits, the previously mentioned behavior modification techniques were applied in depth. The last control appointment took place in mid-November 2017, during which an excellent oral condition was observed. Currently, the patient is considered a poor candidate for treatment with orthodontic appliances, particularly for treating his anterior open bite. In the meanwhile, the eruption process and occlusal development will be continuously assessed.

3. Discussion

The American Academy of Pediatric Dentistry (AAPD) has recognized that "providing both primary and comprehensive preventive and therapeutic oral health care to individuals with Special Health Care Needs (SHCNs) is an integral part of the specialty of pediatric dentistry," and SHCNs are defined as "any physical, developmental, mental, sensory, behavioral, cognitive, or emotional impairment or limiting condition that requires medical management, healthcare intervention, and/or use of specialized services or programs" [11].

In this report, we present a rare case of a mentally challenged pediatric patient with early infantile GS dentally treated under general anesthesia, who exhibited a critical postoperative adverse effect associated with a compromised airway. Due to the rarity of this condition, such clinical case reports are lacking in the dental literature. To the best of our knowledge, this is the first case describing a child with early infantile GS reported in the pediatric dentistry literature.

GS is a condition of metabolism classified as a lysosomal storage disease associated with soft tissue aberrations; some of these present in the orofacial complex, for instance, macroglossia and adenoidal/tonsillar hypertrophy. Also frequent is a decreased airway diameter [1, 10]. This condition can represent a real challenge for diagnosis and clinical care in pediatric dentistry, for example, diverse significant implications during the dental management with general anesthesia, as occurred in the present case. Despite the potential difficulty being detected at the preanesthetic evaluation and in spite of the anticipated preoperative medical measures being taken, the very problematic extubation could not be avoided. This information confirms that general anesthesia cannot be considered by pediatric dentists as an "easy" solution to manage "difficult" children, nor is there a completely safe procedure [12]. However, in the case of our patient, his significant anatomical condition and lack of cooperation were sufficiently justified selection indicators for carrying out the procedure, despite the high risk involved.

4. Conclusions

Pediatric dentists should always pay special attention to and be aware of the potential risks of disorders that can produce life-threatening conditions. Also, a very careful preanesthetic assessment is crucial in children affected by general conditions or syndromes associated with airway anomalies, such as GS.

Acknowledgments

The English-language reviewing of the manuscript by Maggie Brunner has been particularly appreciated. This work was supported partially by PFCE-UASLP 2017 and PRODEP 2018 grants.

References

[1] R. J. Friedhoff, S. H. Rose, M. J. Brown, T. R. Long, and C. T. Wass, "Galactosialidosis: a unique disease with significant clinical implications during perioperative anesthesia management," *Anesthesia and Analgesia*, vol. 97, no. 1, pp. 53–55, 2003.

[2] S. D. Kingma, O. A. Bodamer, and F. A. Wijburg, "Epidemiology and diagnosis of lysosomal storage disorders; challenges of screening," *Best Practice & Research Clinical Endocrinology & Metabolism*, vol. 29, no. 2, pp. 145–157, 2015.

[3] I. Annunziata and A. d'Azzo, "Galactosialidosis: historic aspects and overview of investigated and emerging treatment options," *Expert Opinion on Orphan Drugs*, vol. 5, no. 2, pp. 131–141, 2017.

[4] A. Durante, M. Trini, and R. Spoladore, "Left ventricular "diverticulum" in a patient affected by galactosialidosis," *Case Reports in Medicine*, vol. 2011, Article ID 356056, 3 pages, 2011.

[5] S. Kostadinov, B. A. Shah, J. Alroy, and C. Phornphutkul, "A case of galactosialidosis with novel mutations of the protective protein/cathepsin A gene: diagnosis prompted by trophoblast vacuolization on placental examination," *Pediatric and Developmental Pathology*, vol. 17, no. 6, pp. 474–477, 2014.

[6] Z. K. Timur, S. A. Demir, and V. Seyrantepe, "Lysosomal cathepsin A plays a significant role in the processing of endogenous bioactive peptides," *Frontiers in Molecular Biosciencies*, vol. 3, no. 68, pp. 1–7, 2016.

[7] Genetic Home Reference, Lister Hill National Center for Biomedical Communications (US NLH), "Galactosialidosis," 2017, https://ghr.nlm.nih.gov/condition/galactosialidosis.

[8] A. Caciotti, S. Catarzi, R. Tonin et al., "Galactosialidosis: review and analysis of CTSA gene mutations," *Orphanet Journal of Rare Diseases*, vol. 8, pp. 114–122, 2013.

[9] B. Guzel-Nur, G. Kaya-Aksoy, M. Koyun, S. Akman, and E. Mihci, "Early infantile galactosialidosis presenting with an unusual renal involvement," *Journal of Genetic Syndromes & Gene Therapy*, vol. 5, no. 5, pp. 244–246, 2014.

[10] C. B. Riggs, L. F. Escobar, and M. E. Tucker, "Early-infantile galactosialidosis: clinical and radiographic findings," *Journal of Clinical & Medical Case Reports*, vol. 2, no. 2, pp. 1–4, 2015.

[11] American Academy of Pediatric Dentistry, "Guideline of management of dental patients with special health care needs," *Pediatric Dentistry*, vol. 38, no. 6, pp. 171–176, 2017.

[12] N. Ramazani, "Different aspects of general anesthesia in pediatric dentistry: a review," *Iranian Journal of Pediatrics*, vol. 26, no. 2, p. e2613, 2016.

6

Autotransplantation and Orthodontic Treatment after Maxillary Central Incisor Region Trauma: A 13-Year Follow-Up Case Report Study

Farzad Piroozmand,[1] Hossein Hessari,[2] Mohsen Shirazi,[3] and Pegah Khazaei ⓘ[2]

[1]Department of Orthodontics, School of Dentistry, Tehran University of Medical Sciences, International Campus, Tehran, Iran
[2]Research Center for Caries Prevention, Dentistry Research Institute, Tehran University of Medical Sciences, Tehran, Iran
[3]Department of Orthodontics, School of Dentistry, Tehran University of Medical Sciences, Tehran, Iran

Correspondence should be addressed to Pegah Khazaei; pegahkhazaee@gmail.com

Academic Editor: Daniel Torrés-Lagares

The anterior maxilla is the most prone region to the trauma during childhood, and tooth loss sometimes happens due to trauma. Replacing the missing teeth has always been one of the dentists' challenges in children and adolescents, since their dentofacial growth is not complete. Autotransplantation of mandibular premolars with two-thirds or three-quarters of root formation provides the best prognosis for the tooth survival. This case report describes the management of a 10-year-old boy suffering a severe dental injury who received the autotransplantation of the premolars from mandible to restore the space caused by trauma in maxillary central incisor region and a 13-year follow-up of the autotransplantation.

1. Introduction

Severe dental injuries can lead to the permanent loss of teeth. The anterior maxilla is the most traumatized region and the most accident prone age of trauma is between 8 and 12 years old when the incisors are erupted, and the periodontal ligament has the minimal resistance to the external forces [1–3]. Space maintenance of avulsed tooth is necessary until the completion of dentofacial growth. One of the treatment options is replacing the teeth using implants. However, implants are not recommended in these patients because of their residual facial growth. The other treatment options include prosthetic replacement and orthodontic space closure [4]. On the other hand, if donor teeth are available, autotransplantation can be considered as a possible option. Autotransplantation involves moving the tooth from one site to another in the same individual [5]. In cases with bone loss, transplanted tooth can induce bone formation and reestablishment of alveolar process [6]. Successful tooth transplantation can improve mastication, speech, esthetics, dentofacial growth, and arch form [7]. Transplantation of mandibular premolars with root formation of two-thirds to three-quarters and wide open apex provides the best prognosis for the pulp survival and reduces the risk of resorption [8–11]. This case report describes the management of a 10-year-old boy suffering a severe dental injury who received the autotransplantation of the premolars from mandible to restore the space caused by trauma in maxillary central incisor region.

2. Case Report

A 10-year-old boy was brought to the Shariati hospital emergency department after a car accident. Avulsion of the maxillary central incisors and intrusion of lateral incisors were diagnosed (Figure 1). The avulsed central incisors were not replanted and missed.

Panoramic radiograph showed a permanent dentition except second primary molars (Figure 2).

Four weeks after accident, the boy was examined by an orthodontist. Extraoral examination showed no soft tissue injury probably because of the time of examination. Intraoral examination also showed neither laceration nor alveolar bone fracture. Clinical examination revealed that

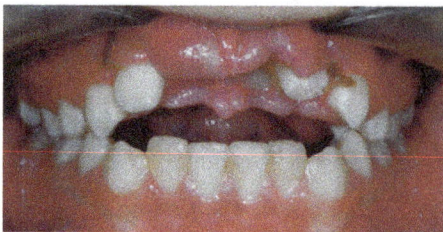

FIGURE 1: Clinical view showing the missing maxillary central incisors and intrusion of the maxillary lateral incisors.

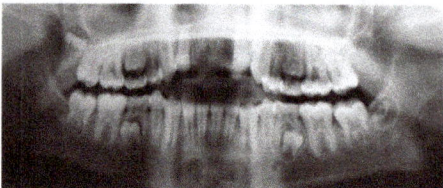

FIGURE 2: Panoramic radiograph before autotransplantation.

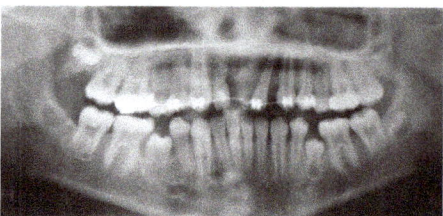

FIGURE 3: Radiographic view showing root resorption of maxillary lateral incisor.

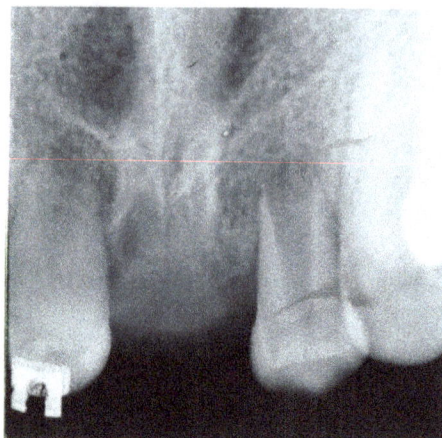

FIGURE 4: Transplanted mandibular second premolars.

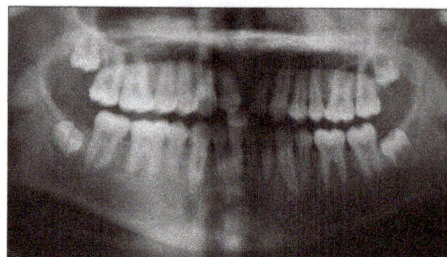

FIGURE 5: Radiographic view after orthodontic treatments.

the patient had an angle's Cl II malocclusion, open bite, and lower jaw space deficiency and crowding. The aim of orthodontic management was to treat the Cl II malocclusion and to relieve crowding by extractions in lower jaw. After the completion of radiographic and clinical examination, mandibular second premolars were selected for the extraction. Due to loss of maxillary incisors, we decided to transplant mandibular second premolars into the place of maxillary incisors at the time of orthodontics extractions.

3. Preliminary Orthodontics Treatment

Preliminary orthodontics treatment was performed to extrude the intruded maxillary lateral incisors and regain the incisal space. Evaluation of maxillary lateral incisors showed severe root resorption. Therefore, we had to extract them (Figure 3).

4. Teeth Preparation for Transplantation and Surgery

The root formation of these premolars was two-thirds of its potential length at the extraction time. Prior to the extraction, with the aid of periapical radiograph, the size and length of premolar roots were measured, and then socket preparation was done in the maxillary central incisor region. A slightly larger socket was prepared, in order to minimize

periodontal ligament damage, which could be happened because of excessive compressive forces or prolonged extra alveolar time for donor teeth. The premolars were extracted under the local anesthesia. A crevicular incision by number 12 scalpel blade was performed before the luxation to preserve the maximum possible periodontal ligament on the root surface. Teeth crowns were also covered by cotton rolls to avoid contacting the beaks of forceps with the root surface. After extraction, donor teeth immediately fitted into the prepared sockets (Figure 4). Proximal surface of premolars formed the labial surface of transplanted teeth in the incisor region.

5. Postsurgery Orthodontics Treatment

Transplanted teeth were splinted to the adjacent teeth using 0.3 mm thick stainless-steel wire and composite for 10 days. Five months after transplantation, transplanted teeth were tested clinically and radiographically. There was no sign of ankylosis, and root development had been initiated. Following that, orthodontics management started including fixing brackets on teeth and moving them as well as transplanted teeth. Root development of transplanted teeth continued, and they moved following orthodontic forces like other teeth. Periapical radiographs of transplanted teeth with 6 months' intervals revealed no sign of root resorption during treatment period. No inflammation of the gingiva or any patient complaint was reported. The treatment was accomplished to a Cl I occlusion with no prosthetic intervention during 23 months (Figures 5 and 6).

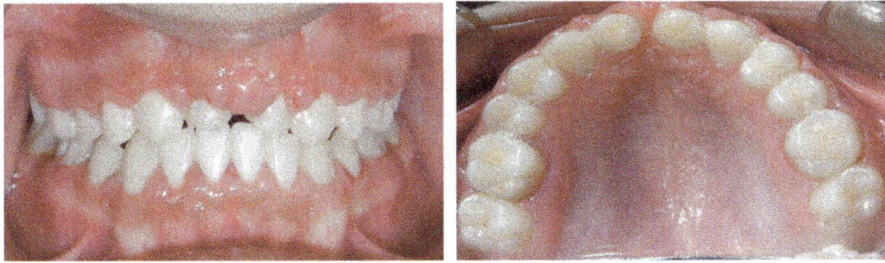

FIGURE 6: Clinical view after orthodontic treatments.

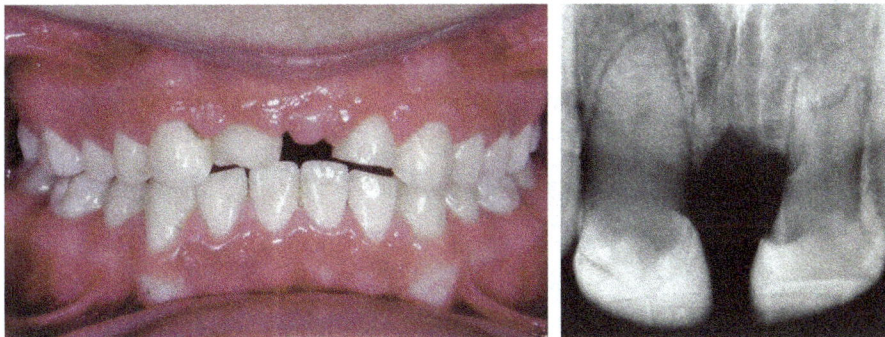

FIGURE 7: Radiographic and clinical view at the 6-year follow-up.

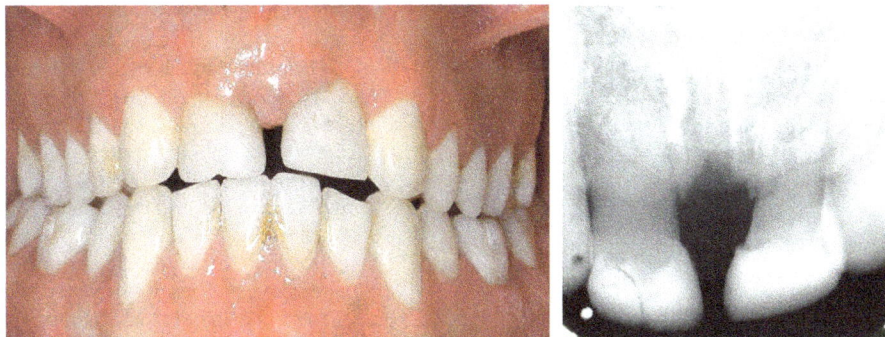

FIGURE 8: Radiographic and clinical view at the 13-year follow-up.

6. Follow-ups

Six- and thirteen-year follow-ups confirmed complete health of transplanted teeth. The teeth were clinically vital, radiographically normal, with no pulp obliteration, and had no signs and symptoms of ankylosis or root resorption (Figures 7 and 8). Root development and the crown/root ratio were not similar in the transplanted teeth, although, periodontal ligament and pulpal health were acceptable in both. The alveolar ridge levels of transplanted teeth were parallel with that in adjacent teeth. However, there was a resorbed area in the midline due to large diastema between the transplanted teeth. No sign of mobilization was seen.

Further prosthodontic treatments or periodontal esthetic surgery could be performed at the later ages.

7. Discussion

Loss of maxillary incisors due to severe dental injuries is common, especially in ages between 8 and 12 years [1, 2]. Tooth loss during the growth time period can lead to the horizontal and vertical deficiencies of bone and soft tissue [10, 12].

There are several options to replace the missing tooth such as orthodontic treatment or implants. However, using implants is contraindicated until completion of the facial growth. When the implants are planned for the treatment, extensive surgeries like bone and soft tissue augmentation may be required [13].

Another possible treatment option is autotransplantation if the donor tooth is present. Transplanted tooth preserves alveolar bone until growth completion, even if future failure of transplantation occurred. Preservation of the bone will facilitate provision of implants. Also, the transplanted tooth can recover the proprioceptive function and normal periodontal healing. Therefore, a natural chewing feeling and natural biological response will occur. Additionally, the transplanted tooth can be used as a bridge abutment or orthodontic anchorage [14, 15].

The stage of root development is one of the main factors affecting the prognosis of the transplanted tooth [11, 16]. The chance of revascularization and reinnervation of the dental pulp is increasing when the apex is open. Transplantation of tooth with root development of more than 50% has shown high success rate [17]. Survival rate of transplanted premolars with incomplete roots is reported 95% to 98% up to 13 years by Andreasen et al. [18–20].

Ideally, when the donor tooth exhibits three-quarters development of full root length and diameter of apical opening is more than 1 mm at the time of auto-transplantation, transplantation shows the most favorable prognosis [6, 16, 21]. In premolars, this developmental stage can be seen between ages of 10 and 13 years.

Regarding the transplantation stage, the results of Northway study [22] showed two-thirds and three-fourths completion of root development is the preferred stage for transplantation. The incidence of pulp necrosis and root resorption is greater when the apex of transplanted premolars is closed [10, 18, 19]. Transplantation of fully formed root decreases the potential for pulp regeneration, but an adequate endodontic therapy can ensure good prognosis of transplantation. In our case, transplantation was done when the root formation completed by three-quarters of its full length; and pulp healing and regeneration was achieved, as the root was immature. Transplanted tooth had a wide apical opening, and therefore, there was no need for endodontic treatment.

Another factor that affects the prognosis of transplantation is surgical procedure. A minimal handling and an atraumatic extraction to preserve the intact periodontal ligaments and Hertwig's root sheath should be considered. If not, ankylosis or root resorption and attachment loss might be occurred [10, 17, 21]. It is also important to minimize the implantation time after extraction. The donor tooth should be transplanted immediately after extraction to avoid drying out. However, Kim et al. showed no relationship between extraoral time and root resorption or ankylosis with a prolonged experimental time of 7.8 minutes [23]. In our case, the donor tooth was transplanted immediately after extraction, and maximum care was done to preserve the intact periodontal ligaments and Hertwig's root sheath.

Immobilization of the transplanted tooth is another factor that can influence the outcome of transplantation. However, long term and rigid immobilization can adversely affect the periodontal ligaments and pulpal healing of the transplanted tooth.

Orthodontic treatments can be initiated after confirmation of the presence of the lamina dura in radiographs and regeneration of periodontal space [24]. In our case, we started orthodontic treatment 5 months after transplantation.

Orthodontic treatment ended 23 months after initiation. Pogrel [25] recommended that the final success or failure of transplanted tooth can usually be predicted at 2 years after transplantation. In our case, thirteen years after transplantation, no ankylosis or root resorption was observed.

8. Conclusion

In growing individuals, autotransplantation of immature premolar with open apex root can be considered as a predictable method to replace the missing teeth. Transplanted tooth can reestablish a normal alveolar process after loss of the bone due to dental injury.

References

[1] A. B. Skaare and I. Jacobsen, "Dental injuries in Norwegians aged 7–18 years," *Dental Traumatology*, vol. 19, no. 2, pp. 67–71, 2003.

[2] U. Glendor, "Epidemiology of traumatic dental injuries–a 12 year review of the literature," *Dental Traumatology*, vol. 24, no. 6, pp. 603–611, 2008.

[3] K. Almpani, S. N. Papageorgiou, and M. A. Papadopoulos, "Autotransplantation of teeth in humans: a systematic review and meta-analysis," *Clinical Oral Investigations*, vol. 19, no. 6, pp. 1157–1179, 2015.

[4] F. M. Andreasen, "Replacement of lost anterior teeth in young individuals: autotransplantation of premolars: the joint role of the paediatric dentist, oral surgeon and orthodontist," *Annals of the Royal Australasian College of Dental Surgeons*, vol. 22, p. 74, 2014.

[5] J. A. Asif, T. Y. Noorani, and M. K. Alam, "Tooth auto-transplantation: an alternative treatment," *Bulletin of Tokyo Dental College*, vol. 58, no. 1, pp. 41–48, 2017.

[6] M. Gilijamse, J. A. Baart, J. Wolff, G. K. Sándor, and T. Forouzanfar, "Tooth autotransplantation in the anterior maxilla and mandible: retrospective results in young patients," *Oral Surgery, Oral Medicine, Oral Pathology and Oral Radiology*, vol. 122, no. 6, pp. e187–e192, 2016.

[7] S. B. Kotha, "Intra-alveolar auto-transplantation to correct a single tooth rotation: a case report with four years of follow-up," *Saudi Journal of Oral Sciences*, vol. 1, no. 2, p. 110, 2014.

[8] E. M. Czochrowska, A. Stenvik, B. Album, and B. U. Zachrisson, "Autotransplantation of premolars to replace maxillary incisors: a comparison with natural incisors," *American Journal of Orthodontics and Dentofacial Orthopedics*, vol. 118, no. 6, pp. 592–600, 2000.

[9] E. M. Czochrowska, A. Stenvik, and B. U. Zachrisson, "The esthetic outcome of autotransplanted premolars replacing maxillary incisors," *Dental Traumatology*, vol. 18, no. 5, pp. 237–245, 2002.

[10] M. Ruano, A. Lopez, G. Lin, and N. McDonald, "Factors influencing the long-term prognosis of auto-transplanted teeth with complete root formation: a systematic review," *International Journal of Oral and Dental Health*, vol. 2, no. 7, 2016.

[11] I. Michl, D. Nolte, C. Tschammler, M. Kunkel, R. Linsenmann, and J. Angermair, "Premolar auto-transplantation in juvenile dentition: quantitative assessment of vertical bone and soft tissue growth," *Oral Surgery, Oral Medicine, Oral Pathology and Oral Radiology*, vol. 124, no. 1, pp. e1–e12, 2017.

[12] D. Schwartz-Arad and L. Levin, "Post-traumatic use of dental implants to rehabilitate anterior maxillary teeth," *Dental Traumatology*, vol. 20, no. 6, pp. 344–347, 2004.

[13] B. Thilander, J. Ödman, K. Gröteborg, and B. Friberg, "Osseointegrated implants in adolescents. An alternative in replacing missing teeth?," *European Journal of Orthodontics*, vol. 16, no. 2, pp. 84–95, 1994.

[14] T. Jonsson and T. J. Sigurdsson, "Autotransplantation of premolars to premolar sites. A long-term follow-up study of 40 consecutive patients," *American Journal of Orthodontics and Dentofacial Orthopedics*, vol. 125, no. 6, pp. 668–675, 2004.

[15] R. Wang, C. Wan, and Y. Leung, "Autotransplantation of teeth: a case report," *International Journal of Oral Maxillofacial Surgery*, vol. 46, p. 281, 2017.

[16] W. Harzer, D. Rüger, and E. Tausche, "Autotransplantation of first premolar to replace a maxillary incisor–3D-volume tomography for evaluation of the periodontal space," *Dental Traumatology*, vol. 25, no. 2, pp. 233–237, 2009.

[17] A. L. M. Aas and A. B. Skaare, "Management of a 9-year-old boy experiencing severe dental injury–a 21-year follow-up of three autotransplants: a case report," *Dental Traumatology*, vol. 27, no. 6, pp. 468–472, 2011.

[18] J. Andreasen, H. Paulsen, Z. Yu, and T. Bayer, "A long-term study of 370 autotransplanted premolars. Part IV. Root development subsequent to transplantation," *European Journal of Orthodontics*, vol. 12, no. 1, pp. 38–50, 1990.

[19] J. Andreasen, H. Paulsen, Z. Yu, T. Bayer, and O. Schwartz, "A long-term study of 370 autotransplanted premolars. Part II. Tooth survival and pulp healing subsequent to transplantation," *European Journal of Orthodontics*, vol. 12, no. 1, pp. 14–24, 1990.

[20] J. Andreasen, H. Paulsen, Z. Yu, and O. Schwartz, "A long-term study of 370 autotransplanted premolars. Part III. Periodontal healing subsequent to transplantation," *European Journal of Orthodontics*, vol. 12, no. 1, pp. 25–37, 1990.

[21] A. K. Singh and L. Shrestha, "Auto-transplantation of teeth: our experience," *Journal of College of Medical Sciences-Nepal*, vol. 12, no. 3, pp. 99–102, 2016.

[22] W. Northway, "Autogenic dental transplants," *American Journal of Orthodontics and Dentofacial Orthopedics*, vol. 121, no. 6, pp. 592-593, 2002.

[23] E. Kim, J.-Y. Jung, I.-H. Cha, K.-Y. Kum, and S.-J. Lee, "Evaluation of the prognosis and causes of failure in 182 cases of autogenous tooth transplantation," *Oral Surgery, Oral Medicine, Oral Pathology, Oral Radiology, and Endodontology*, vol. 100, no. 1, pp. 112–119, 2005.

[24] B. I. Aslan, N. Üçüncü, and A. Doğan, "Long-term follow-up of a patient with multiple congenitally missing teeth treated with autotransplantation and orthodontics," *Angle Orthodontist*, vol. 80, no. 2, pp. 396–404, 2010.

[25] M. Pogrel, "Evaluation of over 400 autogenous tooth transplants," *Journal of Oral and Maxillofacial Surgery*, vol. 45, no. 3, pp. 205–211, 1987.

7

Nonsyndromic Bilateral Posterior Maxillary Supernumerary Teeth: A Report of Two Cases and Review

Ravi Kumar Mahto ⑩,[1] **Shantanu Dixit,**[2] **Dashrath Kafle,**[1] **Aradhana Agarwal,**[1] **Michael Bornstein,**[3] **and Sanad Dulal**[4]

[1]*Department of Orthodontics, Dhulikhel Hospital, Kathmandu University School of Medical Sciences, Dhulikhel, Nepal*
[2]*Department of Oral Medicine and Radiology, Dhulikhel Hospital, Kathmandu University School of Medical Sciences, Dhulikhel, Nepal*
[3]*Oral and Maxillofacial Radiology, Applied Oral Sciences, Faculty of Dentistry, University of Hong Kong, Pokfulam, Hong Kong*
[4]*Department of Oral and Maxillofacial Surgery, Dhulikhel Hospital, Kathmandu University School of Medical Sciences, Dhulikhel, Nepal*

Correspondence should be addressed to Ravi Kumar Mahto; drravimahto@gmail.com

Academic Editor: Gavriel Chaushu

Supernumerary tooth/hyperdontia is defined as those teeth which are present in excess of the usual distribution of twenty deciduous and thirty-two permanent teeth. It can be seen in both syndromic and nonsyndromic patients. In Nepalese population, prevalence of supernumerary tooth is documented to be 1.6%. To the best of our knowledge, no studies from Nepal have reported the incidence of bilateral maxillary paramolars or the combination of unilateral maxillary paramolar and distomolar till date. Hence, we are reporting these two cases with a brief review of literature to put emphasis on incidence, prevalence, proposed hypothesis for etiology, and management of supernumerary teeth.

1. Introduction

Supernumerary tooth (ST) is defined as a tooth or a structure resembling tooth which forms from dental lamina in addition to the normal dental formula [1, 2]. It can occur both in the maxillae and/or mandible, unilaterally or bilaterally, solitary or in multiples, and erupted or unerupted. It can be seen in both syndromic and nonsyndromic patients. Previous researches had documented the prevalence rate of ST to be 0.2%–0.8% and 0.5%–5.3% in deciduous and permanent dentition, respectively. The male-to-female ratio for the incidence of ST was reported to range in between 1.18 : 1 and 1.5 : 1. Supernumerary teeth are also associated with larger than average teeth which reflect their multifactorial etiology. Various hypothesis were postulated by different authors to explain the phenomena of ST development, but

the exact etiology is still unknown [3]. However, Brook [4] had hypothesized an interaction of environmental and genetic factors.

ST can be classified on the basis of the morphology (conical, tuberculate, supplemental, and odontomes), location (mesiodens, paramolar, distomolar, and parapremolar), position (buccal, palatal, and transverse), and orientation (vertical or normal, inverted, transverse, or horizontal). Mesiodens is the most prevalent supernumerary teeth which is seen in premaxilla. ST in the molar region is comparatively very rare [3]. Also, a very few cases have been reported about the bilateral presence of ST in the molar region [5].

Hence, we are reporting two cases of bilateral ST in the molar region. Our first case is of bilateral maxillary paramolars, whereas the other case is a combination of unilateral maxillary paramolar and distomolar. In addition, we have

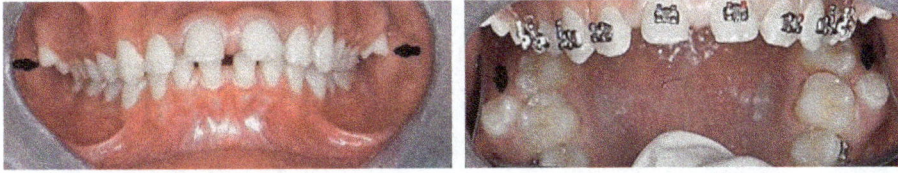

FIGURE 1: Intraoral images of Case 1 depicting bilateral maxillary paramolars (shown by arrows).

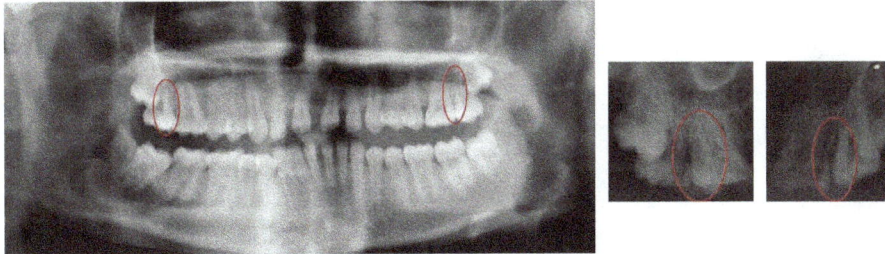

FIGURE 2: Panoramic and intraoral radiographs showing bilateral maxillary paramolars (encircled).

reviewed the existing literature to focus on incidence, prevalence, proposed hypothesis for etiology, and management of supernumerary teeth.

2. Case Report 1

A 17-year-old male patient visited to the department of orthodontics and dentofacial orthopedics with a chief complaint of malalignment of teeth. His medical and family histories were not significant. On intraoral examination, buccally placed bilateral paramolars were present in between first and second maxillary molars (Figure 1). No clinical complications were present secondary to paramolars. Radiological investigations (intraoral periapical radiographs and panoramic radiograph) were advised to determine the root orientation (Figure 2). Both the paramolars were vertically oriented. Extractions were advised for both the paramolars to prevent any interruption in the orthodontic treatment. Extracted paramolars showed supplemental shape and form with well-defined transverse and marginal ridges resembling maxillary premolars (Figure 3). It was followed by initiation of the orthodontic treatment.

3. Case Report 2

A 23-year-old female patient visited to the department of orthodontics and dentofacial orthopedics with a chief complaint of forwardly placed upper front teeth. No significant medical and family histories were reported. On intraoral examination, fourteen teeth were present in maxillary arch (Figure 4). Clinically, maxillary third molars were missing bilaterally. She was advised for routine radiological investigations required for the orthodontic treatment. Panoramic radiograph revealed presence of a distomolar on the right side and a paramolar between left second and third molars (Figure 5). Computed tomographic scan was advised to know the accurate orientation of these impacted supernumerary teeth to formulate the treatment

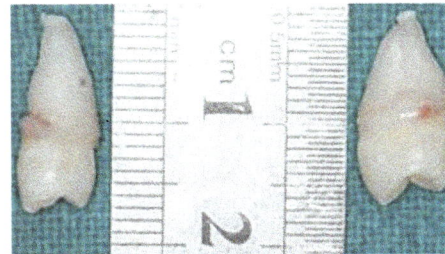

FIGURE 3: Extracted paramolars resembling maxillary premolars.

plan. It revealed the vertical orientation of both the impacted supernumerary teeth. Extraction of supernumerary teeth followed by the orthodontic treatment was advised to the patient.

4. Discussion

ST or hyperdontia as defined earlier are those teeth which are present in excess of the usual distribution of twenty deciduous and thirty-two permanent teeth [6]. Singh et al. had reported the prevalence of ST in Nepalese population to be 1.6%, which was in accordance with Hungarian (1.53%), Swedish (1.6%), and Brazilian (1.7%) population. The same study had showed the male predilection for ST with male: female ratio of 1.3:1 which was similar to Hungarian (1.4:1), British (1.4:1), and Brazilian (1.45:1) population [7–11]. Similarly, this study had also documented the prevalence of the single ST to be the most commonest (82.60%) followed by paired (15.21%) and triple ones (2.17%). Maxillary arch (98.8%) with the anterior medial region (mesiodens) and conical form was found to be the most common location and form of the supernumerary teeth in this study [7].

To the best of our knowledge, no studies from Nepal have reported the incidence of bilateral maxillary paramolars or the combination of unilateral maxillary paramolar and distomolar till date. The documented incidences similar to

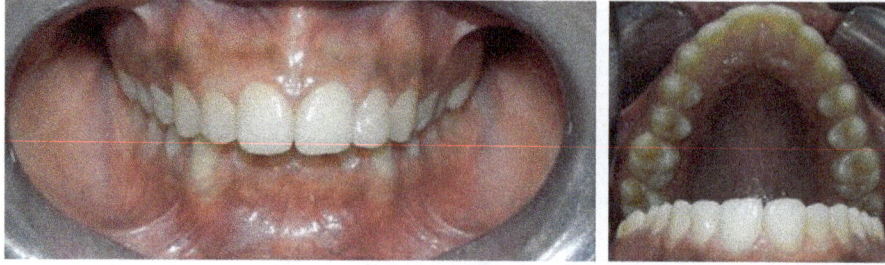

Figure 4: Intraoral images of Case 2.

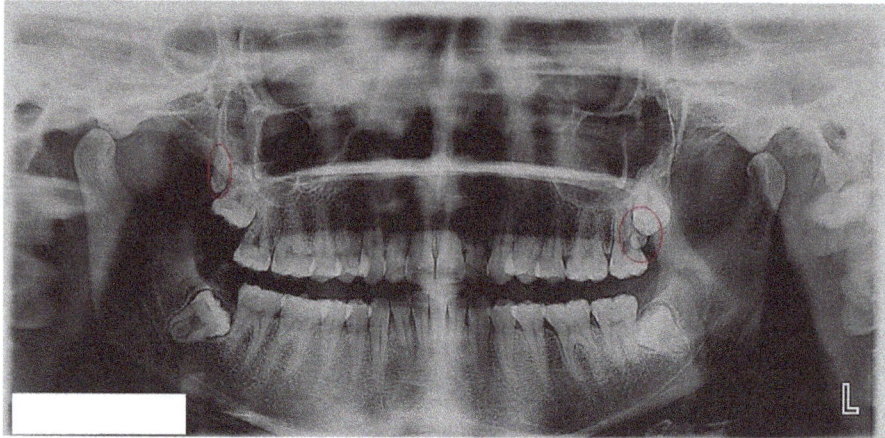

Figure 5: Panoramic radiograph showing maxillary the right distomolar and left paramolar (encircled).

our cases reported in other population are briefed in Tables 1 and 2 [12, 13]. Hou et al. [14], Dhull et al. [15], Shetty [16], and Sulabha and Sameer [17] had reported the presence of bilateral maxillary paramolars similar to our first case report. Nirmala and Tirupathi [12] had documented the combination of unilateral maxillary paramolar and distomolar similar to our second case report.

The exact etiology of occurrence of ST is not known. Numerous theories have been postulated to understand their existence along with the normal dentition. Atavism theory stated the occurrence of supernumerary teeth as the phylogenetic reversion to the extinct ancestral human dentition [33]. Dichotomy theory suggested that a developing tooth bud can divide into two teeth, giving rise to ST and a normal tooth [34]. Dental lamina hyperactivity theory, the most accepted one, suggests the localized and independent hyperactivity of the dental lamina to be the cause for the development of ST [7, 35]. Niswander and Sujaku [36] also proposed the presence of an autosomal recessive gene which explains the familial tendency to ST. It have been reported in patients with syndromes like cleft lip and palate, cleidocranial dysplasia, Ehlers–Danlos syndrome type III, Fabry–Anderson's syndrome, Ellis–van Creveld syndrome, Gardner's syndrome, Goldenhar syndrome, Hallermann–Streiff syndrome, orofaciodigital syndrome type I, incontinentia pigmenti, Marfan syndrome, Nance–Horan syndrome, and trichorhinophalangeal syndrome 1 [12].

ST may be associated with different clinical complications. These can result into clinical problems like midline diastema; crowding; malocclusion due to insufficient space; dilaceration, delayed, or failure of eruption of permanent teeth; root resorption of adjacent teeth; cyst formation; cheek bite; periodontal problems; dental caries, and other difficulties related to ectopic position. These complications occur rarely, but earlier diagnosis can help to prevent these complications [4, 13].

Radiographic screening plays a significant role in identification and localization of ST, especially when they are impacted or need surgical intervention. Two-dimensional imaging modalities (periapical radiographs, occlusal radiographs, and orthopantomographs) do provide sufficient information to the clinicians, but accurate position of buccally or lingually placed ST is difficult to determine due to the superimposition by the surrounding structures [4, 13, 37]. Clark and Richards had suggested horizontal and vertical tube shift technique, respectively, to determine exact location of ST using conventional radiography. Both of these are widely accepted due to their simplicity [4, 38, 39]. Recently, Toureno et al. proposed a guideline to use three-dimensional imaging modalities (cone beam computerized tomography) along with two-dimensional imaging modalities for better assessment of ST, planning surgical intervention with minimal treatment errors [40].

There are two different school of thoughts about the management of ST. Some authors recommended the removal of ST as soon as detected, whereas others emphasized the periodic monitoring and removal only in the case of any

TABLE 1: Reported cases of paramolars.

Arch/side		Unilateral				Bilateral		
	Author	Year	Population	Location	Author	Year	Population	Location
Maxillae	Puri et al. [18]	2013	Indian	Bucally placed between second and third molars	Sulabha and Sameer et al. [17]	2015	Indian	Buccally placed between first and second molars
	Nayak et al. [19]	2012	Indian	Palatally placed between left first and second molars	Dhull et al. [15]	2012	Indian	Between first and second molars
	Nagaveni et al. [13]	2010	Indian	Buccally placed between right first and second molars	Shetty et al. [16]	2012	Indian	Palatally placed between first and second molars
					Hou et al. [14]	1995	Taiwanese	Buccally placed between first and second molars
Mandible	Ghogre and Gurav [20]	2014	Indian	Fused with the second molar	Dhull et al. [15]	2014	Indian	Mesial and lingual to the second molar
	Venugopal et al. [21]	2013	Indian	Fused with the right second molar	Nunes et al. [22]	2002	Brazil	Fused with the second molar
	Rudagi et al. [23]	2012	Indian	Fused with the left second molar				
	Salem et al. [24]	2010	Iran	Fused with the left second molar				
	Rosa et al. [25]	2010	Brazil	Fused with the right first molar				
	Ballal et al. [26]	2007	Indian	Fused with the second molar				
	Ghoddusi et al. [27]	2006	Iran	Fused with the left second molar				
	Dubuk et al. [28]	1996	Japanese	Mesial to the right second molar				
	Kumasaka et al. [29]	1988	Japanese	Two impacted paramolar on the right side				

TABLE 2: Reported cases of combination of paramolar and distomolar/bilateral paramolars.

Arch	Author	Year	Population	Location
Maxillae	Present case	2017	Nepalese	Buccally placed bilateral paramolars in between first and second molars; combination of a distomolar on the right side and a paramolar between left second and third molars
	Nirmala and Tirupathi [12]	2015	Indian	Combination of developing unerupted paramolar on the right side and distomolar on the left side
	Omal et al. [30]	2011	Indian	Bilateral paramolar between second and third molars; bilaterally impacted distomolar
	Mayfield and Casamassimo [31]	1990	Hispanic	Bilateral paramolars and distomolars
Mandible	Reddy et al. [32]	2013	Indian	Bilateral paramolar between first and second molars; bilateral distomolar with impacted second molar

associated pathology or hindrance to any dental treatment especially the orthodontic treatment [41–43]. Hogstrom and Andersson also suggested two different options for ST removal. According to them, ST either should be removed as early as it is identified or after completion of the adjacent tooth's root formation. However, former option could result into creation of dental phobia in young children and can disturb the growth of adjacent teeth [44]. Recently, Omer et al. suggested the optimal time for the removal of ST during 6 to 7 years, based upon their retrospective analysis. According to them, during this age interval, ST removal can be done with minimal disturbances to the adjacent teeth [1].

5. Conclusion

Supernumerary teeth are uncommon and generally present without causing any complications like our cases. Our cases required surgical intervention for future orthodontic treatment and planning. Although complications are rare, clinicians should be aware of early identification, proper management, and associated complications with the same.

References

[1] R. S. Omer, R. P. Anthonappa, and N. M. King, "Determination of the optimum time for surgical removal of

unerupted anterior supernumerary teeth," *Pediatric Dentistry*, vol. 32, no. 1, pp. 14–20, 2010.

[2] M. T. Cobourne and P. T. Sharpe, "Making up the numbers: the molecular control of mammalian dental formula," *Seminars in Cell & Developmental Biology*, vol. 21, no. 3, pp. 314–324, 2010.

[3] X.-P. Wang and J. Fan, "Molecular genetics of supernumerary tooth formation," *Genesis*, vol. 49, no. 4, pp. 261–277, 2010.

[4] A. H. Brook, "A unifying aetiological explanation for anomalies of human tooth number and size," *Archives of Oral Biology*, vol. 29, no. 5, pp. 373–378, 1984.

[5] S. K. Mallineni, "Supernumerary teeth: review of the literature with recent updates," *Conference Papers in Science*, vol. 2014, Article ID 764050, 6 pages, 2014.

[6] C. Schulze, "Developmental abnormalities of the teeth and jaws," in *Toma's Oral Pathology*, R. J. Gorlin and H. M. Goldman, Eds., pp. 112–122, C.V. Mosby, St. Louis, MI, USA, 1970.

[7] V. P. Singh, A. Sharma, and S. Sharma, "Supernumerary teeth in Nepalese children," *Scientific World Journal*, vol. 2014, Article ID 215396, 5 pages, 2014.

[8] K. Gabris, G. Fabian, M. Kaan, N. Rozsa, and I. Tarjan, "Prevalence of hypodontia and hyperdontia in paedodontic and orthodontic patients in Budapest," *Community Dental Health*, vol. 23, no. 2, pp. 80–82, 2006.

[9] I. Bodin, P. Julin, and M. Tomsson, "Hyperdontia. I. Frequency and distribution of supernumerary teeth among 21,609 patients," *Dentomaxillofacial Radiology*, vol. 7, no. 1, pp. 15–17, 1978.

[10] F. X. P. C. Simoes, I. Crusoe-Rebello, F. S. Neves, C. Oliveira Santos, A. L. Ciamponi, and O. G. da Silva Filho, "Prevalence of supernumerary teeth in orthodontic patients from South Western Brazil," *International Journal of Odontostomatology*, vol. 5, no. 2, pp. 199–202, 2011.

[11] A. H. Brook, "Dental anomalies of number, form and size: their prevalence in British school children," *Journal of the International Association of Dentistry for Children*, vol. 5, no. 2, pp. 37–53, 1974.

[12] S. V. S. G. Nirmala and S. P. Tirupathi, "Rare combination of developing unerupted paramolar and distomolar in maxilla: a case report and review of literature," *Journal of Interdisciplinary Medicine and Dental Science*, vol. 4, no. 4, pp. 1–6, 2016.

[13] N. B. Nagaveni, K. V. Umashankara, N. B. Radhika, B. Praveen Reddy, and S. Manjunath, "Maxillary paramolar: report of a case and literature review," *Archives of Orofacial Sciences*, vol. 5, no. 1, pp. 24–28, 2010.

[14] G. L. Hou, C. C. Lin, and C. C. Tsai, "Ectopic supernumerary teeth as a predisposing cause in localized periodontitis. Case report," *Australian Dental Journal*, vol. 40, no. 4, pp. 226–228, 1995.

[15] K. S. Dhull, S. Acharya, P. Ray, S. Yadav, and S. D. Prabhakaran, "Bilateral maxillary paramolars: a case report," *Journal of Dentistry for Children*, vol. 79, no. 2, pp. 84–87, 2012.

[16] Y. N. Shetty, "A rare case of bilateral maxillary paramolars between 1st and 2nd molars," *Journal of Orofacial Research*, vol. 2, no. 1, pp. 52–55, 2012.

[17] A. N. Sulabha and C. Sameer, "Unusual bilateral paramolars associated with clinical complications," *Case Reports in Dentistry*, vol. 2015, Article ID 851765, 4 pages, 2015.

[18] K. Puri, M. Bansal, D. Jain et al., "Nonsyndromic multiple supernumerary premolars and paramolars: an overview and report of 2 cases," *Indian Journal of Dental Sciences*, vol. 5, pp. 54–56, 2013.

[19] G. Nayak, S. Shetty, I. Singh, and D. Pitalia, "Paramolar - A supernumerary molar: a case report and an overview," *Dental Research Journal*, vol. 9, pp. 797–803, 2012.

[20] P. Ghogre and S. Gurav, "Non-invasive endodontic management of fused mandibular second molar and a paramolar, using cone beam computed tomography as an adjunctive diagnostic aid: a case report," *Journal of Conservative Dentistry*, vol. 17, pp. 483–486, 2014.

[21] S. Venugopal, B. V. Smitha, and S. P. Saurabh, "Paramolar concrescence and periodontitis," *Journal of Indian Society of Periodontology*, vol. 17, pp. 383–386, 2013.

[22] E. Nunes, I. G. de Moraes, P. M. de Novaes, and S. M. de Sousa, "Bilateral fusion of mandibular second molars with supernumerary teeth: case report," *Brazilian Dental Journal*, vol. 13, pp. 137–141, 2002.

[23] K. Rudagi, B. M. Rudagi, S. Metgud, and R. Wagle, "Endodontic management of mandibular second molar fused to a supernumerary tooth, using spiral computed tomography as a diagnostic aid: a case report," *Case Reports in Dentistry*, vol. 2012, p. 614129, 2012.

[24] A. S. Milani, "Endodontic management of a fused mandibular second molar and paramolar: a case report," *Iranian Endodontic Journal*, vol. 5, pp. 131–134, 2010.

[25] F. M. Rosa, A. Stankiewicz, and I. M. Faraco, "Impaction of mandibular molar by supernumerary tooth: case report," *Journal of Dentistry for Children*, vol. 75, pp. 181–184, 2008.

[26] S. Ballal, G. S. Sachdeva, and D. Kandaswamy, "Endodontic management of a fused mandibular second molar and paramolar with the aid of spiral computed tomography: a case report," *Journal of Endodontics*, vol. 33, pp. 1247–1251, 2007.

[27] J. Ghoddusi, M. Zarei, and H. Jafarzadeh, "Endodontic treatment of a supernumerary tooth fused to a mandibular second molar: a case report," *Journal of Oral Science*, vol. 48, pp. 39–41, 2002.

[28] A. N. Dubuk, K. A. Selvig, G. Tellefsen, and U. M. Wikesjo, "Atypically located paramolar. Report of a rare case," *European Journal of Oral Sciences*, vol. 104, pp. 138–140, 1996.

[29] S. Kumasaka, K. Hideshima, H. Shinji et al., "A case of two impacted paramolar in lower right molar dentition," *Kanagawa Shigaku*, vol. 23, pp. 417–423, 1988.

[30] P. Omal, V. Jacob, J. Lonapan, and A. Kurian, "Bilateral fourth molars with paramolars in maxilla," *Kerala Dental Journal*, vol. 34, pp. 277–279, 2011.

[31] A. Mayfeld and P. S. Casamassimo, "Bilateral paramolars and fourth molars," *Oral Surgery, Oral Medicine, Oral Pathology, Oral Radiology*, vol. 69, p. 394, 1990.

[32] G. S. Reddy, G. V. Reddy, I. V. Krishna, and S. K. Regonda, "Nonsyndromic bilateral multiple impacted supernumerary mandibular third molars: a rare and unusual case report," *Case Reports in Dentistry*, vol. 2013, p. 857147, 2013.

[33] R. P. Anthonappa, N. M. King, and A. B. Rabie, "Aetiology of supernumerary teeth: a literature review," *European Archives of Paediatrc Dentistry*, vol. 14, pp. 279–288, 2013.

[34] W. Bateson, "On numerical variation in teeth, with a discussion of conception of homology," *Proceedings of Zoological Society of London*, vol. 102, no. 4, p. 115, 1982.

[35] G. V. Black, "Supernumerary teeth," *Dental Summary*, vol. 29, pp. 83–110, 1909.

[36] J. D. Niswander and C. Sujaku, "Congenital anomalies of teeth in Japanese children," *American Journal of Physical Anthropology*, vol. 21, no. 4, pp. 569–574, 1963.

[37] M. Dojs and A. Roicka, "The usefulness of pantomographic x-ray pictures in estimating the position of the paramolar and distomolar teeth," *Annales Academiae Medicae Stetinensis*, vol. 53, no. 1, pp. 83–85, 2007.

[38] C. A. Clark, "A method of ascertaining the relative position of unerupted teeth by means of film radiographs," *Proceedings of Royal Society of Medicine*, vol. 3, pp. 87–90, 1910.

[39] A. G. Richards, "Roentgenographic localization of the mandibular canal," *Journal of Oral Surgery*, vol. 10, pp. 325–329, 1952.

[40] L. Toureno, J. H. Park, R. A. Cederberg, E. H. Hwang, and J. W. Shin, "Identification of supernumerary teeth in 2D and 3D: review of literature and a proposal," *Journal of Dental Education*, vol. 77, no. 1, pp. 43–50, 2013.

[41] S. Rotberg and H. M. Kopel, "Early vs late removal of mesiodens: a clinical study of 375 children," *Compendium of Continuing Education in Dentistry*, vol. 5, pp. 115–119, 1984.

[42] D. Munns, "A case of partial anodontia and supernumerary tooth present in the same jaw," *Dental Practitioner and Dental Record*, vol. 18, no. 1, pp. 34–37, 1967.

[43] P. J. Scanlan and S. J. Hodges, "Supernumerary premolar teeth in siblings," *British Journal of Orthodontics*, vol. 24, no. 4, pp. 297–300, 1997.

[44] A. Hogstrom and L. Andersson, "Complications related to surgical removal of anterior supernumerary teeth in children," *Journal of Dentistry for Children*, vol. 54, no. 5, pp. 341–343, 1987.

8

Cheilitis Glandularis of Both Lips: Successful Treatment with a Combination of an Intralesional Steroid Injection and Tacrolimus Ointment

Norberto Sugaya ⓘD and Dante Migliari ⓘD

Division of Oral Medicine Clinic, Department of Stomatology, School of Dentistry, University of Sao Paulo, Sao Paulo, SP, Brazil

Correspondence should be addressed to Norberto Sugaya; nnsugaya@usp.br

Academic Editor: Noam Yarom

Cheilitis glandularis (CG) is an inflammatory condition of unknown cause that predominantly affects the minor salivary glands of the lips. Although a diagnosis of CG is not difficult, its treatment is a challenge. This article highlights the clinical presentation of the disease together with a case of successful management of this disease using a combination of a steroid injection followed by a topical immunosuppressor.

1. Introduction

Cheilitis glandularis (CG) is a rare inflammatory condition that predominantly affects the minor salivary glands and surrounding tissues of the lips. It affects adults (over 40 years old) to a greater extent than young people and almost exclusively white individuals. The ratio of male/gender involvement is 3 : 1. To date, no specific factor or cause has been associated with the disease onset [1].

The clinical features of CG lend to its diagnosis. The labial mucosa exhibits dilation of the orifices of the minor salivary glands through which thick saliva (mucin-rich) flows more intensely due to the inflammatory process inside the glandular parenchyma. This excessive salivary flow eventually dries out, leading to the development of yellowish plaques (or crusts) that cover the labial mucosa surface. These plaques are easily removed but form again, mainly during sleep. In addition to this main feature, the patient also develops enlargement and eversion of the lips. The vermilion border is typically not affected [2].

Although a diagnosis of CG is not difficult, its treatment is a challenge. The present article reports the successful management of a case treated with a combination of steroid injection followed by a topical immunosuppressor.

2. Case Report

A 16-year-old white male was referred to our oral medicine clinic for investigation of an enlargement of the lower and upper lips ongoing for approximately one year. His primary complaint was yellowish crusts on the mucosa surface of both lips but particularly the lower one (Figures 1(a) and 1(b)). Despite removal, the crusts reappeared mostly in the morning. He underwent previous treatments with topical corticosteroids to no avail. The patient was healthy with no history of substantive medical treatment.

Based on the aspect of the lesions, the diagnosis was cheilitis glandularis. The initial treatment was two intralesional injections of 10 mg triamcinolone suspension in both lips with a one-month interval between the applications. Two months following the second injection, an improvement was noticed with a reduction in the enlargement and eversion of the lips. Recurrent appearance of the crusts was also reduced but not to the extent that the patient felt comfortable. Instead of administering another steroid injection, a topical immunosuppressor (0.1% tacrolimus ointment) was applied twice daily for two weeks based on two effective management reports on CG found in the literature [3, 4] Before application, the patient was instructed to (1) wash his hands, (2) remove

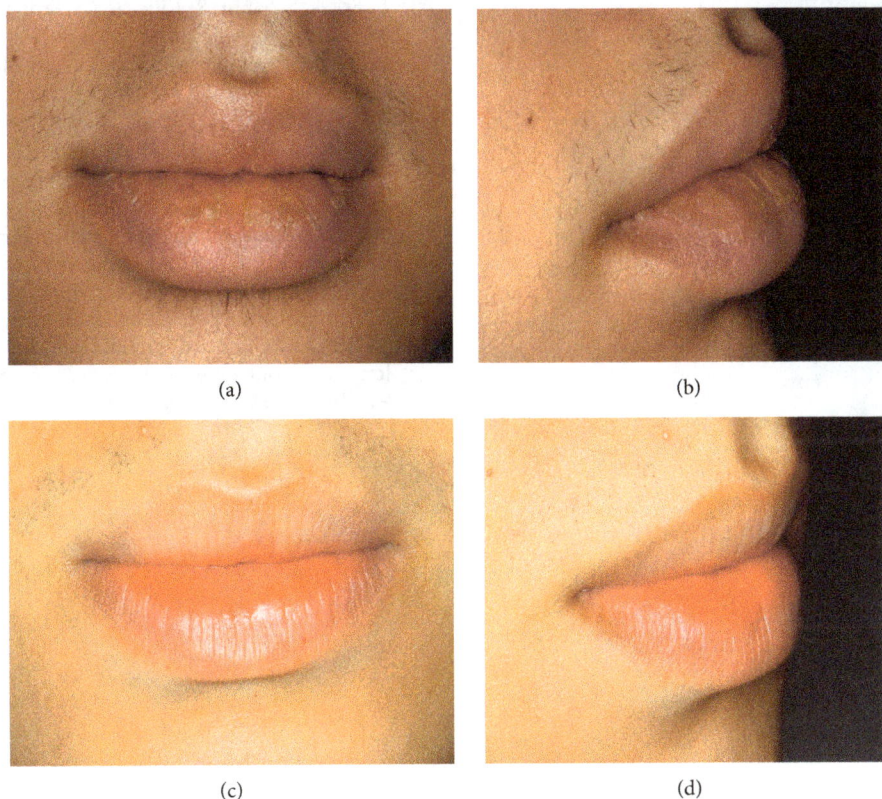

FIGURE 1: (a, b) Initial consultation with the patient exhibiting yellowish crusts on the labial mucosa. The lips (mainly the lower one) are also swollen and everted, whereas the vermilion border appears unaffected. (c, d) After treatment, both lips regained normal contour and aspect. A discreet redness of the lip mucosae remained unchanged throughout the follow-up.

the labial crusts and apply 2% chlorhexidine gluconate on lip surfaces for disinfection, (3) allow the mucosa surfaces to dry and then apply the tacrolimus ointment, and (4) wash his hands again. This management procedure succeeded in completely resolving the lesions with no recurrence after a one-year follow-up (Figures 1(c) and 1(d)).

3. Discussion

CG is a rare disease but may occasionally be observed by the clinician. The lesion appears mainly through a process of renewed yellowish-plaque formation that is puzzling to health professionals. It seems that topical corticosteroids alone are not effective. Intralesional steroid injection has received some acceptance, but there is no consensus that it works in all cases. The mainstream treatment for CG has been vermilionectomy, but this treatment produces collateral effects, such as permanent itching and paresthesia.

Our patient did not require a biopsy. Biopsy was judged unnecessary because there was no clear-cut evidence that a biopsy would constructively help diagnose CG. Based on two relevant studies [1, 2], the histopathological findings were nonspecific, consisting mainly of chronic inflammation with various degrees of nonspecific sialadenitis and ductal ectasia of the minor salivary glands and fibrosis within the glands.

Possible differential diagnoses of CG may include contact cheilitis and cheilitis granulomatosa [1, 2, 5]. The first condition is attributed to irritants or allergic contactants. In these cases, apart from disclosing the contactant agent, the clinical features of contact cheilitis differ substantially from those of CG. For example, in the former, the lesions appear more prominent on the lip vermilion and are characterized mostly by the presence of adherent scales. Cheilitis granulomatosa shares some similarities to CG concerning lip swelling and eversion but lacks inflammation in the labial salivary glands, which leads to an increase of the salivary secretion and subsequent crust formation, a feature commonly observed in CG cases.

In the event of a difficulty in making a differential diagnosis between CG and cheilitis granulomatosa, a biopsy can be helpful as the latter can exhibit noncaseating granulomas; however, this feature is only observed in 40 to 50% of the cases. In either disease, the exact etiopathogenesis remains unknown. In a few cases of cheilitis granulomatosa, the development of this disease is potentially associated with food allergy (mainly cinnamon and benzoate compounds) [6].

Although one case of CG is not sufficient to judge the performance of a therapy, the treatment used in the present case appears to be effective. Tacrolimus was instrumental in preventing crust formation, possibly due to its effective action in controlling glandular inflammation by curbing the production of proinflammatory cytokines inside the minor salivary glands.

References

[1] S. Reiter, M. Vered, N. Yarom, C. Goldsmith, and M. Gorsky, "Cheilitis glandularis: clinico-histopathological diagnostic criteria," *Oral Diseases*, vol. 17, no. 3, pp. 335–339, 2011.

[2] M. M. Nico, J. Nakano de Melo, and S. V. Lourenço, "Cheilitis glandularis: a clinicopathological study in 22 patients," *Journal of the American Academy of Dermatology*, vol. 62, no. 2, pp. 233–238, 2010.

[3] E. Erkek, S. Sahin, R. Kilic, and S. Erdogan, "A case of cheilitis glandularis superimposed on oral lichen planus: successful palliative treatment with topical tacrolimus and pimecrolimus," *Journal of the European Academy of Dermatology and Venereology*, vol. 21, no. 7, pp. 999-1000, 2007.

[4] H. J. Bovenschen, "Novel treatment for cheilitis glandularis," *Acta Dermato Venereologica*, vol. 89, no. 1, pp. 99-100, 2009.

[5] P. R. Carrington and T. D. Horn, "Cheilitis glandularis: a clinical marker for both malignancy and/or severe inflammatory disease of the oral cavity," *Journal of the American Academy of Dermatology*, vol. 54, no. 2, pp. 336-337, 2006.

[6] K. A. Al Johani, D. R. Moles, T. A. Hodgson, S. R. Porter, and S. Fedele, "Oralfacial granulomatosis: clinical features and long-term outcome of therapy," *Journal of the American Academy of Dermatology*, vol. 62, no. 4, pp. 611–620, 2010.

9

Management of Retrograde Peri-Implantitis Using an Air-Abrasive Device, Er,Cr:YSGG Laser, and Guided Bone Regeneration

Nikolaos Soldatos ⓘ,[1] Georgios E. Romanos,[2,3] Michelle Michaiel,[1] Ali Sajadi,[1] Nikola Angelov,[1] and Robin Weltman ⓘ[1]

[1]Department of Periodontics and Dental Hygiene, School of Dentistry, University of Texas Health Science Center at Houston, Houston, TX, USA
[2]Department of Periodontology, School of Dental Medicine, Stony Brook University, Stony Brook, NY, USA
[3]Department of Oral Surgery and Implant Dentistry, Johann Wolfgang Goethe University of Frankfurt, Frankfurt, Germany

Correspondence should be addressed to Nikolaos Soldatos; nikolaos.k.soldatos@uth.tmc.edu

Academic Editor: Gerardo Gómez-Moreno

Background. The placement of an implant in a previously infected site is an important etiologic factor contributing to implant failure. The aim of this case report is to present the management of retrograde peri-implantitis (RPI) in a first maxillary molar site, 2 years after the implant placement. The RPI was treated using an air-abrasive device, Er,Cr:YSGG laser, and guided bone regeneration (GBR). *Case Description.* A 65-year-old Caucasian male presented with a draining fistula associated with an implant at tooth #3. Tooth #3 revealed periapical radiolucency two years before the implant placement. Tooth #3 was extracted, and a ridge preservation procedure was performed followed by implant rehabilitation. A periapical radiograph (PA) showed lack of bone density around the implant apex. The site was decontaminated with an air-abrasive device and Er,Cr:YSGG laser, and GBR was performed. The patient was seen every two weeks until suture removal, followed by monthly visits for 12 months. The periapical X-rays, from 6 to 13 months postoperatively, showed increased bone density around the implant apex, with no signs of residual clinical or radiographic pathology and probing depths ≤4 mm. *Conclusions.* The etiology of RPI in this case was the placement of an implant in a previously infected site. The use of an air-abrasive device, Er,Cr:YSGG, and GBR was utilized to treat this case of RPI. The site was monitored for 13 months, and increased radiographic bone density was noted.

1. Introduction

Retrograde peri-implantitis (RPI) is termed as a symptomatic periapical lesion, developed after implant placement, while the coronal portion of the implant remains fully osseointegrated [1]. It was initially described in 1992 by McAllister et al. where they described two cases of RPI caused by bacteria remained in the extraction socket [2]. In 1993, Sussman and Moss defined it as "localized osteomyelitis secondary due to endodontic pathology" [3]. In 1995, Reiser and Nevins described it as "active implant periapical lesion" [4]. Piattelli et al., in 1998, histologically examined an implant that was removed due to periapical radiolucency.

They discovered the presence of necrotic bone inside the antirotational hole and the demineralization of the bordered trabecular bone [5]. Esposito et al. in 1998 considered the placement of an implant in a previously infected site to be an important factor contributing to implant failure [6].

Etiological factors of RPI are divided to those which occur at the time of implant placement and those due to a preexisting disease (Table 1) [7–9]. Moreover, an HIV-related infection was described as an etiological factor for RPI as well [7].

Bacteria can be encapsulated in edentulous areas, up to 1 year after the extraction [10]. Therefore, many implants that developed RPI, where previously root canal treated teeth,

TABLE 1: Etiological factors of RPI.

At the time of implant placement	Preexisting disease related to a tooth
(1) Contamination of the surgical bed	(1) Endodontic pathology associated with an extracted tooth
(2) Excessive heat or compression over the time of implant placement	(2) Retained root tip
(3) Presence of remnants of milling	(3) Preexisting bone disease
(4) Overextended osteotomy	(4) Adjacent tooth with periapical radiolucency
(5) Presence of a foreign body	(5) Remaining cells from a cyst or granuloma
(6) Premature loading leading to bone microfractures	

were present [10]. The reported prevalence of RPI is very low (0.26%), but it can be increased up to 7.8% when there is a history of a root canal treatment of an adjacent tooth, next to the implant site [11]. Studies support the launch of symptoms from 1 week after implant placement, up to 4 years later [12–15]. The symptoms vary from presence of a fistula tract to pain and swelling. The presence of a fistula tract has shown the highest prevalence (65.6%) [9, 12, 15, 16]. Maxillary implant sites (78%) seem to be more exposed to RPI compared to mandibular (18%) [12, 15, 16]. Reiser and Nevins connected that finding to the higher frequency of radicular cysts in the maxilla [4]. Bhaskar connected the higher frequency of maxillary radicular cysts with the epithelial rests of Malassez, which seem to be more numerous in the maxilla than in the mandible [17].

The aim of this case report was to present the management of RPI in a first maxillary molar site, 2 years after the implant placement. The implant apex was located in close proximity to where the periapical radiolucency of tooth #3 was in 2013. The diagnosis was RPI, and the affected implant was treated successfully using the combination of an air-abrasive device, Er,Cr:YSGG laser, and guided bone regeneration (GBR).

2. Case Presentation

A 65-year-old Caucasian male, nonsmoker, ASA II with a significant medical history for hypertension, was referred in 2016 to the Graduate Periodontics Clinic at the University of Texas Health Science Center at Houston. His chief complaint was "they said I have an abscess around my implant." The patient had been prescribed clindamycin 300 mg for a week by his referring predoctoral student of the same University. Clinically, a draining fistula was present at the tooth #3 implant site, just apical to the mucogingival junction, measuring approximately 3 × 3 mm. Comprehensive periodontal and radiographic evaluations were performed. The patient was very meticulous with oral hygiene, and there was absence in bleeding on probing and mobility, with thick gingival biotype. The periodontal pocket measurements around the implant were ≤4 mm. The diagnosis associated with the implant at the area of tooth #3 was RPI.

The dental history of tooth #3 revealed periapical radiolucency in 2013, on the mesial buccal root (Figure 1), measuring ~5.4 × 8.7 mm in a cone beam CT (Figure 2). A Seibert Class I ridge deformity was noted at the buccal wall of #3. Upon flap reflection, a fenestration was noted

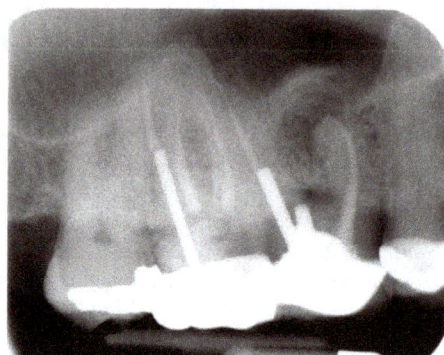

FIGURE 1: Radiograph of tooth #3 showed periapical radiolucency on the mesial buccal root.

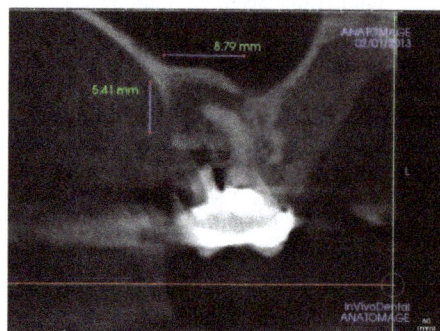

FIGURE 2: A cone beam CT of tooth #3 in 2013 showed periapical radiolucency of the mesial buccal root (~5.4 × 8.8 mm).

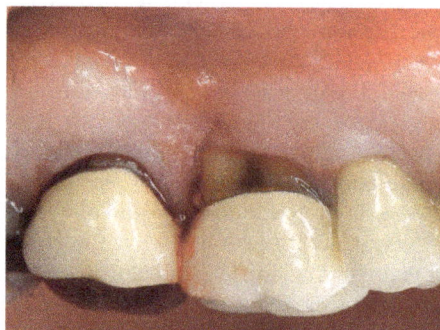

FIGURE 3: Intraoral picture of tooth #3 at the time of tooth extraction. A draining fistula was noted on the distal surface of #3.

penetrating the buccal wall at the site of the mesiobuccal root apex. The tooth was sectioned, extracted, and a thorough debridement of the socket was performed. Valsava testing was performed to exclude the possibility of communication with the sinus cavity. Freeze-dried bone allograft (FDBA), a collagen membrane, and a nonresorbable high density PTFE membrane were used for ridge preservation and grafting of the buccal plate of area #3 (Figures 3–5). The site was healed by secondary intention. A periapical X-ray was taken with the surgical guide before the implant placement, showing no residual radiographic pathology (Figure 6). The implant osteotomy was prepared with the use of osteotome sinus floor elevation technique [18]. A 4.7 × 11.5 mm Zimmer TSV implant (Zimmer Biomet, Palm Beach Gardens, FL) was placed. The implant was torqued in 35 N/cm, and a healing abutment was placed (Figures 7–9). The implant was referred to the predoctoral clinic for final restoration with cement-retained porcelain fused to metal (PFM) crown (Figure 10). The same surgical and restorative approach was uneventfully followed for site #2, as well (Figure 11). The patient was given an occlusal stabilization splint and was placed on a 6-month maintenance protocol in 2014.

3. Case Management

The patient presented for surgical implant debridement with a nondraining fistula (Figure 12) in July of 2016. The patient understood the benefits and the risks of the surgical approach and signed a consent form. The site #3 implant showed ~5.5 mm lack of radiographic bone density around the apex (Figure 13). The site was anesthetized by means of local infiltrations, on the buccal and palatal aspects of tooth #3. Intrasulcular incisions extending from #2–4 were performed with a vertical releasing incision placed at the mesial line angle of #4. Upon reflection of a full thickness flap, a fenestration of 2 × 2 mm and 7 mm depth was revealed around the apex of implant #3 (Figure 14). Fibrous granulation tissue was present on the mesial, palatal, and distal aspects of the implant. The bone defect was degranulated using Gracey curettes. No communication with the maxillary sinus was found. The implant surface was initially decontaminated utilizing an air-abrasive device with amino acid glycine powder avoiding direct contact with the implant surface and copious amounts of sterile saline to remove the powder from the implant surface and bone defect (Figure 15). After degranulation, seven threads of the implant were exposed (Figure 16). Before the first laser pass, the patient and the operating staff wore special protective glasses according to U.S. Food and Drug Administration rules [19]. Implant surface decontamination continued utilizing Er,Cr:YSGG laser (with a wavelength of 2,780 nm) at 1.5 W/25 Hz and a radially firing fiber tip (500 μm, RFPT5-14 mm, Biolase Technology, Irvine, CA) (Figure 17). The laser tip was placed perpendicular to the implant surface and 5 mm away from the implant surface. The area was irrigated with saline, and the sequence was repeated (air-abrasive device, sterile saline irrigation, and Er,Cr:YSGG application). Each laser irradiation occurred approximately for 2 minutes. Cortical perforations

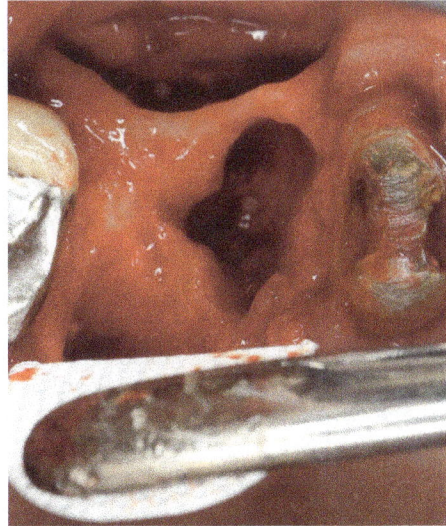

Figure 4: Intraoral picture of the extraction site of #3. The buccal plate showed horizontal deficiency. The nonresorbable high density PTFE membrane was placed on the lingual aspect of #3.

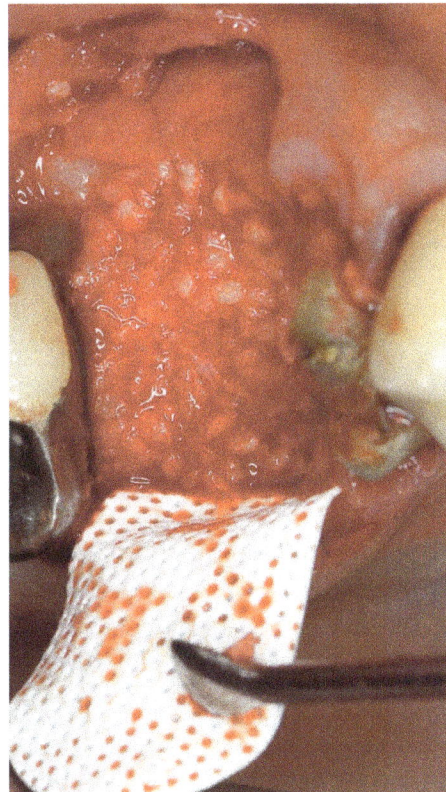

Figure 5: The collagen membrane was placed on the buccal aspect to cover the grafted buccal plate. The nonresorbable high density PTFE membrane was placed on the lingual aspect to cover the grafted socket.

were performed with a finishing round carbide bur, and FDBA was placed around the implant apex, covered with a collagen membrane (Figures 18 and 19). The flap was repositioned and sutured, without tension, with 4–0

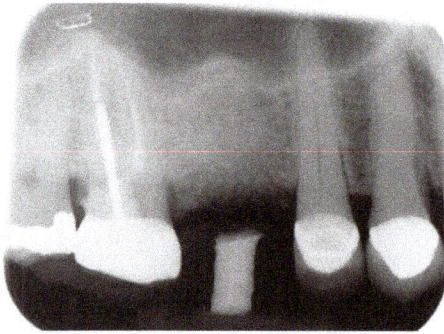

FIGURE 6: A periapical radiograph 3 months after the extraction and ridge preservation showed no signs of residual pathology.

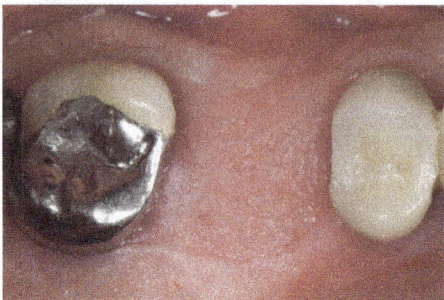

FIGURE 7: The site of #3, 3 months after the ridge preservation showed complete epithelization.

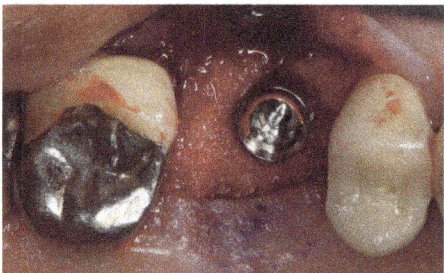

FIGURE 8: A 4.7/11 mm endosseous implant was placed at site #3 with the use of osteotome sinus floor elevation technique.

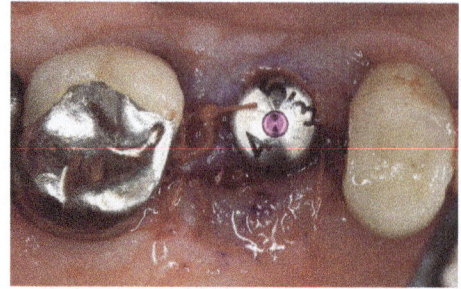

FIGURE 9: The implant was torqued in 35 N/cm, and a healing abutment was placed. The site was sutured with three 5–0 chromic gut single-interrupted sutures.

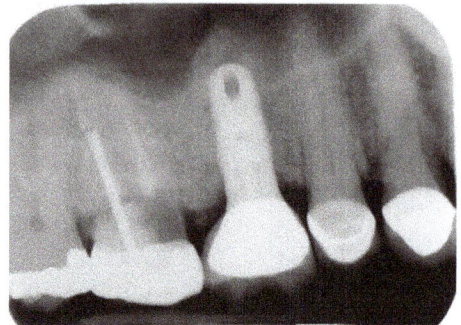

FIGURE 10: A periapical radiograph was taken after the implant placement. Bone condensation is noted apical to implant #3 due to the use of the osteotome sinus floor elevation technique. Mesial of #2, a deep unrestorable decay was observed.

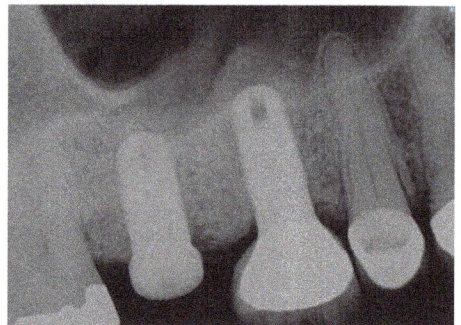

FIGURE 11: The same protocol of extraction, ridge preservation and subsequent implant placement, was followed successfully for site #2. The implant at site #3 did not show any signs of infection or inflammation, radiographically nor clinically.

nonabsorbable monofilament sutures. The patient was prescribed amoxicillin 500 mg three times daily for a week, codeine/acetaminophen 30 mg/300 mg every 6 hours as needed for pain management, and a 0.12% chlorhexidine oral rinse twice daily. The postoperative protocol was very strict with biweekly appointments, until the suture removal in 4 weeks. After the initial phase of healing, the patient returned monthly, for the next 12 months in the clinic, for clinical evaluation of the surgical site and radiographic evaluation. The patient healed uneventfully, without any signs of infection or inflammation. Postoperative periapical radiographs from 6 to 13 months showed the increased density of the bone around the implant apex (Figures 20 and 21). The intraoral picture, 13 months postoperatively, displayed no signs of pathology and the probing depths around the implant measured ≤4 mm (Figure 22).

4. Discussion

Bacteria associated with failing implants due to infection are similar to those found in chronic periodontitis cases. Therefore, the disruption of the biofilm is a prerequisite for successful treatment [20, 21]. Any peri-implant radiolucency should be addressed immediately to prevent further loss of osseointegration [14].

Reiser and Nevins [4] suggested a classification system for implant periapical lesions differentiating them as either

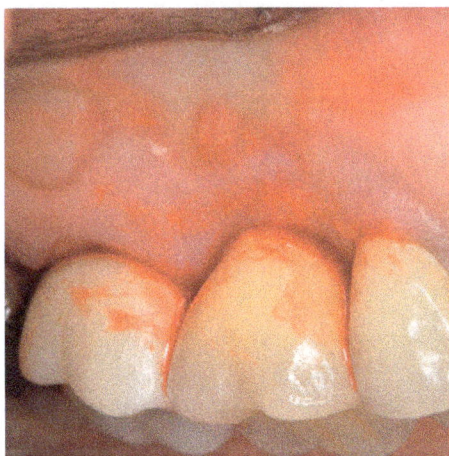

FIGURE 12: The patient presented at the day of surgical debridement of site #3 with a nondraining fistula at the same site where the fistula was noted before the extraction of #3. The picture is taken after the intrasulcular incisions were performed, with the use of a 15c blade.

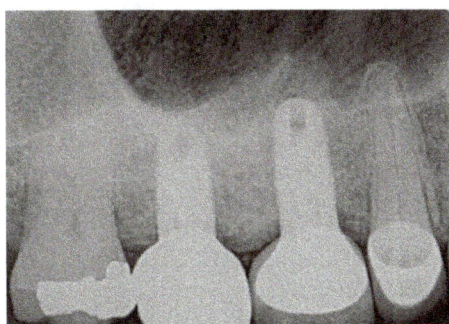

FIGURE 13: A periapical radiograph on the day of surgical debridement showing a 5×5 mm lack of bone density around the implant apex.

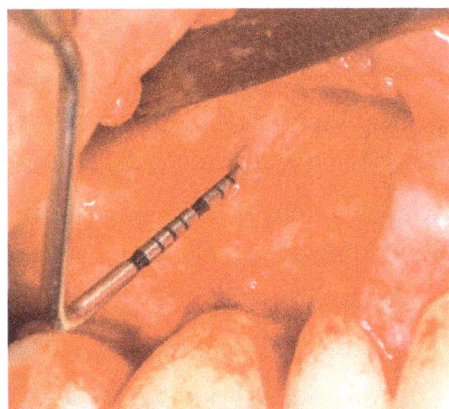

FIGURE 14: Following reflection of full thickness mucoperiosteal flap, a fenestration of 2×2 mm width and 7 mm depth was revealed.

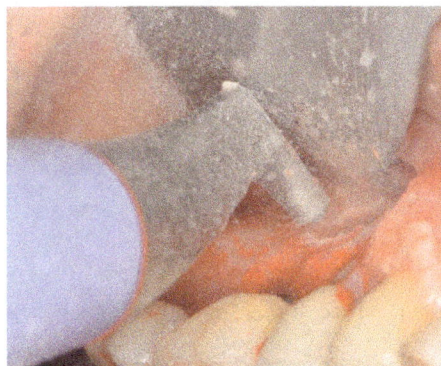

FIGURE 15: The air powder flow was used to decontaminate the implant surface.

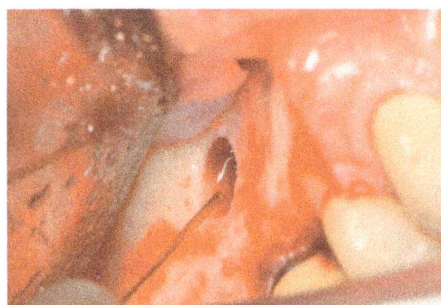

FIGURE 16: An Er,Cr:YSGG laser with the radially firing periodontal tip used to decontaminate the implant surface.

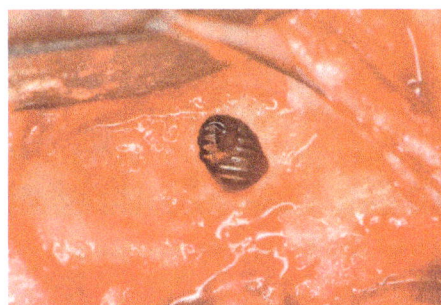

FIGURE 17: Exposed 7 threads of the implant.

This classification has 4 classes. Class 1 is when the implant placement results in devitalization of an adjacent previously vital tooth. Class 2 is when an implant apex is infected by a persistent periapical lesion on an adjacent tooth or implant. Class 3 is when an implant apex is placed labial or lingual, outside the alveolar housing. Class 4 is when an implant apex develops a lesion due to residual infection at the placement site. Our case belongs to class 4, which is an implant apical lesion developed due to residual infection. The treatment associated with this class is surgical debridement of the implant site with possible grafting [22]. The management of our case is in accordance with the suggested treatment.

To date, there is no consensus for the treatment of RPI; therefore, the treatment is empiric. Romanos et al., based on

"infected" or "inactive" [22]. The authors suggested a surgical intervention for the infected type and monitoring for the inactive lesion. Recently, a new classification scheme was proposed for RPI with treatment strategies for each class.

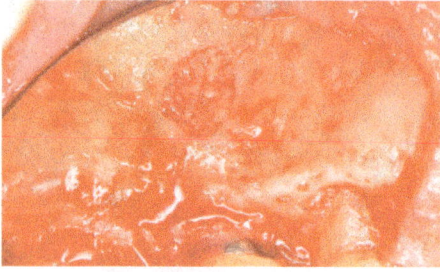

FIGURE 18: Mineralized cortical bone placed around the apex of the implant.

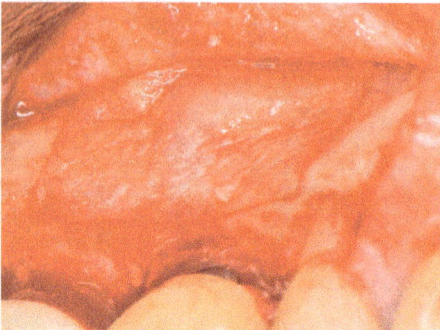

FIGURE 19: A collagen membrane placed over the grafted site.

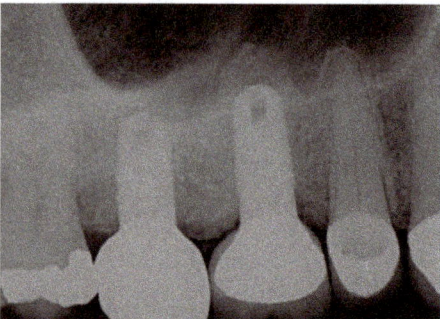

FIGURE 20: A periapical radiograph at 6 months postoperatively demonstrated an increased density around the implant apex.

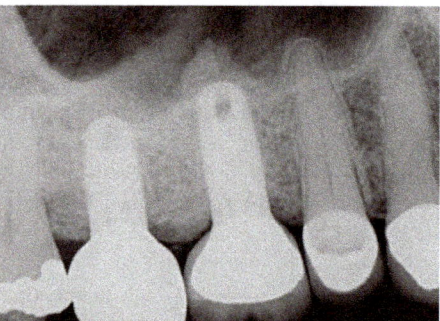

FIGURE 21: Radiograph at 13 months postoperatively presented increased bone density around the implant apex.

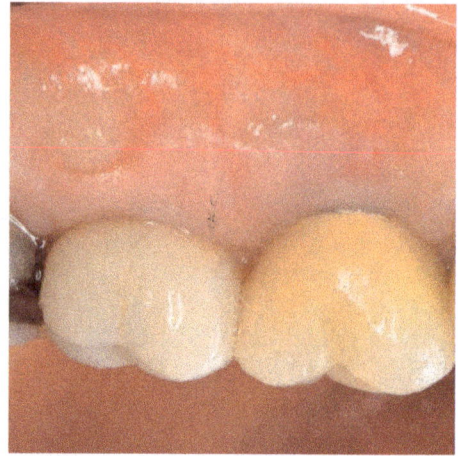

FIGURE 22: Clinical evaluation 13 months postoperatively showed no signs of pathology.

a systematic evaluation of clinical case reports, showed that the use of antimicrobials only was not successful in any case for the treatment of implant periapical lesions [12]. The use of an air-abrasive device for the treatment of peri-implantitis compared to mechanical debridement showed significantly better results in BOP reduction after 12 months [23]. Application of air-abrasive powders seems to be an efficacious modality for the decontamination of implant surfaces and is ranking very high, among the other treatment modalities for the removal of the plaque biofilm. Nevertheless, it has an increased risk for emphysema [24]. The preservation of implants' surface integrity is essential even though Ayangco et al. claimed that any scratching during the surgical debridement is not critical [25].

Mohamed et al. presented a case report where a patient was referred for implant placement at the upper lateral incisor (#10) [26]. Both, the central and lateral incisors (#9, 10) had periapical lesions and were treated endodontically. The tooth #10 was extracted due to fracture, and an immediate implant was placed. Four months postoperatively, the implant was diagnosed with RPI due to radiographic and clinical signs of periapical pathology. The implant site was treated surgically with debridement and placement of anorganic bovine bone and platelet-rich fibrin. The authors followed up the case for 12 months. The periapical lesion around the implant apex showed radiographic signs of resolution on the distal aspect, whereas on the mesial aspect, the lesion was still present [26].

Quaranta et al. presented a similar case report of an implant which was placed immediately in a postextraction socket [27]. The extracted premolar (#13) was symptomatic, but further information was not given, nor a radiograph. Three months after the placement, the implant showed both radiographic and clinical signs of RPI. The site was surgically debrided, and a pericardium membrane was placed over the defect without the addition of any grafting material. Five years postoperatively, the implant had no radiographic or clinical signs of residual pathology, and new bone formation was noted around the apex [27].

Ataullah et al. displayed a case where an endodontically treated central incisor (#9) had class III mobility, a post and core and a large periapical lesion [28]. The authors performed extraction and ridge preservation with mixed anorganic bovine bone mineral and autogenous bone. Six months later, an implant was placed successfully on site #9. Two months after the implant placement, the patient presented with a sinus tract between #9 and 10 and a periapical lesion around #9. Implant #9 was diagnosed with RPI, and tooth #10 was vital. The site was surgically debrided and anorganic bovine bone with a collagen membrane was placed. Three months postoperatively, the implant showed no signs of periapical pathology. No further information was given after the first three months postoperatively [28].

Case reports showed that RPI was diagnosed after immediate implant placement in a previously infected area [26, 27]. Therefore, ridge preservation seemed to be a safer approach, when the extracted tooth showed periapical lesions. Nevertheless, like our case, implants were diagnosed with RPI, even if a ridge preservation procedure preceded the implant placement. Implant apicoectomy was suggested in two case reports by Dahlin et al. [29]. Follow-up in both cases showed uneventful healing and absence of clinical symptoms [29]. Quirynen et al. suggested that implant apicoectomy is not required for the treatment of RPI [9]. To achieve complete bone regeneration around peri-implant defects, the use of augmentation materials is required. The concurrent use of GBR following implant decontamination provides stabilization of the blood clot and space maintenance [30, 31]. Implants with periapical lesions that were treated successfully showed a survival rate of 75%, ranging from 4 months to 7 years postoperatively [12].

Different types of lasers are available in surgical dentistry, in various wavelengths, such as carbon dioxide (CO_2); diode (810–980 nm); neodymium-doped: yttrium, aluminum, and garnet (Nd:YAG); erbium-doped: yttrium, aluminum, and garnet (Er:YAG); and erbium, chromium-doped: yttrium, scandium, gallium, and garnet (Er,Cr:YSGG) [32–34]. During their application, caution is advised not to overheat the implant and therefore compromise the implants' surface integrity. Er,Cr:YSGG laser ablates tissue through a hydrokinetic process and can be used with radially firing periodontal tip and energy settings up to 2.5 W. It does not increase the temperature in critical levels to affect implant surfaces. Furthermore, it successfully removes the plaque biofilm over roughened surfaces, compared to plastic curettes and chlorhexidine [32–34].

Azzeh, showed in a peri-implantitis case report that the use of Er,Cr:YSGG laser enabled the regenerative osseous surgery around an implant. In his case report, the laser was used for flap reflection, as well as for cortical perforations. The results were comparable to our clinical case report, achieving bone regeneration without any complications and with high patient satisfaction [35]. Al-Falaki et al. used Er,Cr:YSGG in a case series of nonsurgical management of peri-implantitis. They treated 28 implants with a mean PD of 6.64 ± 1.48 mm. Six months after the treatment, the PDs were decreased to 2.97 ± 0.7 mm, and the BOP reduction was

significantly reduced compared to baseline [36]. Like Er,Cr:YSGG, the use of a CO_2 laser helps avoid implant surface damage, and the temperature is not increased in critical levels [37, 38]. On the contrary, the use of a Nd:YAG laser could lead to detrimental effects and melting of the implant surface due to overheating since it is being absorbed by the implant surface [39].

Schwarz et al. performed a controlled clinical study comparing Er:YAG versus mechanical debridement with chlorhexidine, in moderate and advanced peri-implantitis cases. The results in terms of reduction of PD and CAL were not significant at 12 months. The most interesting result of this study is that 12 months postoperatively, all patients were discontinued from the study and received further laser treatment and GBR. The reason for that decision was the increased BOP after 12 months of healing [40].

To the best of the authors' knowledge, this is the first case report to describe the concurrent use of an air-abrasive device, Er,Cr:YSGG, and GBR for the treatment of RPI. Implant #3 was placed one year after extraction of tooth #3 and ridge preservation. The implant was placed according to the restorative needs of this site; however, the apex of the implant was positioned in the approximate location of the previous periapical radiolucency of the mesial buccal root of tooth #3. Even though no signs of infection or inflammation were present at the site before and/or after implant placement, RPI was diagnosed 2 years after the implant placement. Dahlin et al. suggested a more aggressive debridement due to the rough surface of the implants. The implants with rough surfaces create an environment where further progression of the RPI or peri-implantitis occurs. Our treatment was in accordance with this suggestion, with the use of an air-abrasive device and Er,Cr:YSGG. The aim of our approach was, due to limited surgical access, to avoid leaving any locus minoris, allowing the bacteria to nevertheless reside in the implant surface after the end of the surgical debridement phase [29]. The subsequent use of GBR was to allow the stabilization of the blood clot and the space maintenance to facilitate the regeneration of the bone around the implant apex. Our results demonstrated radiographic bone fill around the apex of the implant, without radiographic or clinical signs of residual pathology during 13 months of follow-up. Further clinical and radiographic follow-ups are required to provide evidence of this combined surgical approach.

5. Conclusions

The etiology of RPI in this case was the placement of an implant in a previously infected site. This case of RPI was treated through a surgical approach utilizing an air-abrasive device, Er,Cr:YSGG, and GBR. The site was monitored for 13 months, and increased radiographic bone density was noted.

References

[1] M. Quirynen, F. Gijbels, and R. Jacobs, "An infected jawbone site compromising successful osseointegration," *Periodontology 2000*, vol. 33, no. 1, pp. 129–144, 2003.

[2] B. S. McAllister, D. Masters, and R. M. Meffert, "Treatment of implants demonstrating periapical radiolucencies," *Practical Periodontics and Aesthetic Dentistry*, vol. 4, no. 9, pp. 37–41, 1992.

[3] H. I. Sussman and S. S. Moss, "Localized osteomyelitis secondary to endodontic-implant pathosis. A case report," *Journal of Periodontology*, vol. 64, no. 4, pp. 306–310, 1993.

[4] G. M. Reiser and M. Nevins, "The implant periapical lesion: etiology, prevention and treatment," *Compendium of Continuing Education in Dentistry*, vol. 16, no. 8, pp. 786–772, 1995.

[5] A. Piattelli, A. Scarano, B. Balleri, and G. A. Favero, "Clinical and histologic evaluation of an active "implant periapical lesion": a case report," *International Journal of Oral & Maxillofacial Implants*, vol. 13, no. 5, pp. 713–716, 1998.

[6] M. Esposito, J. M. Hirsch, U. Lekholm, and P. Thomsen, "Biological factors contributing to failures of osseointegrated oral implants. (II). Etiopathogenesis," *European Journal of Oral Sciences*, vol. 106, no. 3, pp. 721–764, 1998.

[7] N. Sarmast, H. H. Wang, N. K. Soldatos et al., "A novel treatment decision tree and literature review of retrograde peri-implantitis," *Journal of Periodontology*, vol. 87, no. 12, pp. 1458–1467, 2016.

[8] M. Peñarrocha-Diago, M. Peñarrocha-Diago, and J. A. Blaya-Tárraga, "State of the art and clinical recommendations in periapical implant lesions. 9th Mozo-Grau Ticare Conference in Quintanilla, Spain," *Journal of Clinical and Experimental Dentistry*, vol. 9, no. 3, pp. 471–473, 2017.

[9] M. Quirynen, R. Vogels, G. Alsaadi, I. Naert, R. Jacobs, and D. van Steenberghe, "Predisposing conditions for retrograde peri-implantitis, and treatment suggestions," *Clinical Oral Implants Research*, vol. 16, no. 5, pp. 599–608, 2005.

[10] J. D. Kassolis, M. Scheper, B. Jham, and M. A. Reynolds, "Histopathologic findings in bone from edentulous alveolar ridges: a role in osteonecrosis of the jaws?," *Bone*, vol. 47, no. 1, pp. 127–130, 2010.

[11] W. Zhou, C. Han, D. Li, Y. Li, Y. Song, and Y. Zhao, "Endodontic treatment of teeth induces retrograde peri-implantitis," *Clinical Oral Implants Research*, vol. 20, no. 12, pp. 1326–1332, 2009.

[12] G. E. Romanos, S. Froum, S. Costa-Martins, S. Meitner, and D. P. Tarnow, "Implant periapical lesions: etiology and treatment options," *Journal of Oral Implantology*, vol. 37, no. 1, pp. 53–63, 2011.

[13] T. F. Tozum, M. Sencximen, K. Ortakoglu et al., "Diagnosis and treatment of a large periapical implant lesion associated with adjacent natural tooth: a case report," *Oral Surgery, Oral Medicine, Oral Pathology, Oral Radiology, and Endodontology*, vol. 101, no. 6, pp. 132–138, 2006.

[14] D. Flanagan, "Apical (retrograde) peri-implantitis: a case report of an active lesion," *Journal of Oral Implantology*, vol. 28, no. 2, pp. 92–96, 2002.

[15] A. Ramanauskaite, G. Juodzbalys, and T. Tözüm, "Apical/retrograde periimplantitis/implant periapical lesion: etiology, risk factors, and treatment options," *Implant Dentistry*, vol. 25, no. 5, pp. 684–697, 2016.

[16] M. G. Newman and T. F. Flemmig, "Bacterial-host interaction," in *Advanced Osseointegration Surgery*, P. Worthington and P. I. Brånemark, Eds., Quintessence, Berlin, Germany, 1992.

[17] S. Bhaskar, "Periapical lesions–types, incidence and clinical features," *Oral Surgery, Oral Medicine, Oral Pathology*, vol. 21, no. 5, pp. 657–671, 1966.

[18] P. Rosen, R. Summers, J. Mellado et al., "The bone-added osteotome sinus floor elevation technique: multicenter retrospective report of consecutively treated patients," *International Journal of Oral & Maxillofacial Implants*, vol. 14, no. 6, pp. 853–858, 1999.

[19] U.S. Food and Drug Administration, *Waterlase expanded indications for use*, 2006, http://www.fda.gov/cdrh/pdf3/k030523.pdf.

[20] E. S. Rosenberg, J. P. Torosian, and J. Slots, "Microbial differences in 2 clinically distinct types of failures of osseointegrated implants," *Clinical Oral Implants Research*, vol. 2, no. 3, pp. 135–144, 1991.

[21] A. Leonhardt, S. Renvert, and G. Dahlen, "Microbial findings at failing implants," *Clinical Oral Implants Research*, vol. 10, no. 5, pp. 339–345, 1999.

[22] N. Sarmast, H. W. Wang, A. Sajadi, N. Angelov, and S. O. Dorn, "Classification and clinical management of retrograde peri-implantitis associated with apical periodontitis: a proposed classification system and case report," *Journal of Endodontics*, vol. 43, no. 11, pp. 1–4, 2017.

[23] G. John, N. Sahm, J. Becker, and F. Schwarz, "Non-surgical treatment of peri-implantitis using an air-abrasive device or mechanical debridement and local application of chlorhexidine. Twelve-month follow-up of a prospective, randomized, controlled clinical study," *Clinical Oral Investigations*, vol. 19, no. 8, pp. 1807–1814, 2015.

[24] E. van de Velde, P. Thielens, H. Schautteet, and R. Vanclooster, "Subcutaneous emphysema of the oral floor during cleaning of a bridge fixed on an IMZ implant. Case report," *Revue Belge de Médecine Dentaire*, vol. 46, pp. 64–71, 1991.

[25] L. Ayangco and P. J. Sheridan, "Development and treatment of retrograde peri-implantitis involving a site with a history of failed endodontic and apicoectomy procedures: a series of reports," *International Journal of Oral & Maxillofacial Implants*, vol. 16, no. 3, pp. 412–417, 2001.

[26] J. Mohamed, N. Alam, G. Singh, and C. Chandrasekaran, "The management of retrograde peri-implantitis: a case report," *Journal of Clinical and Diagnostic Research*, vol. 6, no. 9, pp. 1600–1602, 2012.

[27] A. Quaranta, S. Andreana, G. Pompa, and M. Procaccini, "Active implant peri-apical lesion: a case report treated via guided bone regeneration with a 5-year clinical and radiographic follow-up," *Journal of Oral Implantology*, vol. 40, no. 3, pp. 313–319, 2014.

[28] K. Ataullah, L. Chee, L. Peng, and H. Kim Lung, "Management of retrograde peri-implantitis: a clinical case report," *Journal of Oral Implantology*, vol. 32, no. 6, pp. 308–312, 2006.

[29] D. Dahlin, H. Nikfarid, B. Alsen, and H. Kashani, "Apical peri-implantitis: possible predisposing factors, case reports, and treatment suggestions," *Clinical Implant Dentistry and Related Research*, vol. 11, no. 3, pp. 222–227, 2009.

[30] L. G. Persson, I. Ericsson, T. Berglundh, and J. Lindhe, "Guided bone regeneration in the treatment of peri-implantitis," *Clinical Oral Implants Research*, vol. 7, no. 4, pp. 366–372, 1996.

[31] C. Dahlin, L. Sennerby, U. Lekholm et al., "Generation of new bone around titanium implants using a membrane technique an experimental study in rabbits," *International Journal of Oral & Maxillofacial Implants*, vol. 4, no. 1, pp. 19–25, 1989.

[32] F. Schwarz, E. Nuesry, K. Bieling et al., "Influence of an erbium, chromium-doped yttrium, scandium, gallium, and

garnet (Er,Cr:YSGG) laser on the reestablishment of the biocompatibility of contaminated titanium implant surfaces," *Journal of Periodontology*, vol. 77, no. 11, pp. 1820–1827, 2006.

[33] F. Schwarz, A. Sculean, G. Romanos et al., "Influence of different treatment approaches on the removal of early plaque biofilms and the viability of $SAOS_2$ osteoblasts grown on titanium implants," *Clinical Oral Investigations*, vol. 9, no. 2, pp. 111–117, 2005.

[34] R. J. Miller, "Treatment of the contaminated implant surface using the Er,Cr:YSGG laser," *Implant Dentistry*, vol. 13, no. 2, pp. 165–170, 2004.

[35] M. Azzeh, "Er,Cr:YSGG laser-assisted surgical treatment of peri-implantitis with 1-year reentry and 18-month follow-up," *Journal of Periodontology*, vol. 79, no. 10, pp. 2000–2005, 2008.

[36] R. Al-Falaki, M. Cronshaw, and F. J. Hughes, "Treatment outcome following use of the erbium, chromium: yttrium, scandium, gallium and garnet in the non-surgical management of peri-implantitis: a case series," *British Dental Journal*, vol. 217, no. 8, pp. 453–457, 2014.

[37] H. Deppe, H. H. Horch, and A. Neff, "Conventional versus CO_2 laser-assisted treatment of peri-implant defects with the concomitant use of pure-phase beta-tricalcium phosphate: a 5-year clinical report," *International Journal of Oral & Maxillofacial Implants*, vol. 22, no. 1, pp. 79–86, 2007.

[38] G. E. Romanos and G. H. Nentwig, "Regenerative therapy of deep peri-implant infrabony defects after CO_2 laser implant surface decontamination," *International Journal of Periodontics & Restorative Dentistry*, vol. 28, no. 3, pp. 245–255, 2008.

[39] G. E. Romanos, H. Everts, and G. H. Nentwig, "Effects of diode and Nd:YAG laser irradiation on titanium discs: a scanning electron microscope examination," *Journal of Periodontology*, vol. 71, no. 5, pp. 810–815, 2000.

[40] F. Schwarz, K. Bieling, M. Bonsmann, T. Latz, and J. Becker, "Nonsurgical treatment of moderate and advanced peri-implantitis lesions: a controlled clinical study," *Clinical Oral Investigations*, vol. 10, no. 4, pp. 279–288, 2006.

10

Alveolar Ridge Preservation Using a Novel Synthetic Grafting Material: A Case with Two-Year Follow-Up

Peter Fairbairn [iD],[1] **Minas Leventis** [iD],[2] **Chas Mangham,**[3] **and Robert Horowitz**[4]

[1]*Department of Periodontology and Implant Dentistry, School of Dentistry, University of Detroit Mercy, 2700 Martin Luther King Jr. Boulevard, Detroit, MI 48208, USA*
[2]*Department of Oral and Maxillofacial Surgery, Dental School, National and Kapodistrian University of Athens, 2 Thivon Street, Goudi, Athens 115 27, Greece*
[3]*Manchester Molecular Pathology Innovation Centre, The University of Manchester, Nelson Street, Manchester M13 9NQ, UK*
[4]*Departments of Periodontics, Implant Dentistry, and Oral Surgery, New York University College of Dentistry, 345 E. 24th Street, New York, NY 10010, USA*

Correspondence should be addressed to Minas Leventis; dr.minasleventis@gmail.com

Academic Editor: Eduardo Hochuli-Vieira

This case report highlights the use of a novel in situ hardening synthetic (alloplastic), resorbable, bone grafting material composed of beta tricalcium phosphate and calcium sulfate, for alveolar ridge preservation. A 35-year-old female patient was referred by her general dentist for extraction of the mandibular right first molar and rehabilitation of the site with a dental implant. The nonrestorable tooth was "atraumatically" extracted without raising a flap, and the socket was immediately grafted with the synthetic biomaterial and covered with a hemostatic fleece. No membrane was used, and the site was left uncovered without obtaining primary closure, in order to heal by secondary intention. After 12 weeks, the architecture of the ridge was preserved, and clinical observation revealed excellent soft tissue healing without loss of attached gingiva. At reentry for placement of the implant, a bone core biopsy was obtained, and primary implant stability was measured by final seating torque and resonance frequency analysis. Histological analysis revealed pronounced bone regeneration while high levels of primary implant stability were recorded. The implant was successfully loaded 12 weeks after placement. Clinical and radiological follow-up examination at two years revealed stable and successful results regarding biological, functional, and esthetic parameters.

1. Introduction

Clinical and experimental studies have shown that grafting the postextraction sockets at the time of tooth extraction with a bone grafting material constitutes a predictable and reliable way to limit the resorption of the alveolar ridge [1–3]. Such alveolar ridge preservation measures involve the use of a wide variety of bone substitutes, barrier membranes, and biologically active materials, and many different surgical techniques and protocols have been proposed [4–6].

According to Yip et al. [7], the ideal grafting material should have specific attributes. It should be osteoconductive, osteoinductive, and biocompatible. It is important to be totally replaced by host bone having an appropriate resorption time in relation to new bone formation. Moreover,

it should be able to maintain the volume stability of the augmented site, have satisfactory mechanical properties, and have no risk of disease transmission.

Allografts, xenografts, and synthetic particulate materials, with or without a membrane, have been extensively used and documented, showing adequate results in the preservation of the ridge dimensions [5]. It is important that these bone substitutes vary in terms of origin, composition and biological mechanism of function regarding graft resorption and new bone formation, each having their own advantages and disadvantages [8, 9].

Alloplasts represent a group of synthetic osteoconductive, biocompatible bone substitutes that are free of any risk of transmitting infections or diseases by themselves, and their availability is unlimited [10–12]. One of the most promising groups of synthetic bone substitutes is calcium phosphate ceramics, and among them beta tricalcium phosphate (β-TCP) is commonly used [13–15]. Apart from being osteoconductive, there is strong experimental evidence that calcium phosphates also have osteoinductive properties. Although the underlying mechanism remains largely unknown, it has been shown that these alloplastic materials can stimulate osteogenic differentiation of stem cells in vitro and bone induction in vivo [16, 17].

The ability of the bacteriostatic calcium sulfate (CS) to set and hence be stable is well documented. Adding CS to β-TCP produces an in situ hardening grafting material that binds directly to the host bone, maintains the space and shape of the grafted site, and acts as a stable scaffold [18–23]. The improved stability throughout the graft material seems to further improve the quality of the bone that will be regenerated due to reduced micromotion of the material, which may lead to mesenchymal differentiation to fibroblasts instead of osteoblasts. It is known that micromovements between bone and any implanted grafted material prevent bone formation, resulting in the development of fibrous tissue [24, 25]. Moreover, the CS element creates a nanoporous cell occlusive membrane that may prevent the early stage invasion of unwanted soft tissue cells into the graft [26, 27].

Both CS and β-TCP are fully resorbable materials leading to the regeneration of high-quality vital host bone without the long-term presence of residual graft particles. The CS element will resorb over a 3–6-week period, depending on patient physiology, thus increasing porosity in the β-TCP scaffold for improved vascular ingrowth and angiogenesis, while the β-TCP element will resorb by hydrolysis and cellular resorption over a period of 9–16 months, again dependent on host physiology [13].

The purpose of this report is to present a case that highlights the clinical, radiological, and histological outcomes of socket grafting with an in situ hardening β-TCP/CS synthetic bone substitute following a minimally invasive procedure.

2. Case Presentation

A 35-year-old female patient, nonsmoker, with noncontributory medical history, presented with a nonconservable mandibular right first molar due to extensive caries and periapical pathology (Figure 1). After thorough clinical and radiological examination, a delayed implant placement treatment plan was decided, consisting of extraction of the failing tooth with simultaneous socket grafting and implant placement after a 12-week healing period.

Tooth extraction was performed under local anesthesia without flap elevation. In order to minimize surgical trauma, the tooth was sectioned with a Lindemann burr (Komet Inc., Lemgo, Germany) under copious irrigation with sterile saline, and each root was independently mobilized and carefully luxated using periotomes and elevators. Attention was given not to injure the surrounding soft and hard tissues, especially in the buccal aspect. After extraction, the socket was thoroughly debrided from granulation tissue, using bone curettes, and rinsed with sterile saline. A periodontal probe was then utilized to explore the site which revealed

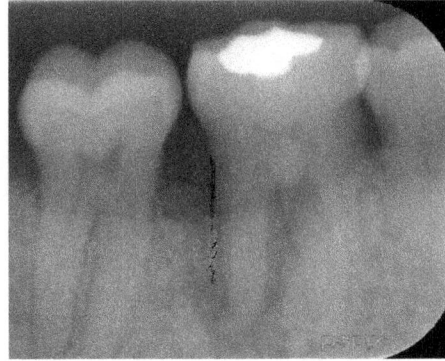

FIGURE 1: Preoperative periapical X-ray.

that the septal bone and the buccal bone wall were completely missing (Figure 2).

A fully resorbable alloplastic in situ hardening bone substitute (EthOss®, Ethoss Regeneration Ltd., Silsden, UK) was used to graft the site. The material consists of β-TCP (65%) and CS (35%), preloaded in a plastic sterile syringe. In accordance with the manufacturer's instructions prior to injecting the material into the socket, the particles of the biomaterial were mixed in the syringe with sterile saline. After application of the graft into the postextraction site, a bone plunger was used to condense the moldable graft particles, in order to occupy all the volume of the socket up to the level of the surrounding host bone (Figure 3). Attention was given not to overfill the socket as this could result in subsequent sequestration of the exposed coronal particles or displacement of the entire graft mass after mechanical irritation during the first phases of healing. A saline-wet gauze was used to further compact the graft particles and accelerate the in situ hardening of the CS element of the graft. As a result, after a few minutes, the alloplastic bone substitute formed a stable, porous scaffold for the host osseous regeneration. The site was then covered with a hemostatic dressing material (Jason® Collagen Fleece, Botiss Biomaterials GmbH, Germany), and a cross-mattress tension-free 5/0 suture (Vicryl®, Ethicon, Johnson & Johnson, Somerville, NJ, USA) was placed over to achieve soft tissue stability (Figure 4). The site was left uncovered without obtaining primary closure in order to heal by secondary intention. The patient did not wear any prosthesis during the healing period. Antibiotic therapy consisting of 500 mg amoxicillin every 8 hours for 5 days, and a 0.2% chlorhexidine mouthwash for 7 days were prescribed. The suture was removed 1 week postoperatively.

The postoperative healing was uneventful, and the site was gradually covered by newly formed soft tissue with no loss of bone graft particles. After 12 weeks, the area was completely covered with newly formed keratinized epithelium, while the volume and architecture of the ridge were adequately preserved. A periapical X-ray at this point in time showed the consolidation of the grafting material, resulting in bone regeneration at the site (Figure 5). A site-specific full thickness flap was elevated revealing that the grafted area was filled with regenerated hard tissue (Figure 6). Prior to implant placement, a bone core biopsy was taken (Figure 7) with a depth of 7 mm from the center of the site using a trephine drill with

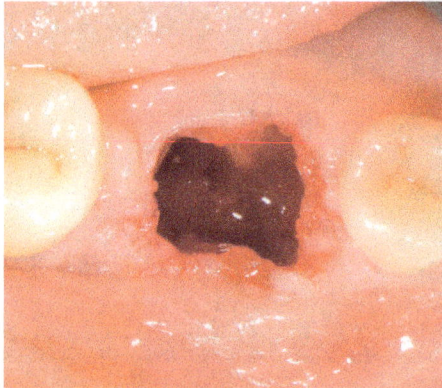

(a)

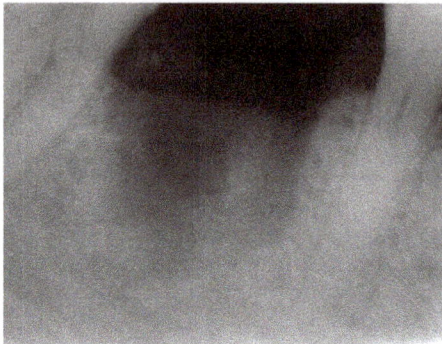

(b)

FIGURE 2: Clinical view and periapical X-ray of the site immediately after the "atraumatic" flapless extraction. The septal bone is completely missing, and the buccal bone was defective. Note the shortage of buccal keratinized soft tissue.

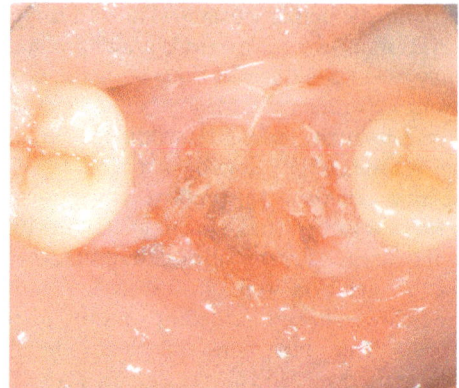

(a)

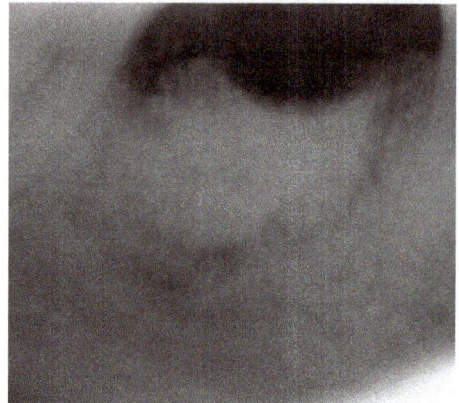

(b)

FIGURE 4: Clinical view and periapical X-ray of the grafted site.

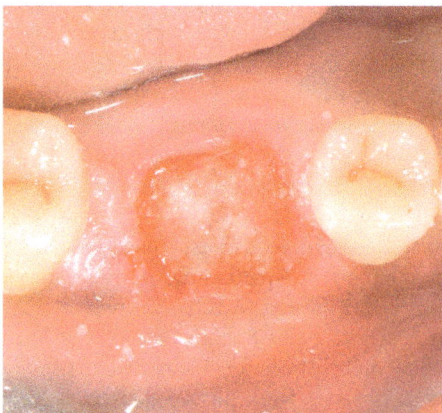

FIGURE 3: Grafting of the site with the in situ hardening synthetic bone substitute. Attention was given not to overfill the socket.

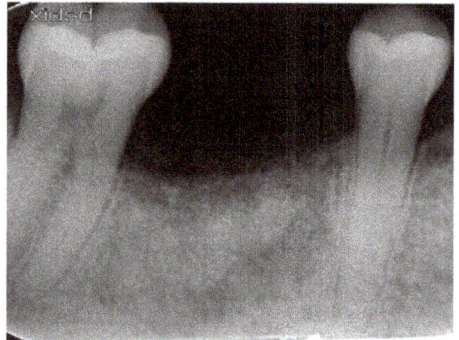

FIGURE 5: Periapical X-ray at 12 weeks showing that the site is occupied by newly formed hard tissue.

a diameter of 2.3 mm (Komet Inc., Lemgo, Germany). Following the harvesting of the bone sample, the preparation of the bony bed was completed at the same site and a tapered implant (Dio Co., Busan, Korea), of 4.5 mm in diameter and 10 mm in length, was then placed at the optimal position (Figure 8). Immediately after implant placement, the final seating torque was recorded using the manufacturer's hand ratchet (Dio Co., Busan, Korea). The ISQ was also measured by resonance frequency analysis (Osstell ISQ™, Göteborg, Sweden) showing excellent initial stability (35 Ncm and 69/70 resp.). The cover screw was placed, and the mucoperiosteal flap was repositioned and closed, without tension, using interrupted resorbable 4-0 sutures (Vicryl, Ethicon, Johnson & Johnson, Somerville, NJ, USA).

The bone specimen was fixed in 10% formalin for 2 days and subsequently decalcified in bone decalcification solution for 14 days. After routine tissue processing the entire core was embedded into paraffin wax, orientated for

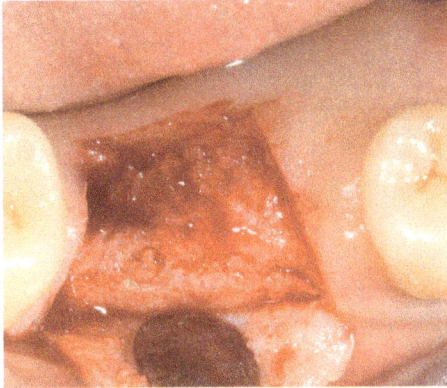

FIGURE 6: Clinical reentry after 12 weeks of healing. The site is occupied by newly formed hard tissue.

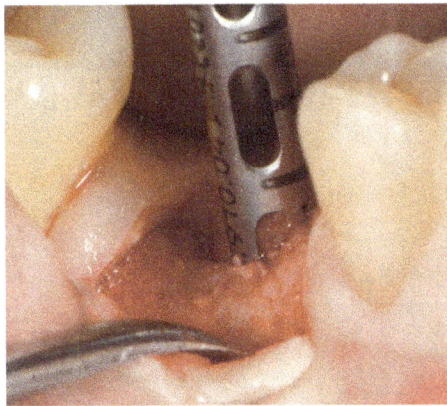

(a)

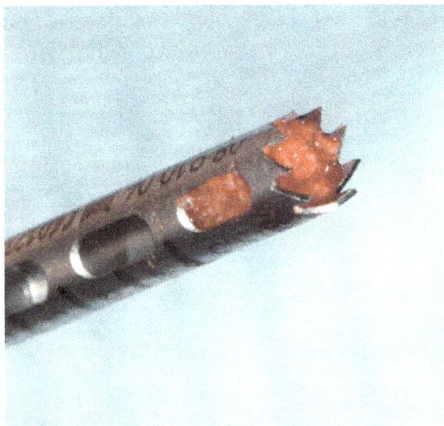

(b)

FIGURE 7: Trephine bone biopsy taken at the center of the regenerated site.

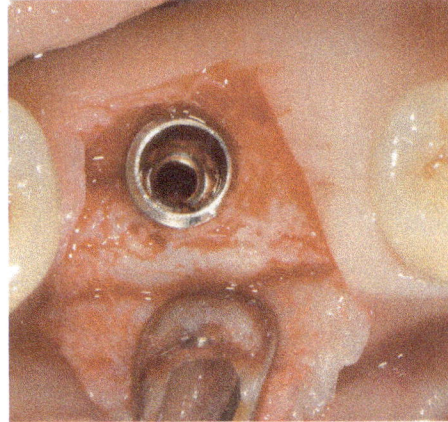

(a)

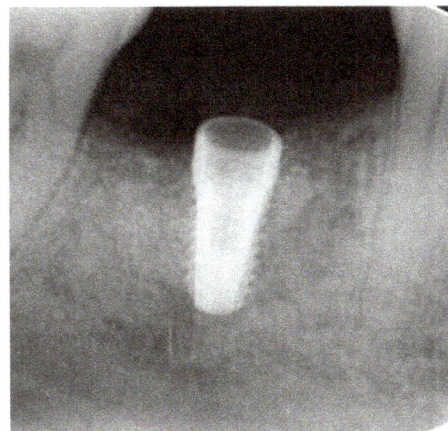

(b)

FIGURE 8: Implant placement at the optimal positioning.

graft particles were surrounded by or in contact with trabecular bone, while active osteoblasts forming osteoid and new woven bone could be identified, demonstrating persistent osteogenesis (Figure 9). Histomorphometric analysis was performed "blind" by one independent observer using the ImageJ imaging analysis software (NIH Image, National Institutes of Health, Maryland, USA). The reference area was the entire area in the biopsy. Histomorphometric analysis revealed that after 12 weeks of healing, the grafted site was occupied by 50.28% of new bone, 12.27% of residual grafting material, and 37.45% of connective tissue.

After allowing 10 weeks for osseointegration, the implant was accessed using a tissue punch, and a higher ISQ (77) was measured (Figure 10). Two weeks later, the implant was restored with the final stock titanium abutment (Dio Co., Busan, Korea) and a cement-retained lithium-disilicate glass-ceramic crown (PS e.max Press; Ivoclar Vivadent AG, Schaan, Liechtenstein), achieving pleasant clinical and radiological results (Figure 11).

Follow-up clinical examination two years after loading revealed stable peri-implant keratinized soft tissues with excellent preservation of the volume and architecture of the ridge (Figure 12). A periapical X-ray and CBCT showed

longitudinal sectioning. 4 μm-thick tissue sections were cut and stained with hematoxylin and eosin (H&E) for light microscopical examination. Histologically, the analyzed biopsy contained newly formed bone, residual grafting material, and vascularized uninflamed connective tissue. No necrosis or foreign body reactions were detected. The

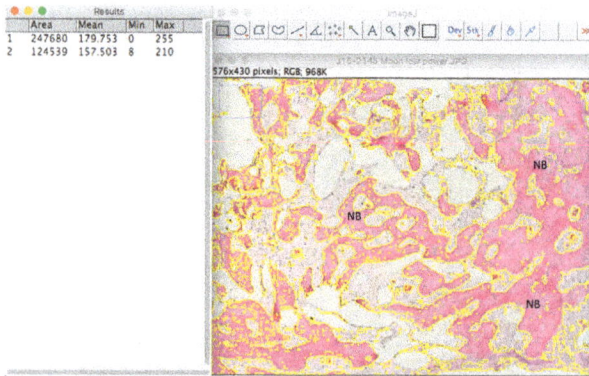

(a)

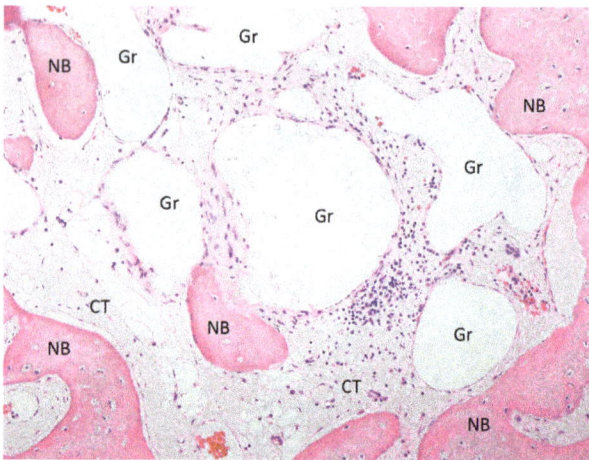

(b)

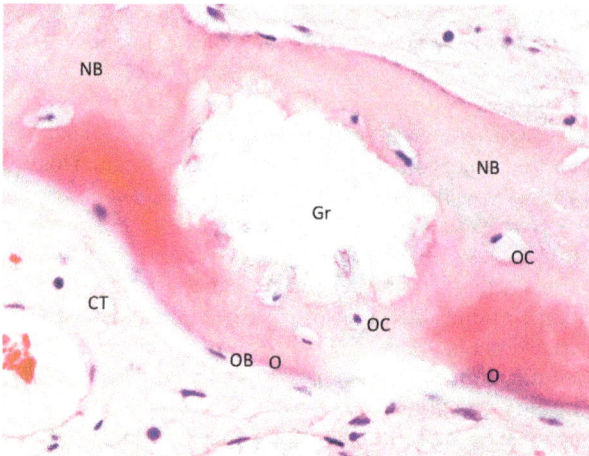

(c)

FIGURE 9: Histological sections of bone core biopsy harvested from the regenerated site using a trephine burr. (a) Overview image of the coronal-apical cut through the entire core biopsy showing new bone (NB) formation in the extraction socket. The new bone is marked, and its surface was calculated in accordance to the overall surface of the specimen, revealing a 50.28% percentage of new bone (H&E stain, original magnification ×20). (b) EthOss particles (Gr) are embedded in well-perfused connective tissue (CT) and newly formed bone (NB) (H&E stain, original magnification ×200). (c) High magnification showing new bone (NB) in contact with a graft particle (Gr). Osteocytes (OC) can be detected inside the new bone and osteoblasts (OB) forming osteoid (O) on its outer surface (H&E stain, original magnification ×400).

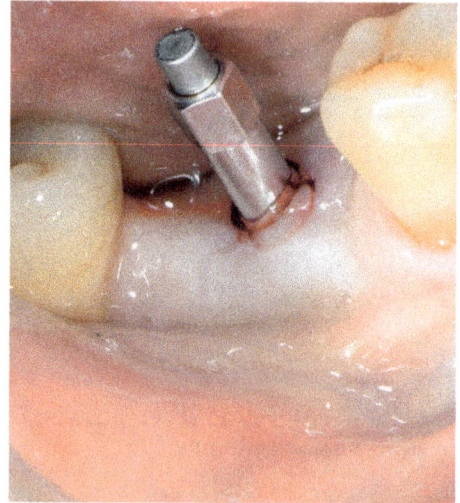

FIGURE 10: ISQ measurement at uncovering of the implant.

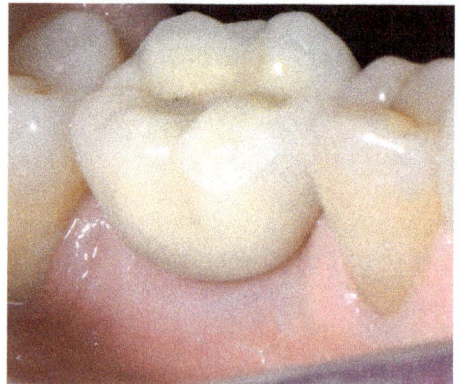

FIGURE 11: Clinical view of the restoration immediately after fitting the restoration.

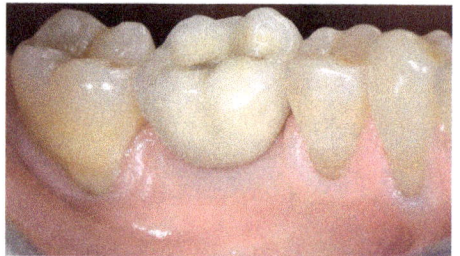

FIGURE 12: Clinical view two years after loading the implant.

further functional remodeling of the bone around the loaded implant with no radiological findings of residual biomaterial (Figure 13).

3. Discussion

In this case, a minimally invasive protocol was followed. Extraction and socket grafting were performed without raising a flap, and the augmented site was not covered with a barrier membrane nor a flap. This approach was selected in order to

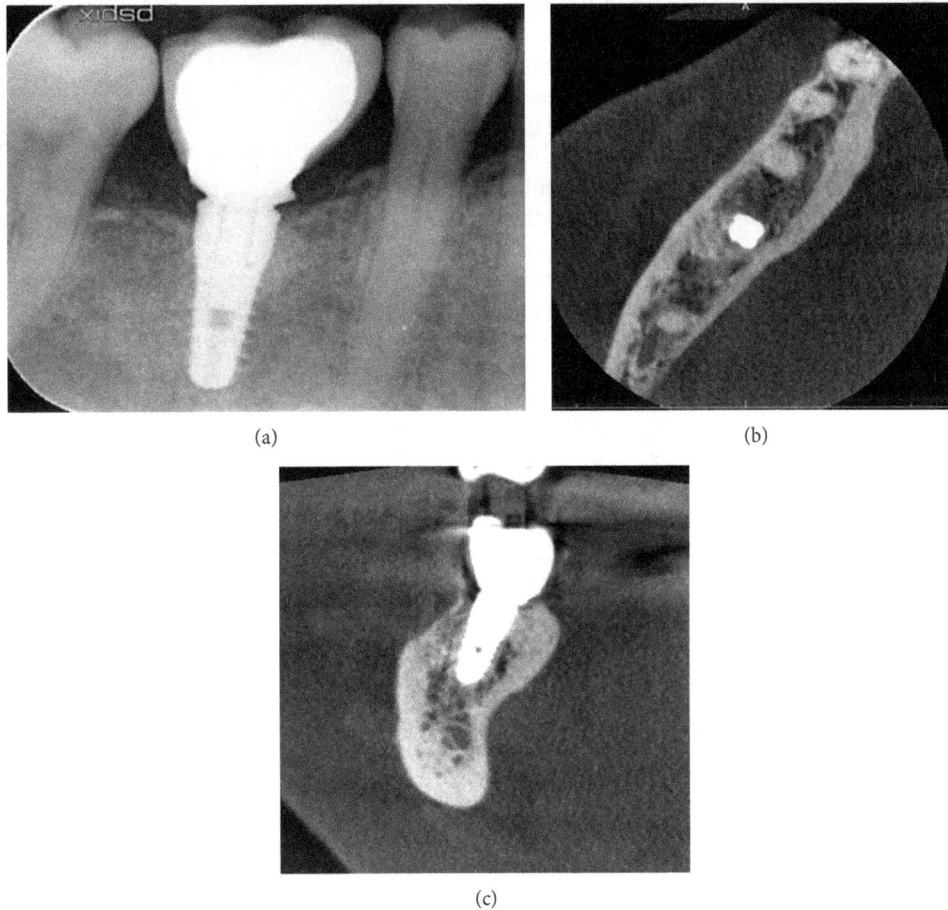

(a)

(b)

(c)

FIGURE 13: Radiological examination two years after loading of the implant: periapical X-ray and axial and coronal planes of the CBCT showing the preservation of the dimensions of the regenerated bone.

minimize patient morbidity, surgical time, and cost, but mostly in an attempt not to displace the mucogingival junction and to allow for the spontaneous formation of new soft tissue over the postextraction grafted site, as described in similar studies using self-hardening synthetic bone grafting materials [11, 28]. The biomechanical stability of the β-TCP/CS graft used in the presented case allowed the site to heal gradually by secondary intention, without loss of the exposed biomaterial in the oral environment. Elevating and advancing a full thickness flap for covering the socket will protect the grafting material. However, it is shown that achieving primary closure does not present beneficial effects on preserving the ridge width. In addition, patients experience more discomfort, and the distortion of the vestibule and the coronal displacement of the buccal keratinized gingiva may lead to esthetic problems, alter the soft tissue profile of the site, and influence in a negative way the health status of the supporting tissues around dental implants [4, 29].

It is without doubt that bone quality is of paramount importance in successful implant therapy. According to Horváth et al. [2], it is doubtful whether an alveolar ridge preservation method should be claimed successful, if it only preserves the external contour of the alveolar ridge, but the newly formed hard tissue is of inferior quality and quantity (percentage of matured trabecular bone) to what is spontaneously achieved following a tooth extraction. Contemporary literature reports conflicting results with the use of the widely used xenografts, with changes in the percentage of vital bone ranging from −22% (decrease) to 9.8% (increase), while considerable residual hydroxyapatite and xenogenic particles (15% to 36%) remained at a mean of 5.6 months after socket grafting procedures [9]. Although it remains unknown whether these changes in bone quality will affect implant success and peri-implant tissue stability in the long term, there is a concern that firstly the long-term, presence of residual nonresorbable or slowly resorbable graft particles might interfere with normal bone healing and remodeling, secondly it may reduce the bone-to-implant contacts, and thirdly it can have a negative effect on the overall quality and architecture of the bone that surrounds implants. In a recent systematic review of randomized controlled clinical trials analyzing the outcomes of flapless socket grafting, Jambhekar et al. [30] reported that, after a minimum healing period of 12 weeks, sockets filled with synthetic biomaterials had the maximum amount of vital bone (45.53%) and the least amount of remnant graft material (13.67%) compared to xenografts and allografts. The results of the present case are in accordance with the above findings as histomorphometry revealed 50.28% of new bone and 12.27% of residual graft 12 weeks after a flapless socket grafting procedure.

Augmenting the bone around implants using fully resorbable grafting materials like β-TCP and CS may raise concerns regarding the long-term volume stability of the site. However, the placement of the implant at 12 weeks will increase the metabolic activity of the regenerated bone, while the subsequent loading of the implant will trigger the remodeling, and gradually enhance the density of the surrounding hard tissues [31, 32]. Assuming that the newly formed hard tissue around the implants is high-quality vital bone with low content or no residual graft particles at all, it might be able to adapt successfully to the placement and loading of the implant and thus maintain its dimensions in a functional way. In the present case where resorbable synthetic materials were used, the ridge did not collapse and retained adequately the architecture and the volume of the hard tissues two years after loading of the implant.

Overall, bone quality is important and might influence in several ways the outcome of implant therapy [9]. However, clinicians should be aware that the remodeling of the regenerated bone around implants might not be affected only by the nature and presence of residual graft particles, but also by other factors like optimal 3D positioning of the implant, type of implant (bone/tissue level), opposing dentition, and occlusal forces, while success of socket grafting can also be influenced by many other parameters like healing time, smoking status, local and systemic factors, socket location, and surgical technique.

4. Conclusions

In the presented case, a novel synthetic resorbable grafting material composed of β-TCP and CS was utilized for alveolar ridge preservation, resulting in pronounced regeneration of high-quality bone capable to support implant placement after a 12-week healing period. In parallel, placing the implant 12 weeks after extraction and socket grafting, and subsequent loading of the implant at 12 weeks resulted in a functional preservation of the volume and dimensions of the site, as shown clinically and radiologically two years after loading in this case. The mechanical stability of self-hardening synthetic biomaterials may also enable clinicians to utilize minimally invasive flapless procedures without primary wound closure for socket grafting that reduce the patient's morbidity, while preserving the attached keratinized gingiva and allowing for further production of newly formed keratinized soft tissue. Additional studies, including larger samples, comparison of different materials, quantitative measurements of the ridge dimensional changes, and inclusion of different sites, like the anterior region, that might show more pronounced changes, are needed in order to confirm and supplement the present findings.

References

[1] G. Vittorini Orgeas, M. Clementini, V. De Risi et al., "Surgical techniques for alveolar socket preservation: a systematic review," *International Journal of Oral & Maxillofacial Implants*, vol. 28, no. 4, pp. 1049–1061, 2013.

[2] A. Horváth, N. Mardas, L. A. Mezzomo et al., "Alveolar ridge preservation. A systematic review," *Clinical Oral Investigations*, vol. 17, no. 2, pp. 341–363, 2013.

[3] G. Pagni, G. Pellegrini, W. V. Giannobile et al., "Post-extraction alveolar ridge preservation: biological basis and treatments," *International Journal of Dentistry*, vol. 2012, Article ID 151030, 13 pages, 2012.

[4] R. E. Wang and N. P. Lang, "Ridge preservation after tooth extraction," *Clinical Oral Implants Research*, vol. 23, no. 6, pp. 147–156, 2012.

[5] R. Horowitz, D. Holtzclaw, and P. S. Rosen, "A review on alveolar ridge preservation following tooth extraction," *Journal of Evidence-Based Dental Practice*, vol. 12, no. 3, pp. 149–160, 2012.

[6] J. D. Keith and M. A. Salama, "Ridge preservation and augmentation using regenerative materials to enhance implant predictability and esthetics," *Compendium of Continuing Education in Dentistry*, vol. 28, no. 11, pp. 614–621, 2007.

[7] I. Yip, L. Ma, N. Mattheos, M. Dard, and N. P. Lang, "Defect healing with various bone substitutes," *Clinical Oral Implants Research*, vol. 26, no. 5, pp. 606–614, 2015.

[8] R. A. Horowitz, M. D. Leventis, M. D. Rohrer et al., "Bone grafting: history, rationale, and selection of materials and techniques," *Compendium of Continuing Education in Dentistry*, vol. 35, no. 4, pp. 1–6, 2014.

[9] H.-L. Chan, G.-H. Lin, J.-H. Fu, and H.-L. Wang, "Alterations in bone quality after socket preservation with grafting materials: a systematic review," *International Journal of Oral & Maxillofacial Implants*, vol. 28, no. 3, pp. 710–720, 2013.

[10] N. Harel, O. Moses, A. Palti, and Z. Ormianer, "Long-term results of implants immediately placed into extraction sockets grafted with β-tricalcium phosphate: a retrospective study," *Journal of Oral and Maxillofacial Surgery*, vol. 71, no. 2, pp. e63–e68, 2013.

[11] A. Kakar, B. H. Rao, S. Hegde et al., "Ridge preservation using an in situ hardening biphasic calcium phosphate (β-TCP/HA) bone graft substitute—a clinical, radiological, and histological study," *International Journal of Implant Dentistry*, vol. 3, no. 1, p. 25, 2017.

[12] Y. Kim, A. E. Rodriguez, and H. Nowzari, "The risk of prion infection through bovine grafting materials," *Clinical Oral Implants Research*, vol. 18, no. 6, pp. 1095–1102, 2016.

[13] Z. Artzi, M. Weinreb, N. Givol et al., "Biomaterial resorption rate and healing site morphology of inorganic bovine bone and beta-tricalcium phosphate in the canine: a 24-month longitudinal histologic study and morphometric analysis," *International Journal of Oral & Maxillofacial Implants*, vol. 19, no. 3, pp. 357–368, 2004.

[14] P. Trisi, W. Rao, A. Rebaudi, and P. Fiore, "Histologic effect of pure-phase beta-tricalcium phosphate on bone regeneration in human artificial jawbone defects," *International Journal of Periodontics and Restorative Dentistry*, vol. 23, no. 1, pp. 69–78, 2003.

[15] R. A. Horowitz, Z. Mazor, C. Foitzik, H. Prasad, M. Rohrer, and A. Palti, "β-tricalcium phosphate as bone substitute material: properties and clinical applications," *Journal of Osseointegration*, vol. 2, no. 2, pp. 61–68, 2010.

[16] H. Yuan, H. Fernandes, P. Habibovic et al., "Osteoinductive ceramics as a synthetic alternative to autologous bone grafting," *Proceedings of the National Academy of Sciences*, vol. 107, no. 31, pp. 13614–13619, 2010.

[17] R. J. Miron, Z. Qiao, A. Sculean et al., "Osteoinductive potential of 4 commonly employed bone grafts," *Clinical Oral Investigations*, vol. 20, no. 8, pp. 2259–2265, 2016.

[18] E. Ruga, C. Gallesio, L. Chiusa, and P. Boffano, "Clinical and histologic outcomes of calcium sulfate in the treatment of postextraction sockets," *Journal of Craniofacial Surgery*, vol. 22, no. 2, pp. 494–498, 2011.

[19] D. Anson, "Using calcium sulfate in guided tissue regeneration: a recipe for success," *Compendium of Continuing Education in Dentistry*, vol. 21, no. 5, pp. 365–370, 2000.

[20] E. Eleftheriadis, M. D. Leventis, K. I. Tosios et al., "Osteogenic activity of β-tricalcium phosphate in a hydroxyl sulphate matrix and demineralized bone matrix: a histological study in rabbit mandible," *Journal of Oral Science*, vol. 52, no. 3, pp. 377–384, 2010.

[21] L. Podaropoulos, A. A. Veis, S. Papadimitriou, C. Alexandridis, and D. Kalyvas, "Bone regeneration using b-tricalcium phosphate in a calcium sulfate matrix," *Journal of Oral Implantology*, vol. 35, no. 1, pp. 28–36, 2009.

[22] M. D. Leventis, P. Fairbairn, I. Dontas et al., "Biological response to β-tricalcium phosphate/calcium sulfate synthetic graft material: an experimental study," *Implant Dentistry*, vol. 23, no. 1, pp. 37–43, 2014.

[23] P. Fairbairn and M. Leventis, "Protocol for bone augmentation with simultaneous early implant placement: a retrospective multicenter clinical study," *International Journal of Dentistry*, vol. 2015, Article ID 589135, 8 pages, 2015.

[24] R. Dimitriou, G. I. Mataliotakis, G. M. Calori, and P. V. Giannoudis, "The role of barrier membranes for guided bone regeneration and restoration of large bone defects: current experimental and clinical evidence," *BMC Medicine*, vol. 10, no. 1, p. 81, 2012.

[25] D. Buser, C. Dahlin, and R. K. Schenk, *Guided Bone Regeneration in Implant Dentistry*, Quintessence Publishing, London, UK, 1995.

[26] G. Pecora, S. Andreana, J. E. Margarone, U. Covani, and J. S. Sottosanti, "Bone regeneration with a calcium sulfate barrier," *Oral medicine, Oral pathology, Oral radiology, and Endodontology*, vol. 84, no. 4, pp. 424–429, 1997.

[27] Z. Mazor, S. Mamidwar, J. L. Ricci, and N. M. Tovar, "Bone repair in periodontal defect using a composite of allograft and calcium sulfate (DentoGen) and a calcium sulfate barrier," *Journal of Oral Implantology*, vol. 37, no. 2, pp. 287–292, 2011.

[28] M. D. Leventis, P. Fairbairn, A. Kakar et al., "Minimally invasive alveolar ridge preservation utilizing an in situ hardening β-tricalcium phosphate bone substitute: a multicenter case series," *International Journal of Dentistry*, vol. 2016, Article ID 5406736, 12 pages, 2016.

[29] A. Bouri Jr., N. Bissada, M. S. Al-Zahrani, F. Faddoul, and I. Nouneh, "Width of keratinized gingiva and the health status of the supporting tissues around dental implants," *International Journal of Oral & Maxillofacial Implants*, vol. 23, no. 2, pp. 323–326, 2008.

[30] S. Jambhekar, F. Kernen, and A. S. Bidra, "Clinical and histologic outcomes of socket grafting after flapless tooth extraction: a systematic review of randomized controlled clinical trials," *Journal of Prosthetic Dentistry*, vol. 113, no. 5, pp. 371–382, 2015.

[31] H. Sasaki, S. Koyama, M. Yokoyama, K. Yamaguchi, M. Itoh, and K. Sasaki, "Bone metabolic activity around dental implants under loading observed using bone scintigraphy," *International Journal of Oral & Maxillofacial Implants*, vol. 23, no. 5, pp. 827–834, 2007.

[32] A. K. Khalifa, M. Wada, K. Ikebe, and Y. Maeda, "To what extent residual alveolar ridge can be preserved by implant? A systematic review," *International Journal of Implant Dentistry*, vol. 2, no. 1, p. 22, 2016.

11

Ceramic Laminate Veneers for Reestablishment of Esthetics in Case of Lateral Incisor Agenesis

Geórgia Silva,[1] Ana Cristina Normandes,[1] Edson Barros Júnior ⓘ,[2] Joyce Gatti ⓘ,[3] Kalena Maranhão ⓘ,[3] Ana Cássia Reis ⓘ,[3] Fernanda Jassé,[3] Lucas Moura,[3] and Thaís Barros ⓘ[3]

[1]School Superior of Amazonia (ESAMAZ), Belém, PA, Brazil
[2]College São Leopoldo Mandic (SLMANDIC), Belém, PA, Brazil
[3]School of Dentistry, School Superior of Amazonia (ESAMAZ), Belém, PA, Brazil

Correspondence should be addressed to Ana Cássia Reis; anacassiareis@gmail.com

Academic Editor: Daniel Torrés-Lagares

The increasing demand of patients looking for esthetics has resulted in the development of several techniques to restore anterior teeth. Conservative treatments should always be the first therapeutic option for the solution of aesthetic problems involving morphological changes and usually provide the result that the patient expects. In this context, ceramic laminate veneers, also known as "contact lenses," are capable to provide an extremely faithful reproduction of natural teeth with great color stability and periodontal biocompatibility. Minimal or no preparation veneers are heavily advertised as the answer to patients' cosmetic needs, when properly indicated by the dentist. This paper reports a clinical case where lateral incisor agenesis was aesthetically corrected using ceramic laminates.

1. Introduction

Agenesis is defined as a numerical anomaly that expresses the lack of development of one or more teeth, occurring in approximately 25% of the population, and can affect deciduous and permanent dentitions resulting from a dental blade disorder which prevents the formation of the dental germ. It may also be referred to as partial anodony, hypodontia, or oligodontia [1–12].

In the Brazilian population, agenesis affects between 2% and 5% of people depending on the affected tooth and excluding the third molars (wisdom tooth) that ranges around 20% to 30%. According to Santos [13], the most frequently observed agenesis, excluding third molars, is the one that affects the maxillary lateral incisors (ILS) (37.1%), followed by the mandibular second premolars (32.26%) and maxillary second premolars (17.54%).

The esthetic and functional alteration that the agenesis of ILS can provoke is quite relevant, being a concern factor, not only for the patients with the anomaly but also for the dentists responsible for planning the case. This anomaly can generate a change between the dental arches; being an important factor predisposing to malocclusions, it alters the function of the stomatognathic system, besides causing a great aesthetic discomfort, which is the main complaint of the patient [1–12].

Several treatments are suggested in the literature in cases of the absence of one or more ILS. The options range from no treatment or even two possibilities of clinical interventions (1) to create adequate space for inclusion of the missing tooth/teeth [14] or (2) to close the available space in the dental arch, providing the contact of the central incisor with canine, associated to the reanatomization of the canine, transforming it into a lateral incisor [11, 15, 16].

The decision during the treatment planning implies in the identification of alternative procedures, the prediction of the relative probabilities in favor of the long-term desired result, and evaluation of the cost-risk-benefit relation of each alternative [11]. The decision should be understandable to the patient or caregivers and better meet the needs of the patient. Many challenges are involved in obtaining and maintaining optimal results [17–19].

With the evolution of restorative materials and adhesion procedures, ceramic laminates have been used in corrections and dental reconstructions with a high predictability of success, especially because they require less wear or, in many cases, no wear, preserving a greater amount of sound dental structure, contributing to pulp and periodontal health [20, 21]. Besides these advantages, the aesthetic treatment using ceramic laminates also presents other ones such as biocompatibility, color stability, and good optical properties, enabling the dental reestablishment with biomechanical characteristics similar to natural teeth [22–25].

The proper selection of a ceramic system for certain clinical situations may provide greater longevity of these restorations. Although most of these systems promote good esthetic results, some are better suited for anterior regions because of the greater translucency of the material. Several criteria can be used by the professional to select the most appropriate ceramic system, such as esthetics, marginal adaptation, biocompatibility, resistance, cost, and ease of manufacturing [26–32].

Therefore, the objective of this work is to describe the esthetic treatment of a patient affected by ILS agenesis (12 and 22), by means of ceramic laminate veneers.

2. Diagnosis and Etiology

2.1. Clinical Case. A 28-year-old male patient was concerned about the esthetic of his smile. After the anamnesis and clinical and radiographic examinations, it was verified that the patient presented agenesis of dental elements 12 and 22; elements 13 and 23 occupied the lateral incisors' space; and elements 14 and 24 were rotated (Figure 1).

2.1.1. Treatment Plan. After case evaluation by the clinician, the first option of a treatment plan proposed to the patient was correction of the positioning of the canines and premolars by means of orthodontic movement and, later, implantation of the lateral incisors. However, this option was not accepted by the patient who was not interested in undergoing the surgical procedure.

The second treatment planning option proposed was reanatomization of elements 14, 13, 11, 21, 23, and 24, by means of the preparation of ceramic laminates in order to better harmonize the patient's smile. All the advantages and disadvantages of the treatment were exhaustively explained to the patient who, after understanding the proposed treatment, agreed with the execution of the procedure.

2.1.2. Diagnostic Waxing. The first clinical step of the treatment was to perform molding using condensation silicone Zetaplus (Zhermack) to study the case. After the model

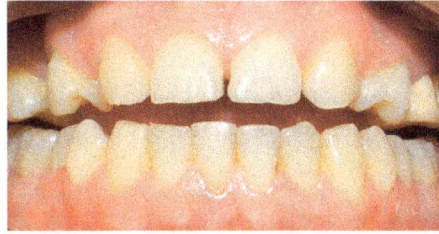

FIGURE 1: Preoperative view of the patient's smile.

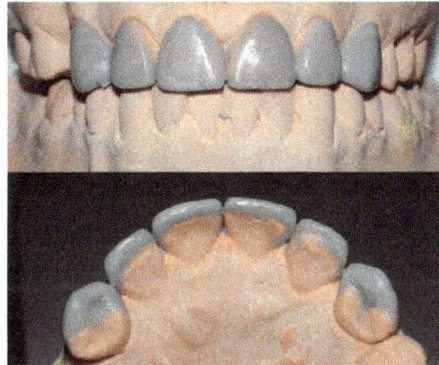

FIGURE 2: Diagnostic waxing proposed to reanatomize and provide harmony to the patient's smile.

was obtained, elements 13 and 23 were waxed so that the anatomy was as close as possible to the anatomy of upper lateral incisors. The elements 14 and 24 had their rotation "corrected" and received anatomical characteristics of canines.

According to the principles of proportionality and in order to maintain the smile harmony, elements 14, 13, 11, 21, 23, and 24 were enlarged both in the mesiodistal and in the cervicoincisal dimensions. Figure 2 shows the proposed waxing model.

2.1.3. Tooth Whitening and Mock-Up. In order to optimize the aesthetic result of the case, the patient underwent an in-office whitening session. Three 15-minute applications of Whiteness HP 35% (FGM) were performed. No sensitivity was reported by the patient, and the result obtained (Figure 3) was considered satisfactory (Initial color: color A3/Final color: A2-VITA Classical scale).

After 7 days, the mock-up was performed so that the patient could visualize the simulation of the proposed treatment, as well as to allow us to detect the need for corrections in the diagnostic waxing.

The waxed model was duplicated, and a silicone tray was made using a vacuum plasticizer, which allowed to "transfer" the proposed waxing to the patient's mouth (Figure 4).

A bisacrylic resin (Protemp 4-3M ESPE) was used to simulate the proposed aesthetic resolution. The tray was loaded with the material (Figure 5) and taken into position after 40 seconds from the start of loading.

After 1 minute, the tray was removed. The "mock-up" was finished with a 15C scalpel blade, 3195 F and FF diamond burs and abrasive papers. Figure 6 illustrates the result obtained after mock-up.

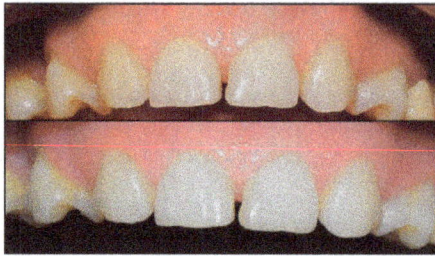

FIGURE 3: Result obtained after bleaching.

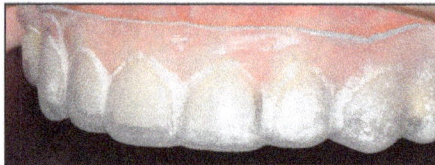

FIGURE 4: Silicone tray in position.

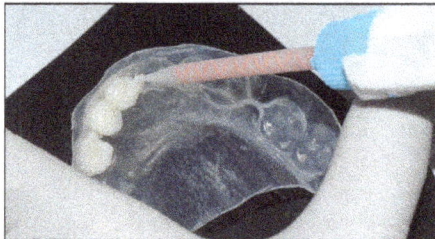

FIGURE 5: Silicone tray being loaded with Protemp 4 (3M ESPE).

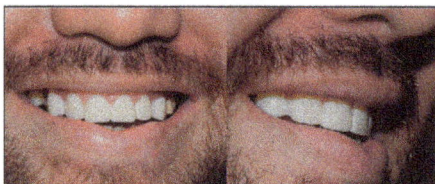

FIGURE 6: Result obtained with mock-up.

The patient was extremely satisfied with the result of the simulation; however, clinically, a small overconfiguration was observed in the mesial region of element 24. The overconfiguration was corrected in the waxed model so that the patient did not present any periodontal changes after finishing of treatment.

2.1.4. Selective Wear. After approval by the patient and adjustments made in the diagnostic waxing, the phase of selective wear was started. It was decided to perform these abrasions only in the areas that presented a thin layer of wax in the waxed model, thus guaranteeing a satisfactory thickness in the future ceramic laminate.

The regions that received selective wear were cervical-mesial of element 13, vestibular-mesial of elements 11 and 21, and cervical-mesial of 23, as shown in Figure 7.

All wear was performed using the 4138F (Poul Sorense) diamond bur and polished with Optimize (TDV) abrasive rubbers and Polimax Felt Disc (TDV). No cervical termination region was established. Figure 8 shows the clinical situation after finishing the wear and polishing steps.

2.1.5. Impressions and Color Selection. In sequence, the impression of preparations was performed using addition silicone (Express-3M ESPE) by means of the double mixing technique and without gingival clearance (Figure 9). The antagonistic arch was molden using alginate (Hydrogun5-Zhermarck), and an interocclusal record was taken using a wax plate 7. Color 1M2 was selected using the VITA 3D Master scale. The laboratory technician was informed that the "preparation" was all in enamel.

2.1.6. Laboratory Steps. The work model was screwed up to obtain a better adaptation of the laminates on the proximal faces (Figure 10). A silicone wall (Zetalabor-Zhemarck) was made based on the waxed model, in order to allow a better visualization of the thickness of the prosthetic pieces (Figure 11).

The porcelain used was the VITA PM-9, which is a feldspathic pottery reinforced by Leucita. The laminates are made by the lost wax technique, in which the ceramic is injected under high temperature (1000°C) and pressure (4, 7 bar) in a coating mold. Figure 12 shows the steps of lost of wax (a), positioning of the mold (b), and inclusion in the coating material (c).

To remove the newly injected ceramic from the coating mold, blasting with glass beads with a 50 μm granulation and a pressure of 2 bar (Figure 13(a)) was used. After the coating is completely removed, the injection channel is separated with a diamond disc, followed by adjustments, finishing, and polishing (Figures 13(b) and 13(c)).

2.1.7. Cementation. The ceramic laminates were tested on the patient to check and adjust the proximal contact points. For cementation, a photoactivated resin cement (AllCem Veneer-FGM) was used, which has a try-in system—it is a color proof paste that mimics the colors of the resin cement after light curing. The selected color for the cement was A3. The adhesive protocol was minutely performed in the dental structure: conditioning with 37% phosphoric acid (Condact 37-FGM) for 30 s, followed by washing for 60 s and removal of moisture. After performing this step, gingival clearance (Figure 14) using retractor wire (Retractor # 00-FGM) was performed to ensure that there is no excess adhesive and/or cement in the gingival sulcus region. Then the adhesive system (Adper SingleBond-3M ESPE) followed by photo-polymerization for 10 s were applied.

The inner surfaces of ceramic laminates were conditioned with 10% hydrofluoric acid (Condac 10%-FGM) for 20 s, followed by rinsing with copious amounts of water, drying, and, afterwards, the application of three layers of silane (Prosil-FGM). After silane evaporation, the adhesive system Adper Single Bond 2 (3M ESPE) was applied.

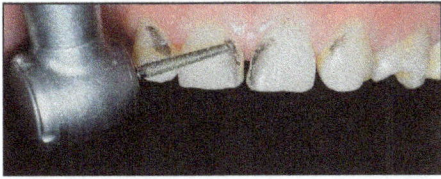

FIGURE 7: Regions selected to receive selective wear.

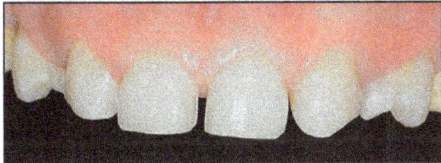

FIGURE 8: Clinical situation after finishing the wear and polishing steps.

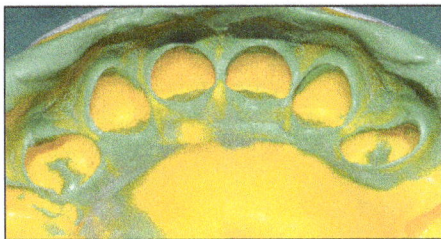

FIGURE 9: Impression of preparations made with addition silicone (Express-3M ESPE).

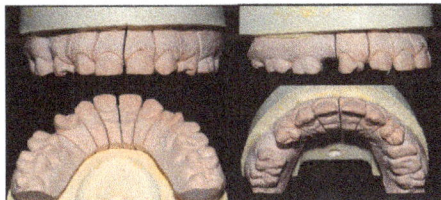

FIGURE 10: Cutting of the plaster work model.

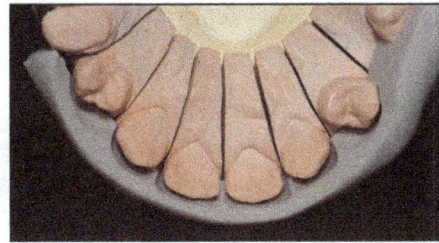

FIGURE 11: Silicone wall in position. The thicknesses of the ceramic laminates can be observed.

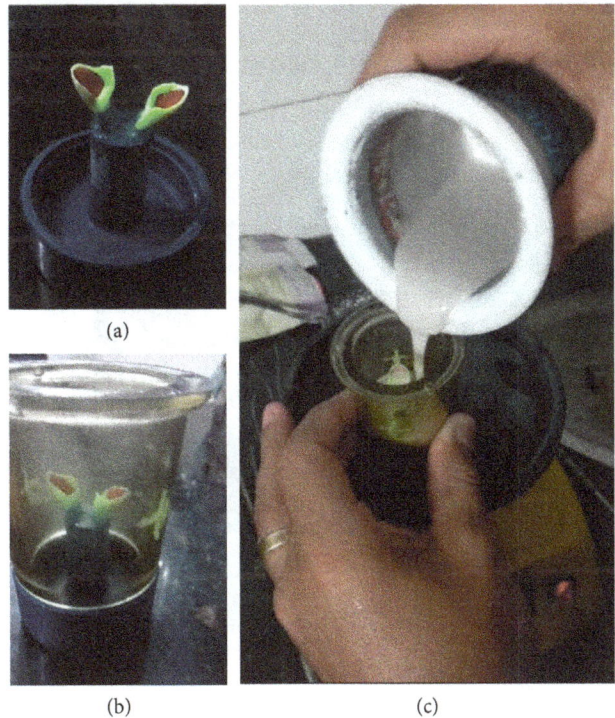

(a)

(b)   (c)

FIGURE 12: Laboratory steps for manufacturing of ceramic laminates. (a) Fixation of the waxed veneers at the base, (b) adaptation of the silicone ring at the base, and (c) addition of the coating liquid.

The cement was applied on the cementation surfaces of ceramic laminates. After that, veneers were positioned with cement until its excess had overflowed (Figure 15).

The cementation sequence adopted was upper central incisors, followed by the premolars and, finally, the canines. After the cementation, the finishing steps were accomplished with fine-grained and extrafine diamond burs, followed by polishing with abrasive rubbers (Exa-cerapol-Edenta). The final result obtained is illustrated in Figure 16.

3. Discussion

Aesthetics has been increasingly required in today's dentistry. With the increase of access to information, through the Internet, books, and magazines, the population becomes more and more demanding.

Therefore, aesthetics should be closely associated with the patient's wishes, respecting the principles of smile harmony, oral rehabilitation, correct diagnosis, treatment plan, and the type of material to be used in the selected treatment.

In the Brazilian population, the prevalence of dental agenesis varies in percentage, depending on the study. The values found were 29.5%, 7.9%, and 2.9% in which agenesis of the third molar is the most common [13]. Opinions vary on the second most commonly affected tooth; some studies show that the second lower premolar has the highest in prevalence while others show that the superior lateral incisor has the highest [1, 3, 5, 13].

The treatment of dental anomalies is always a challenge for the general practitioner. For Alavi et al. [25] and Giordano [28], the best method would be the use of composite resin owing to the preservation of dental structure and the financial cost. For Nathanson and Riis [26], Giordano [28], Van Dijken [29], and Höland et al. [30], ceramic restorative materials would be the best choice since composite restorations undergo time action and require regular

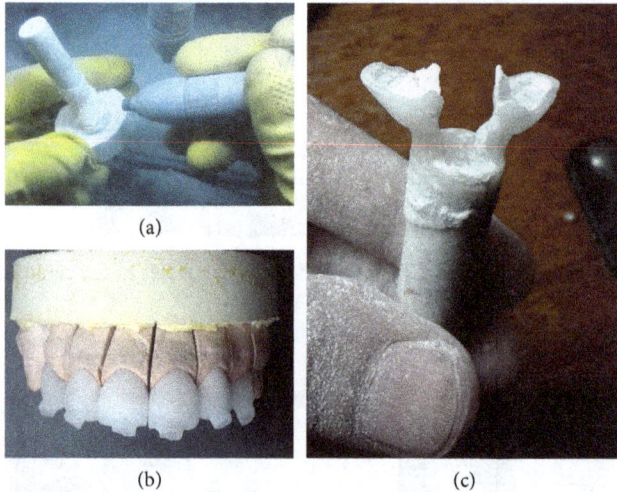

Figure 13: (a) Removal of the laminates from the coating mold using shot blasting with glass microspheres; (b) ceramic pieces placed in the plaster model, still with the remnants of the feed channels; (c) view of the injected parts attached to feed channels.

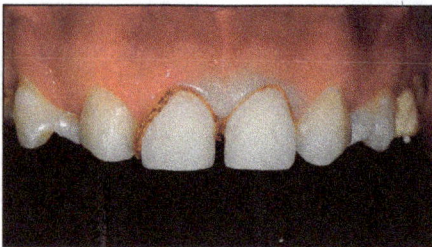

Figure 14: Gingival clearance prior to cementation.

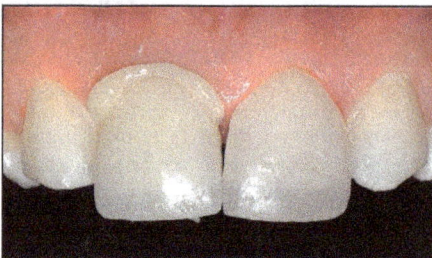

Figure 15: Extravasation of the cementing agent in element 11.

maintenance. In addition, composite resins exhibit lower clinical longevity due to greater susceptibility to pigmentation and marginal fractures [33].

In this clinical report, the use of ceramic laminates was the treatment of choice, in particular, the ceramic system VITA PM-9 because this material presents the following advantages: ability to reproduce the appearance of natural teeth, good translucency, excellent resistance, and similar biomechanical behavior to the tooth structure.

Nowadays the treatment with ceramic laminates rehabilitation is in use in a large scale; this is mainly due to being a very conservative treatment, where the wear of the dental element is minimal preserving the dental structure, especially in young patients [22–32]. However, because they

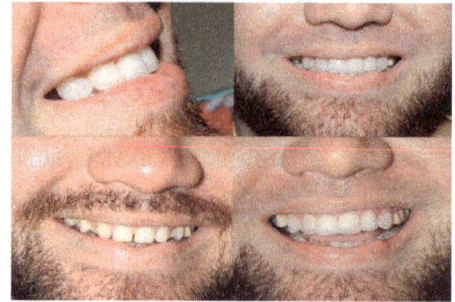

Figure 16: Final result.

are relatively recent techniques, they still do not have a common sense, mainly regarding their indications and limitations [3, 4, 11].

Machry [34] affirms that one must always keep in mind the correct diagnosis to carry out a correct planning and, consequently, an appropriate treatment sequence for each case. Although recent, clinical evaluations have shown a very promising outlook, today they represent an alternative that the clinician needs to employ in selected cases.

4. Conclusion

The diversity of ceramic systems currently available in the world market is due to the increasing search for aesthetic excellence. The systems present advantages and disadvantages when compared to each other.

The most important in clinical cases is to establish a careful and realistic treatment plan, taking into account the patient's wishes. The time factor is often determinant for the selection of the treatment plan, since some patients want to solve their problem in the shortest time possible.

Thus, it can be concluded that the performed procedure corresponded very well with expectations of the patient and that the techniques used to do so were well performed, and it was obtained a satisfactory result.

Authors' Contributions

Ana Cássia de Souza Reis was responsible for study design, manuscript writing, critical review, and final approval; Ana Cristina Néry Normandes and Georgia Marques da Silva performed bibliographic survey, research, and selection of articles from PubMed and Bireme databases; Fernanda Ferreira de Albuquerque Jassé and Lucas Alves Moura wrote and proofread the English language; Edson de Sousa Barros Júnior was responsible for the laboratory stages; Joyce Figueira de Araujo was responsible for preparation and writing of the manuscript; Kalena de Melo Maranhão was responsible for conception, design of the study, preparation, writing of the manuscript, and final approval; and Thaís Andrade de Figueiredo Barros was responsible for the clinical stages and general coordination of the work.

References

[1] E. Argyropoulos and G. Payne, "Techniques for improving orthodontic results in the treatment of missing maxillary lateral incisors. A case report with literature review," *American Journal of Orthodontics and Dentofacial Orthopedics*, vol. 94, no. 2, pp. 150–165, 1988.

[2] B. J. Millar and N. G. Taylor, "Lateral thinking: the management of missing upper lateral incisors," *British Dental Journal*, vol. 179, no. 3, pp. 99–106, 1995.

[3] R. Sabri, "Management of missing maxillary lateral incisors," *Journal of the American Dental Association*, vol. 130, no. 1, pp. 80–84, 1999.

[4] G. Richardson and K. A. Russell, "Congenitally missing maxillary lateral incisors and orthodontic treatment considerations for the single-tooth implant," *Journal-Canadian Dental Association*, vol. 67, no. 1, pp. 25–28, 2001.

[5] V. O. Kokich Jr. and G. A. Kinzer, "Managing congenitally missing lateral incisors. Part I: Canine substitution," *Journal of Esthetic and Restorative Dentistry*, vol. 17, no. 1, pp. 5–10, 2005.

[6] R. Sabri and N. Aboujaoude, "Agenesis of the maxillary lateral incisors: orthodontic and implant approach," *L'Orthodontie Française*, vol. 79, no. 4, pp. 283–293, 2008.

[7] J. H. Park, S. Okadakage, Y. Sato, Y. Akamatsu, and K. Tai, "Orthodontic treatment of a congenitally missing maxillary lateral incisor," *Journal of Esthetic and Restorative Dentistry*, vol. 22, no. 5, pp. 297–312, 2010.

[8] S. Kavadia, S. Papadiochou, I. Papadiochos, and L. Zafiriadis, "Agenesis of maxillary lateral incisors: a global overview of the clinical problem," *Orthodontics*, vol. 12, no. 4, pp. 296–317, 2011.

[9] A. Johal, C. Katsaros, and A. M. Kuijpers-Jagtman, "State of the science on controversial topics: missing maxillary lateral incisors–a report of the Angle Society of Europe 2012 meeting," *Progress in Orthodontics*, vol. 14, no. 20, pp. 14–20, 2013.

[10] B. Mummidi, C. H. Rao, A. L. Prasanna, M. Vijay, K. V. Reddy, and M. A. Raju, "Esthetic dentistry in patients with bilaterally missing maxillary lateral incisors: a multidisciplinary case report," *Journal of Contemporary Dental Practice*, vol. 14, no. 2, pp. 348–354, 2013.

[11] R. R. Almeida, A. C. F. Morandini, R. R. Almeida-Pedrin, M. R. Almeida, R. C. F. R. Castro, and N. M. Insabralde, "A multidisciplinary treatment congenitally missing maxillary lateral incisors: a 14-year follow-up case report," *Journal of Applied Oral Science*, vol. 22, no. 5, pp. 465–471, 2014.

[12] A. Agrawal, N. Jain, N. P. Jose, and S. Shetty, "Interdisciplinary approach for management of congenitally missing maxillary lateral incisors: a case report," *International Journal of Orthodontics*, vol. 26, no. 4, pp. 15–17, 2015.

[13] P. A. Santos, "Tratamento de Ausência Congênita de Incisivo Lateral Superior por meio de Recuperação de Espaço para colocação de Implante Dentário ou Fechamento de Espaço, Relato de Casos," *Revista Dental Press Ortodontia e Ortopedia Facial*, vol. 7, no. 3, pp. 65–77, 2002.

[14] M. Rosa, A. Olimpo, R. Fastuca, and A. Caprioglio, "Perceptions of dental professionals and laypeople to altered dental esthetics in cases with congenitally missing maxillary lateral incisors," *Progress in Orthodontics*, vol. 14, no. 1, p. 34, 2013.

[15] M. Rosa and B. U. Zachrisson, *Integrating Esthetic Dentistry and Space Closure in Patients with Missing Maxillary Lateral Incisors*, vol. 1, no. 1, pp. 41–55, RClin Ortodon Dental Press, Maringá, Brazil, 2002.

[16] V. O. Kokich Jr., "Congenitally missing teeth: orthodontic management in the adolescent patient," *American Journal of Orthodontics and Dentofacial Orthopedics*, vol. 121, no. 6, pp. 594–595, 2002.

[17] B. U. Zachrisson, "Improving orthodontic results in cases with maxillary incisors missing," *American Journal of Orthodontics*, vol. 73, no. 3, pp. 274–289, 1978.

[18] E. Halley, "Direct composite veneers-an aesthetic alternative," *Private Dentistry*, vol. 20, 2012.

[19] A.-H. Muhamad, W. Nezar, A. Azzaldeen, and B. Musa, "Treatment of patients with congenitally missing lateral incisors: is an interdisciplinary task," *Research and Reviews: Journal of Dental Science*, vol. 2, no. 4, 2014.

[20] M. Fradeani, M. Redemagni, and M. Corrado, "Porcelain laminate veneers: 6- to 12-year clinical evaluation—a retrospective study," *International Journal of Periodontics and Restorative Dentistry*, vol. 25, no. 1, pp. 9–17, 2005.

[21] E. Öztürk and S. Bolay, "Survival of porcelain laminate veneers with different degrees of dentin exposure: 2-year clinical results," *Journal of Adhesive Dentistry*, vol. 16, no. 5, pp. 481–489, 2014.

[22] T. S. Liu and X. D. Chen, "Application of all-ceramic laminates veneer with Vita VM9 in clinic," *Huaxi Kouqiang Yixue Zazhi*, vol. 25, no. 5, pp. 447–449, 2007.

[23] S. Turgut and B. Bagis, "Colour stability of laminate veneers: an in vitro study," *Journal of Dentistry*, vol. 39, no. 3, pp. e57–e64, 2011.

[24] S. Turgut and B. Bagis, "Effect of resin cement and ceramic thickness on final color of laminate veneers: an in vitro study," *Journal of Prosthetic Dentistry*, vol. 109, no. 3, pp. 179–186, 2013.

[25] A. A. Alavi, Z. Behroozi, and F. Nik Eghbal, "The shear bond strength of porcelain laminate to prepared and unprepared anterior teeth," *Journal of Dentistry*, vol. 18, no. 1, pp. 50–55, 2017.

[26] D. Nathanson and D. Riis, "Advances and current research in ceramic restorative materials," *Current Opinion in Cosmetic Dentistry*, pp. 34–40, 1993.

[27] D. M. Schneider, "Differing porcelain syste ms," *Current Opinion in Cosmetic Dentistry*, pp. 107–113, 1995.

[28] R. A. Giordano, "Dental ceramic restorative systems," *Compendium of Continuing Education in Dentistry*, vol. 17, no. 8, pp. 779–782, 1996.

[29] J. W. Van Dijken, "All-ceramic restorations: classification and clinical evaluations," *Compendium of Continuing Education in Dentistry*, vol. 20, no. 12, pp. 1115–1124, 1999.

[30] W. Höland, M. Schweiger, R. Watzke, A. Peschke, and H. Kappert, "Ceramics as biomaterials for dental restoration," *Expert Review of Medical Devices*, vol. 5, no. 6, pp. 729–745, 2008.

[31] Y. H. Chun, C. Raffelt, H. Pfeiffer et al., "Restoring strength of incisors with veneers and full ceramic crowns," *Journal of Adhesive Dentistry*, vol. 12, no. 1, pp. 45–54, 2010.

[32] F. J. Burke, "Survival rates for porcelain laminate veneers with special reference to the effect of preparation in dentin: a literature review," *Journal of Esthetic and Restorative Dentistry*, vol. 24, no. 4, pp. 257–265, 2012.

[33] M. E. Miranda, K. A. Olivieri, F. J. Rigolin, and R. T. Basting, "Ceramic fragments and metal-free full crowns: a conservative esthetic option for closing diastemas and rehabilitating smiles," *Operative Dentistry*, vol. 38, no. 6, pp. 567–571, 2013.

[34] L. Machry, *Facetas Em Porcelanas. 44 f. Trabalho de Conclusão de Curso (Especialização em Dentística Restauradora)*, Escola Aperfeiçoamento Profissional–ABO-SC, Florianópolis, Brazil, 2003.

12

Pain Management Associated with Posttraumatic Unilateral Temporomandibular Joint Anterior Disc Displacement: A Case Report and Literature Review

Arturo Garrocho-Rangel (ID), **Andrea Gómez-González, Adriana Torre-Delgadillo,**
Socorro Ruiz-Rodríguez, and Amaury Pozos-Guillén (ID)

Pediatric Dentistry Postgraduate Program, Faculty of Dentistry, San Luis Potosi University, San Luis Potosi, SLP, Mexico

Correspondence should be addressed to Amaury Pozos-Guillén; apozos@uaslp.mx

Academic Editor: Junichi Asaumi

The aim of the present article is to review the etiological risk factors and the general and oral management of anterior disc displacement with reduction caused by a chin trauma, and to describe the diagnostic process and the treatment provided to an affected 7-year-old girl. The patient also experienced frequent and severe cephaleas, which may be related to cervical vertebrae deviation. The patient was successfully treated with an intraoral occlusal splint and analgesics. Pediatric dentists must always be aware of the early signs and symptoms of temporomandibular joint disorders in their patients, especially in cases of orofacial trauma history, with the aim of providing an opportune resolution and preventing its progression later in life. Occlusal splints are strongly recommended for the treatment of anterior disc displacement with reduction in children and adolescents.

1. Introduction

Temporomandibular disorders (TMDs) include a variety of pathological, single or combined, signs or symptoms of the temporomandibular joint and periarticular structures (masticatory muscles, ligaments, bone, and facial skin) [1]. These disorders affect not only adult patients; children also exhibit high incidence/prevalence of TMD, which have been associated with orofacial pain or discomfort, growth abnormalities, and mandibular dysfunction [2–4]. Some cases can course asymptomatic. Misdiagnoses are also frequent, confounding the clinical scenario as a chronic headache or otalgia. In other clinical situations, joint noises such as clicking, popping, snapping, or soft/hard-tissue crepitus are often perceived as normal by the general population and even by general dentists or physicians [2].

The TMD etiology in children and adolescents has been investigated by diverse authors without reaching any definitive consensus [5–7]. However, it is generally accepted that the disorder is of multifactorial origin, in which several genetic and/or environmental factors (e.g., systemic anomalies, parafunctional habits, psychological distress, anatomical factors, malocclusions, and local infection or trauma) can be related [1, 8, 9]. These etiological factors involve abnormal biomechanical forces applied to the mandibular condyle, altering the shape and function of the articular structures [10, 11]. The principal malocclusions related to TMD in children and adolescents are skeletal anterior open bite, steep articular eminence of the temporal bone, overjet > 6-7 mm, Class III malocclusion, and posterior crossbite [12].

Prevalence of TMD in children and adolescents has been estimated to be in the wide range of 16 to 68%, according to epidemiological studies from different countries; this variability is due to each study's methodology and the clinical features examined for determining the presence of the disorder [4, 8, 9]. The American Academy of Orofacial Pain [1, 13] has classified the TMD in children and adolescents into two broad categories: TMJ disorders—joint pain, joint disorders, and joint diseases—and masticatory muscle

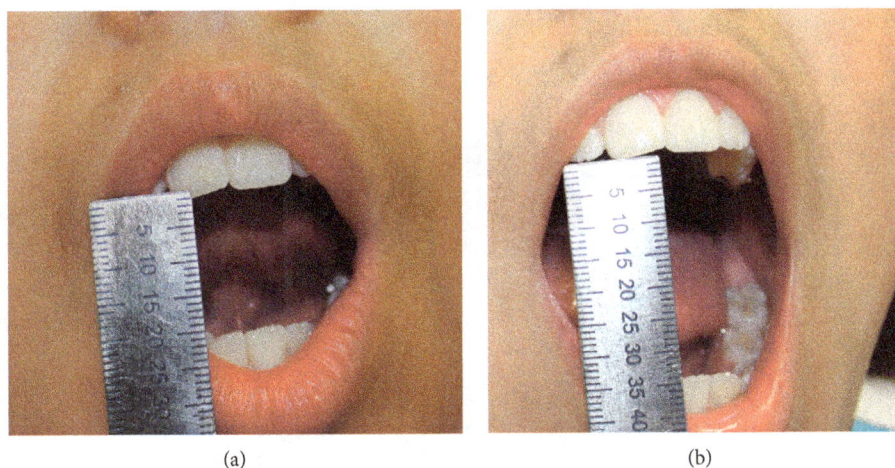

(a)   (b)

FIGURE 1: Oral aperture. Pretreatment (a). Posttreatment, taken after ten months of follow-up (b).

disorders. Joint disorders include the disc-condyle complex position disorders, also called as internal derangements (IDs). ID refers to an abnormal positional relationship of the articular disc in relation to the mandibular condyle and the articular eminence in the glenoid fossa, in the temporal bone [5, 10, 11, 14]. Although there are eight different abnormal disc positions, the anterior and anterior-lateral displacements are the most common. In turn, anterior disc displacements are classified into two main subgroups: displacement with reduction (ADDR) and displacement without reduction [14]; ADDR is the most frequent TMJ disorder found in children, with a prevalence of approximately 6% between 8 and 15 years old, with greater incidence in women [11].

The aim of the present report is to describe the clinical management provided to a 7-year-old girl with a TMD due to a chin trauma, specifically an anteroposterior joint disc displacement with reduction of interarticular space width, and related severe cephalea episodes, and the course of the abnormal condition over a six-month follow-up period.

2. Case Report

2.1. History of Complaints. A 7-year-11-month girl presented with her parents to the Pediatric Dentistry Clinic referred by a local general dentist, complaining of unilateral pain in the left TMJ area. The parents noticed an orofacial trauma episode: the child suffered a chin injury due to a drop from the bicycle at 4 years old, causing a significant skin abrasion/bruise and cervical sprain. The patient was not examined by a dentist, but we can speculate that there were no condylar fractures. An emergency physician indicated to use a semirigid neck collar for two weeks. Thereafter, the child experienced chronic pain in the left side of the face, around the temporomandibular zone, accompanied with recurrent moderate-to-severe cephalea episodes and mild symptoms of anxiety. A severe pinch-type pain during mastication of hard foods was also reported. She received pharmacological treatment, according to the age, weight, and size of the child, consisting in risperidone and imipramine for two weeks. However, the cephalea and intraoral pain had intensified during the last weeks; so, the parents decided to

seek dental treatment. Paranormal habits were informed, particularly diurnal/nocturnal bruxism and onychophagy. Also, a previous event of transient jaw locking while eating was reported.

2.2. Extraoral and Intraoral Examinations. The clinical findings included normal stature and weight for her age. Her face was ovoid and symmetric with normal forehead and normal-set ears, and convex profile due to a retruded chin. Intraorally, the patient exhibited well-shaped arches in mixed dentition stage, multiple nondeep carious lesions, and Class I malocclusion with mild anterior crowding. No dental wear was observed.

The maximum interincisal opening was only 20 mm (Figure 1(a)) (normal = 41–50 mm) [9, 15]. An evaluation of mandible function was carried out, following recommendations [16]; an evident mandibular left displacement was detected during the mouth opening/closure movements. A clicking sound was detected in the same joint, during mandibular opening, on stethoscope auscultation. Articular pain and masticatory muscle tenderness were assessed by bilateral extra and intraoral palpation, according to the Rocabado pain map criteria [17]; left temporomandibular joint manifested a moderate-to-severe posterior inferior synovial pain, radiating to the neck, indicating hurt by compression of the backward-positioned condyle.

2.3. Imaging. Radiographs and a computed tomography (CT) were taken. These images showed a reduction of the left articular condyle-glenoid fossae space width, with no evidence of condyle neck fracture, and a right deviation of first (odontoid process), second, and third cervical vertebrae, regarding the skull base, caused probably by the chin injury (Figure 2). This vertebrae deviation was compressing the spinal cord, giving origin to the moderate-to-severe cephalea episodes (cervicogenic cephalea), and perpetuating the temporomandibular dysfunction.

2.4. Treatment Approach. After performing a careful clinical diagnosis of ADDR, the dental treatment consisted in the placement of an intraoral removable soft occlusal splint

(a)

(b)

(c)

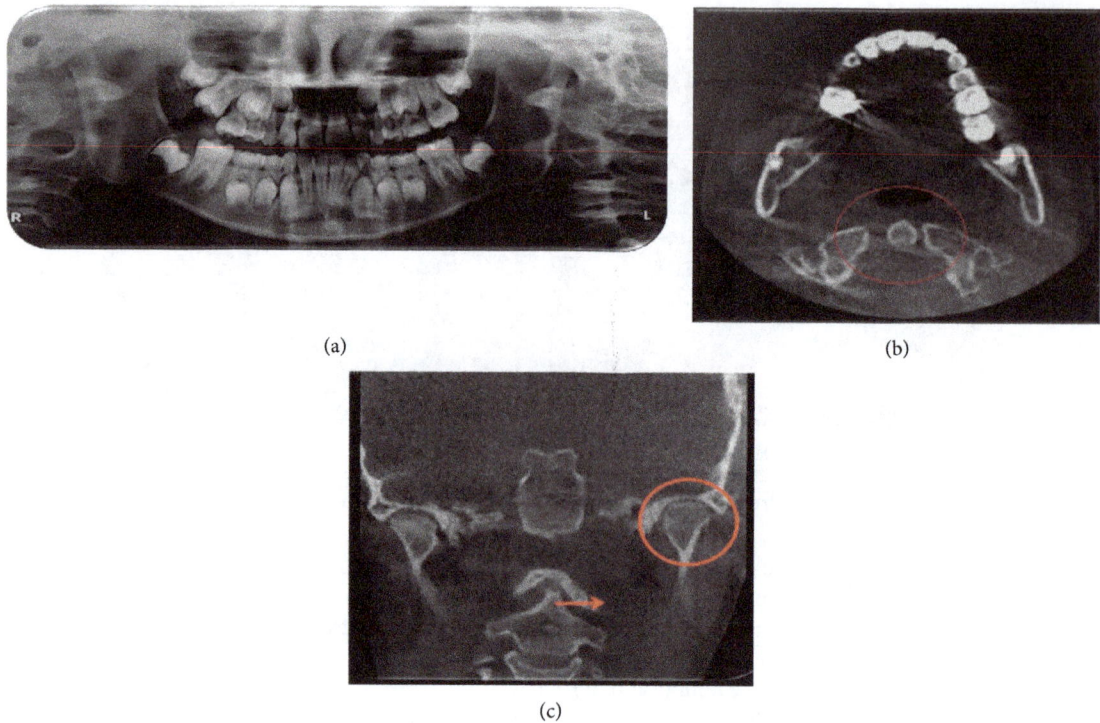

FIGURE 2: (a) Panoramic view. (b) CT of the cranial coronal view. In the circle, it can be observed the coronoid apophysis markedly deviated to the left, maybe caused by the reported craniofacial trauma. (c) CT anteroposterior view of the skull. The cycle shows the reduced interarticular space of the left temporomandibular joint, compared with the right side. The arrow represents the evident left deviation of the coronoid apophysis.

covering the maxilla with an inserted midline bidirectional expansion screw to promote the transverse development. The patient's parents were fully explained about this therapeutic approach, and they agreed to sign a special informed consent form, which included the permission for publishing the clinical case.

The appliance was fabricated with soft polyester and fitted over the upper arch teeth's occlusal and incisal surfaces, with a 2-3 mm thickness, in order to create a precise occlusal contact with the opposite teeth (Figure 3). The fabrication process was as follows: upper and lower stone models were mounted on an AD2 articulator in centric relation. This relation was previously taken in the patient, through adhesive anterior and posterior softened wax discs—for both upper first permanent molars and incisor registry, respectively—placed on a special metallic U-shaped bite plate. The plate was attached to a face bow, which was properly positioned over the patient's forehead. The patient was briefly trained to slowly bite, in centric relation, into the wax discs about 1 mm deep. After seating and fitting the intraoral appliance, simultaneous and symmetric contact points were obtained with maximum intercuspation and flat occlusal plane, according to the recommendations emitted by Restrepo et al. [18]. The patient was instructed to use the splint at least 12 hours a day, especially overnight, and to activate the expansion screw once, two days a week, in order to compensate the natural maxilla transverse growth.

The cervicogenic cephalea was managed with analgesics (Ibuprofen, 10 mg/kg/day orally, every 8 hours), and she was

recommended to maintain a good posture when sitting and standing and avoid sleeping on her front, in order to reduce the strain on the neck muscles and ligaments. The parents were indicated to change their girl's pillow—for a softer one—and to place a rolled towel under her neck while sleeping. After two weeks, analgesic therapy was retired. The parents were instructed to apply a hot water bag wrapped in a towel directly to the affected head area, for 20 min, in case of a cephalea episode.

The patient was scheduled regularly every two weeks. After ten months of follow-up, the parents and patient reported a significant reduction of cephalea attacks—around once per month, usually associated with scholar stress. There had been also lack of pain during chewing or on the cervical area, and no other joint dislocation episode after a maximum mouth opening was mentioned. On auscultation, it was noted that articular noises decreased notably. Paranormal oral habits were also reduced. The maximum interincisal opening is currently between 30 and 35 mm, approximately (Figure 1(b)). New CT was taken, and it showed an evident improvement (Figures 4 and 5). The girl continues under psychological management.

3. Discussion

Temporomandibular joint is considered as a complex synovial articulation and the most used joint in the human body. Therefore, pediatric dentistry should know the

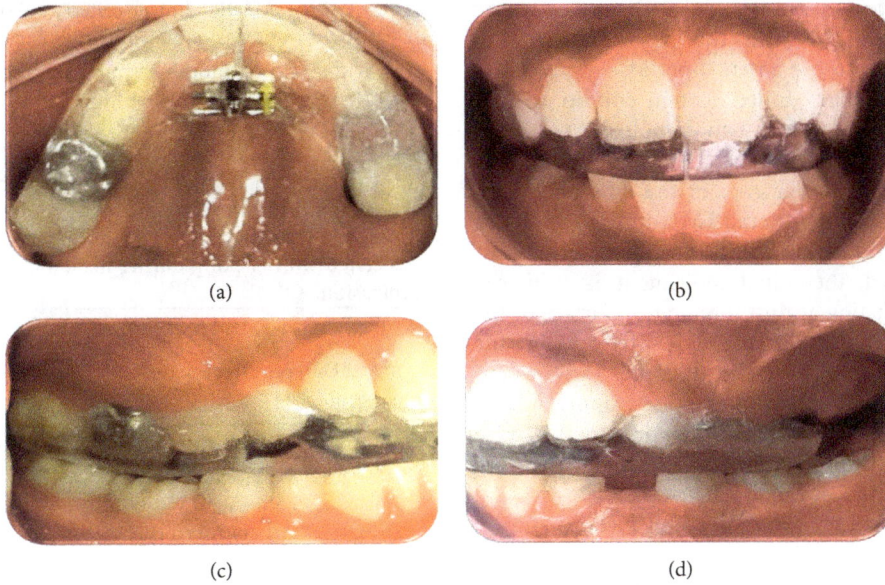

FIGURE 3: Different views of the intraoral appliance.

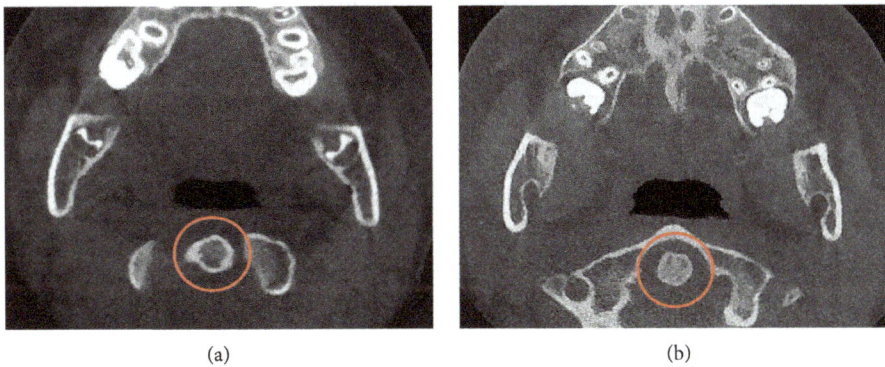

FIGURE 4: Transversal slice CT taken in closed mouth (a) and in maximum oral aperture (b). The circles represent the second cervical vertebrae's body, in the centered position.

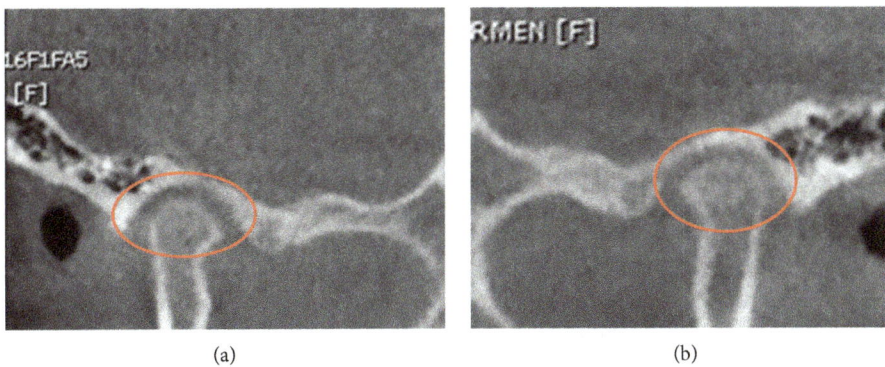

FIGURE 5: Current images of (a) left and (b) right condyles. Observe the adequate articular spaces.

complex physiology and biomechanics of the TMJ in children and adolescents; additionally, they must always be aware of the early signs and symptoms of TMJ disorders in their patients with the aim of providing an opportune resolution and prevent progression [4].

Regarding the first issue, the TMJ is a ginglymoarthrodial joint comprising the mandibular condyle that articulates with the glenoid fossa of the temporal bone [4]. TMJ articular surfaces are in contact with the articular disc, a flexible and biconcave structure composed of a fibrous structure and nourished by synovial fluid. The articular disc is normally positioned between the posterior slope of the articular tubercle and the anterosuperior surface of the mandibular condyle. Thus, under normal conditions, the TMJ is transversely divided into two completely separated compartments [11]. On the other hand, Howard outstandingly summarizes the sequence of the different physiological processes occurring into the TMJ, during the mouth opening in children [9]. This author manifests that when the mouth is opened, the initial movement is primarily the condylar head rotating against the inferior surface of the stationary disc. Then, the disc rotates posteriorly on the condyle, and the disc-condyle system translates forward and downward, guided by contact with the disc's upper surface against the sloped articular tubercle. When the mouth is wide open, the condyle and disc gently translate together to the edge or beyond the apex of the articular tubercle.

In the second place, an exhaustive and focused clinical examination is imperative in those pediatric cases with potential TMD disorders. This examination process in children with suspected TMD, and particularly ADDR, should involve the careful assessment of three main anatomical joint structures: (a) the position of articular disc relative to the mandibular condyle; (b) the location of the condyle relative to the temporal joint surfaces; and (c) the depth of the glenoid fossa. It is also important to collect information about previous direct or indirect trauma (sometimes also called "macrotrauma") in the orofacial area, particularly chin or TMJ injuries [19, 20]. Additionally, it is imperative an exhaustive clinical assessment: mandibular range of motion evaluation, temporomandibular joint palpation including ligaments and capsule structures, masticatory musculature (temporalis and masseter) pain under pressure, load testing, sound detection (clicking, crepitus, and hard-tissue grating); this process should be complemented with diverse auxiliary imaging (e.g., panoramic X-ray, panoramic TMJ images, cone beam computed tomography, and magnetic resonance imaging) [9].

Specifically, ADDR occurs in the closed mouth position. In this position, the articular disc is dislocated anteriorly to the condyle. However, during opening, the disc/condyle relation improves: the disc reduces by slipping back on top of the condyle [5, 10]. The local pain attributed to ADDR is related to a ligament sprain, or to muscle dysfunction, which may limit the mouth opening [5, 11]. Table 1 [11, 21, 22] lists the main different signs and symptoms that make suspicious the presence of ADDR. As in the present case, ADDR are diagnosed by clinical examination combined with diagnostic imaging [1]. According to the collected clinical information, the patient reported here belonged to the category of anterior disc displacement with reduction. The related cephalea attacks, similar to those of tension type headaches, might be caused by stimulating structures that are innervated by nerval roots from C1 to C3 [23, 24].

General and oral treatment of ADDR is still controversial. There is published evidence that has reported a self-resolution tendency even without any clinical treatment or conduct, particularly in cases with absence of pain or severe

TABLE 1: Five ADDR clinical criteria validated by the research diagnostic criteria for temporomandibular disorder [11, 21, 22].

(i) Clicking during mouth opening and closure.
(ii) Interincisal distance when the clicking occurs during opening is at least 5 mm wider than interincisal distance when the clicking occurs during closure.
(iii) Clicking suppression during the mouth opening and closure (with protruded mandible).
(iv) When clicking occurs only during opening or closure, associated with clicking during mandible lateralization or protrusion.

TABLE 2: Different treatment modalities for ADDR in children and adolescents [11].

Noninvasive procedures	Invasive procedures
(i) Cognitive/behavioral therapy	(i) TMJ arthroscopies
(ii) Hot and cold therapy	(ii) Arthrocentesis
(iii) Passive and counter/resistance exercises	(iii) Surgical techniques
(iv) Relaxation techniques	
(v) Repositioning/stabilizing splints	
(vi) Biofeedback	
(vii) Ultrasound	
(viii) Phonophoresis	
(ix) Iontophoresis	
(x) Transcutaneous electrical neural stimulation	
(xi) Drug therapy	
(xii) Tooth selective grinding	
(xiii) Intraoral devices (removable/fix orthodontic appliances and splints)	

articular dysfunction [11]. When pain is present, some type of treatment is necessary, though it has not been definitely established. Different therapeutic procedures are classified as noninvasive or invasive. These treatments are mentioned in Table 2. Conservative treatments are always the first choice. Regarding the pharmaceutical management, to date, there are no approved medications for treating pain caused from TMD in children; however, NSAIDs (e.g., ibuprofen and naproxen) and muscle relaxants can be prescribed, in conjunction with oral corrective/restorative procedures, because of their relatively clinical safety [4, 7]. Additionally, the AAPD recommends the referral to an oral specialist when the following conditions are suspected: primary headaches, otitis media, allergies, abnormal posture, airway congestion, rheumatoid arthritis, connective tissue disease psychiatric disorders, or other medical anomalies [1].

In the patient reported here, the temporomandibular disorder was approached through the use of a removable occlusal splint (or bite guard). In addition, to be indicated for preventing injuries while participating in organized sports and other recreational activities, this appliance may be effective in reducing TMD symptoms and giving more comfort to the patient [1, 4, 7]. The occlusal splint is economical, lightweight, and easy to use; besides, treatment provided with these devices is noninvasive and reversible [25]. The clinical aim of the occlusal splint is to provide orthopedic stability and balance to the affected TMJ, through the modification of the relationship between the mandible and maxilla, raising the vertical dimension, and decreasing the muscle parafunctional activity (e.g. bruxism or jaw clenching) [1, 7, 18, 26]. Occlusal stabilization is achieved because all teeth are in full contact when the mouth is closed; this allows the lateral pterygoid to relax and the elevator muscles to contract, seating the mandibular condyles in centric position [1, 26]. Thus, the pressures over the TMJ are significantly reduced. Also, the device protects teeth from attrition and wear [7, 18, 25].

A possible limitation of the present case report was the lack of an initial MRI for the diagnosis of the anterior disc displacement. This tool is considered the best method to make a diagnostic assessment of the TMJ status [27]; however, MRI cost is high. Thus, in view of evident clinical findings exhibited by the patient, we decided to obtain a CT—a lower cost alternative—after a careful clinical debate between the treating specialists.

The normal function of the temporomandibular joint in children and adolescents is of fundamental importance for a normal development of the oral cavity and craniofacial region. Although the greatest TMJ structural growth takes place during the first 20 years of life, the most rapid growth occurs over the first 10 years [4].

4. Conclusions

Pediatric dentists are obliged to early recognize those characteristic signs and symptoms, proper to the diverse temporomandibular disorders, particularly the anterior disc displacement with reduction. An adequate diagnosis will allow to identify and apply the appropriate treatment option during the primary and mixed dentition stages, in order to avoid the progression of this condition. Among the different treatment options, the use of soft material-based occlusal splints can be recommended. This device reduces the muscular activity, thus giving more comfort to the child; moreover, the therapy relieves symptoms, changes the distribution of traumatic forces, and establish a neuromuscular harmony in the masticatory system.

Acknowledgments

The English-language reviewing of the manuscript by Maggie Brunner has been particularly appreciated. This work was supported partially by PRODEP 2018 Grant.

References

[1] American Academy of Pediatric Dentistry, "Guideline on acquired temporomandibular disorders in infants, children, and adolescents," *Pediatric Dentistry*, vol. 38, no. 6, pp. 308–314, 2016.

[2] M. Mujtarogullari, F. Demirel, and G. Saygih, "Temporomandibular disorders in Turkish children with mixed and primary dentition: prevalence of signs and symptoms," *Turkish Journal of Pediatrics*, vol. 46, no. 2, pp. 159–163, 2004.

[3] P. Toscano and P. Defabianis, "Clinical evaluation of temporomandibular disorders in children and adolescents: a review of the literature," *European Journal Paediatric Dentistry*, vol. 19, no. 4, pp. 188–192, 2009.

[4] L. M. Horton, R. M. John, H. Karibe, and P. Rudd, "Jaw disorders in the pediatric population," *Journal of the American Association of Nurse Practitioners*, vol. 28, no. 6, pp. 294–303, 2016.

[5] J. J. Huddleston-Slater, F. Lobbezoo, N. C. Onland-Moret, and M. Naeije, "Anterior disc displacement with reduction and symptomatic hypermobility in the human temporomandibular joint: prevalence rates and risk factors in children and teenagers," *Journal of Orofacial Pain*, vol. 21, no. 1, pp. 55–62, 2007.

[6] T. H. Hotta, C. E. Sverzut, M. Palinkas et al., "Case report involving temporomandibular dysfunction, eagle's syndrome and torus mandibularis–multidisciplinary approaches," *Open Journal of Stomatology*, vol. 3, no. 7, pp. 338–343, 2013.

[7] A. Hegab, "Pediatric temporomandibular joint disorders," *Journal of Dental Health, Oral Disorders & Therapy*, vol. 2, no. 3, p. 00047, 2015.

[8] M. Fernandes de Sena, K. S. F. De Mesquita, F. R. R. Santos, F. Wanderley-Silva, and K. V. D. Serrano, "Prevalence of temporomandibular disorders in children and adolescents," *Pevista Paulista de Pediatria*, vol. 31, no. 4, pp. 538–545, 2013.

[9] J. A. Howard, "Temporomandibular joint disorders in children," *Dental Clinics of North America*, vol. 57, no. 1, pp. 99–127, 2013.

[10] S. I. Kalaykova, F. Lobbezoo, and M. Naeije, "Risk factors for anterior disc displacement with reduction and intermittent locking in adolescents," *Journal of Orofacial Pain*, vol. 25, no. 2, pp. 153–160, 2011.

[11] M. Lalue-Sánchez, A. R. Gonzaga, A. S. Guimaraes, and E. C. Ribeiro, "Disc displacement with reduction of the temporomandibular joint: the real need for treatment," *Journal of Pain & Relief*, vol. 4, no. 5, pp. 1–5, 2015.

[12] B. Thilander, G. Rubio, L. Pena, and C. De Mayorga, "Prevalence of temporomandibular dysfunction and its association with malocclusion in children and adolescents: an epidemiologic study related to specified stages of dental development," *Angle Orthodontist*, vol. 72, no. 2, pp. 146–154, 2002.

[13] American Academy of Orofacial Pain, *Guidelines for Assessment, Diagnosis, and Management*, R. de Leeuw and G. D. Klasser, Eds., pp. 127–186, Quintessence Publishing, Chicago, IL, USA, 5th edition, 2013.

[14] S. Sener and F. Akgünlü, "MRI characteristics of anterior disc displacement with and without reduction," *Dento Maxillo Facial Radiology*, vol. 33, no. 4, pp. 245–252, 2004.

[15] J. Fatima, R. Kaul, P. Jain, S. Saha, S. Halder, and S. Sarkar, "Clinical measurement of maximum mouth opening in children of Kolkata and its relation with different facial types," *Journal of Clinical and Diagnostic Research*, vol. 10, no. 8, pp. ZC01–ZC05, 2016.

[16] S. G. Cortese, A. M. Biondi, D. E. Fridman, I. Guitelman, and C. L. Farah, "Assessment of mandibular movements in 10 to 15 year-old patients with and without temporomandibular disorders," *Acta Odontológica Latinoamericana*, vol. 28, no. 3, pp. 237–243, 2015.

[17] M. Rocabado, "Rocabado pain map for evaluating TMD," 2017, http://www.treatingtmj.com/cms/tmjcontent/uploads/Rocabado-Pain-Map-for-Evaluating-TMD.pdf.

[18] C. C. Restrepo, I. Medina, and I. Patiño, "Effect of occlusal splints on the temporomandibular disorders, dental wear and anxiety of bruxist children," *European Journal of Dentistry*, vol. 5, no. 4, pp. 441–450, 2011.

[19] H. E. Giannakopoulos, P. D. Quinn, E. Granquist, and J. C. Chou, "Posttraumatic temporomandibular joint disorders," *Craniomaxillofacial Trauma & Reconstruction*, vol. 2, no. 2, pp. 91–101, 2009.

[20] J. C. Türp, A. Schlenker, J. Schröder, M. Essig, and M. Schmitter, "Disk displacement, eccentric condylar position, osteoarthrosis–misnomers for variations of normality? Results and interpretations from an MRI study in two age and cohorts," *BMC Oral Health*, vol. 16, no. 1, pp. 124–133, 2016.

[21] K. Wahlund, T. List, and S. F. Dworkin, "Temporomandibular disorders in children and adolescents: reliability of a questionnaire, clinical examination, and diagnosis," *Journal of Orofacial Pain*, vol. 12, no. 1, pp. 42–51, 1998.

[22] A. C. Mariz, P. S. Campos, V. A. Sarmento, M. O. González, J. Panella, and C. M. Mendes, "Assessment of disk displacements of the temporomandibular joint," *Brazilian Oral Research*, vol. 19, no. 1, pp. 63–68, 2005.

[23] N. Bogduk, "Cervicogenic headache: anatomic basis and pathophysiologic mechanisms," *Current Pain and Headache Reports*, vol. 5, no. 4, pp. 382–386, 2001.

[24] P. Borusiak, H. Biedermann, S. Boberhoff, and J. Opp, "Lack of efficacy of manual therapy in children and adolescents with suspected cervicogenic headache: results of a prospective, randomized, placebo-controlled, and blinded trial," *Headache*, vol. 50, no. 2, pp. 224–230, 2010.

[25] M. S. Lashmi, S. M. Kalkhan, R. Mehta, M. Bhangdia, K. Rathore, and V. Lalwani, "Occlusal splint therapy in temporomandibular joint disorders: an update review," *Journal of International Oral Health*, vol. 8, no. 5, pp. 639–645, 2016.

[26] R. G. Deshpande and S. Mhatre, "TMJ disorders and occlusal splint therapy-a review," *International Journal of Dental Clinics*, vol. 2, no. 2, pp. 22–29, 2010.

[27] T. A. Larheim, "Role of magnetic resonance imaging in the clinical diagnosis of the temporomandibular joint," *Cells Tissues Organs*, vol. 180, no. 1, pp. 6–21, 2005.

13

Miniplate-Aided Mandibular Dentition Distalization as a Camouflage Treatment of a Class III Malocclusion in an Adult

Zaki Hakami ⓘ,[1] Po Jung Chen,[2] Ahmad Ahmida,[2] Nandakumar Janakiraman,[3] and Flavio Uribe[4]

[1]Department of Preventive Dental Sciences, Division of Orthodontics, College of Dentistry, Jazan University, Jazan, Saudi Arabia
[2]Division of Orthodontics, School of Dental Medicine, University of Connecticut, Farmington, CT, USA
[3]Georgia School of Orthodontics, Atlanta, GA, USA
[4]Division of Orthodontics, Department of Craniofacial Sciences, School of Dental Medicine, University of Connecticut, Farmington, CT, USA

Correspondence should be addressed to Zaki Hakami; dr.zhakami@gmail.com

Academic Editor: Maria Beatriz Duarte Gavião

This case report describes orthodontic camouflage treatment for a 32-year-old African American male patient with Class III malocclusion. The treatment included nonextraction, nonsurgical orthodontic camouflage by en masse distalization of the mandibular teeth using skeletal anchorage devices. The total treatment time was 23 months. Normal overjet and overbite with Class I occlusion were obtained despite the compensated dentition to the skeletal malocclusion. His smile esthetics was significantly improved at the completion of his treatment.

1. Introduction

A skeletal Class III malocclusion is an uncommon, yet challenging, orthodontic problem accounting for 8% to 22% of all orthodontic patients [1]. The management of skeletal Class III problems in the late adolescent and adult dentition often involves orthognathic surgery or orthodontic camouflage treatment, which can include differential extraction patterns depending on the severity of the skeletal discrepancy and the patient's expectations and cooperation [2]. Nevertheless, it becomes more challenging when a patient refuses any surgical intervention or extraction treatment options.

Mandibular arch distalization is a nonextraction camouflage treatment modality for Class III malocclusion, and the introduction of skeletal anchorage devices has enabled its use with minimal patient compliance and reciprocal side effects [3–5]. Inter-radicular miniscrews are the most commonly used forms of skeletal anchorage; however, they are often problematic in the mandible because of their high failure rate in the posterior region [6]. Also, the location of miniscrews between the roots limits the extent of distalization

unless relocated periodically [7]. In order to avoid these issues, some clinicians place miniscrews extraradicularly in the buccal shelf area or in the retromolar area [8, 9]. On the other hand, some clinicians prefer mandibular distalization by using indirect anchorage with Class III elastics extending to a miniscrew placed in the posterior region of the maxilla [3, 10].

Miniplates are very stable skeletal anchorage devices as they are supported by two or more miniscrews [11]. Sugawara et al. have placed these behind the mandibular second molars, which allowed sufficient mandibular distalization while using high forces in adult patients [5]. Nevertheless, there is a scarcity of case reports in the literature using this approach, particularly in patients with severe Class III malocclusion and financial concerns.

This case report presents an orthodontic camouflage treatment of an adult patient with a pronounced skeletal Class III malocclusion who did not accept surgical or extraction treatment options. Miniplates were used to retract the lower teeth to achieve acceptable dental occlusion with normal overjet and overbite, and favorable lower lip changes.

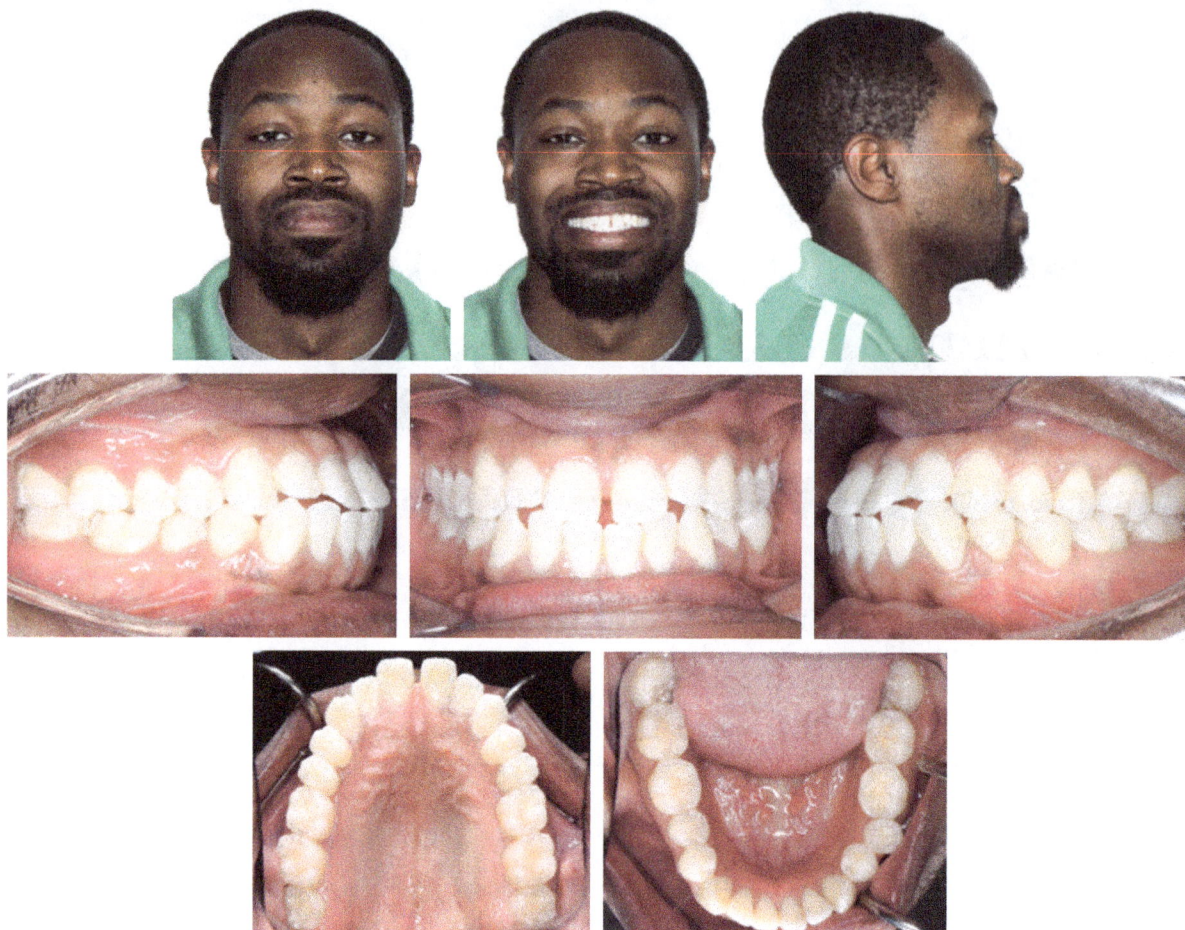

FIGURE 1: Pretreatment facial and intraoral photographs.

2. Diagnosis

A 32-year-old African American male presented to the university clinic with a chief complaint of dissatisfaction with his dental alignment. The patient's medical history was positive for a latex allergy, but there were no other contraindications for orthodontic therapy. The extraoral examination (Figure 1) showed that he had a dolichofacial, symmetrical face and a prognathic mandible with a Class III appearance. The profile showed reduced facial convexity with anterior divergent face, protrusive upper and lower lips, and an acute nasolabial angle (Figure 1). Temporomandibular joint evaluation exhibited normal signs and symptoms, and midline was coincident with the facial midline.

The intraoral examination (Figures 1 and 2) showed a Class III molar relationship (half cusp) and Class III canine tendency bilaterally. Other significant findings included an anterior edge-to-edge relationship and dental crossbite on the lower left second premolar. The dental casts (Figure 2) showed 2 mm maxillary midline diastema and mild crowding (3-4 mm) in the mandible. The panoramic radiograph did not reveal any significant pathology or dental caries, except for a small radiolucent lesion on the distal aspect of the lower right second molar. His mandibular third molars were impacted horizontally (Figure 3(a)). The lateral cephalometric analysis (Figure 3(b) and Table 1) indicated a skeletal Class III jaw relationship (Wits appraisal of −3.5 mm) with bialveolar dental protrusion and increased lower anterior facial height. The maxillary and mandibular incisors were proclined resulting in decreased interincisal angle. In general, the patient was diagnosed with a skeletal Class III malocclusion with bialveolar dental protrusion.

3. Treatment Objectives

Based on the problem lists and the patient's concerns, the treatment objectives were to (1) distalize both arches to improve the protrusive lips profile, (2) achieve Class I molar and canine relationships, (3) establish a normal interincisal relationship, and (4) align the teeth and close upper diastema.

4. Treatment Alternatives

Several treatment options were considered and presented to the patient. The first alternative was combined orthognathic surgical and orthodontic treatment. Maxillary first premolars would be extracted for anterior retraction, and the anterior crossbite would be corrected with a mandibular setback. This approach would have corrected the skeletal discrepancy and improved the facial and dental esthetics.

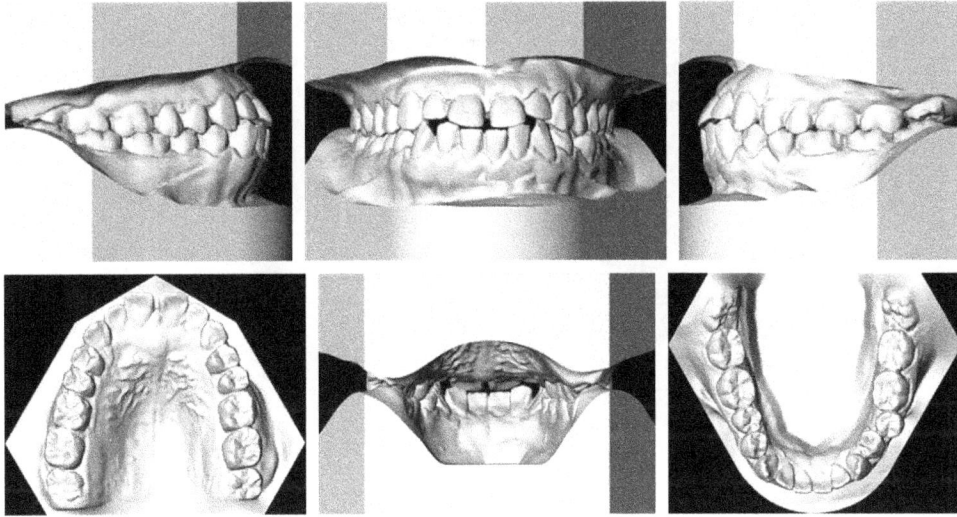

FIGURE 2: Pretreatment dental casts.

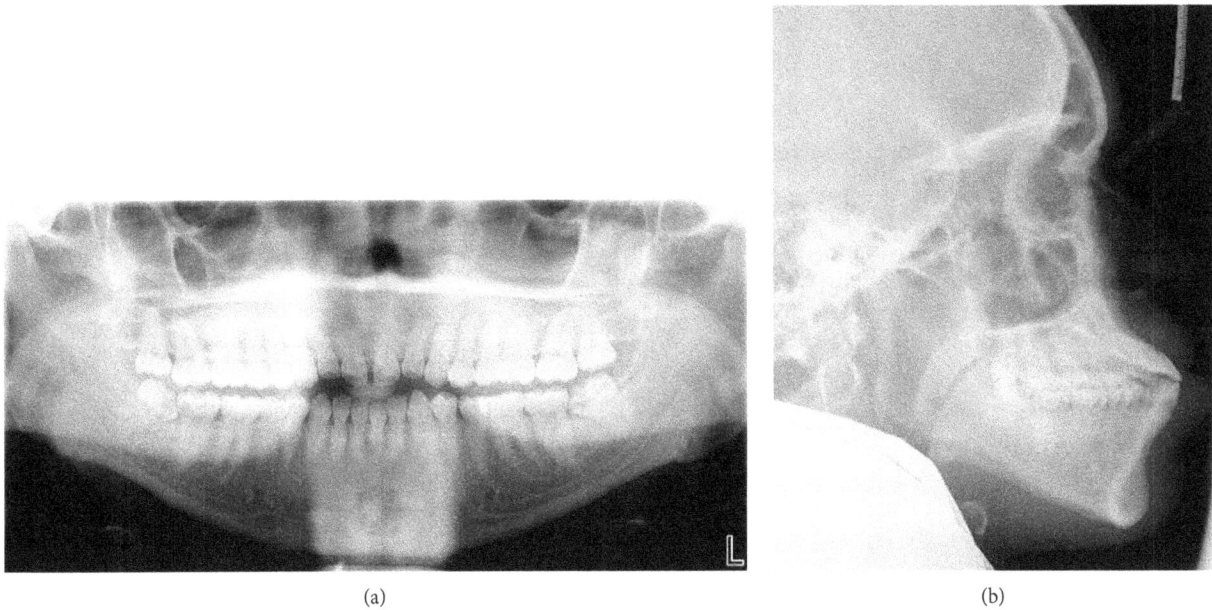

(a)   (b)

FIGURE 3: Pretreatment radiographs: (a) panoramic radiograph; (b) lateral cephalograph.

However, the patient refused this surgical plan due to financial reasons and potential surgical complications.

The second alternative was orthodontic treatment with extraction of four premolars and skeletal anchorage. In this plan, the incisor angulation would be corrected and lip protrusion improved through the retraction of the anterior teeth. However, the patient declined extraction of teeth.

Therefore, the patient's treatment plan would entail nonextraction camouflage treatment by mandibular distalization and skeletal anchorage in both arches or Class III elastics with interproximal reduction on the lower anterior teeth. After discussing these options with the patient, camouflage treatment with skeletal anchorage for distalization on both arches was adopted. Therefore, the treatment plan involved correcting the incisal relationships, reducing anterior proclination, and improving the lip protrusion by distalization with skeletal anchorage.

5. Treatment Progress

Prior to initiating the orthodontic treatment, the patient was referred to his general dentist for extraction of third molars and assessment of caries on the lower second molars. Preadjusted appliance with 0.022×0.028-inch slots were bonded and banded on both arches for leveling and alignment. Both arches were leveled with continuous archwires, starting with 0.016-inch nickel-titanium and working up to 0.019×0.025-inch stainless steel in 9 months. The lower left second premolar crossbite was corrected with X-elastics during the leveling stage. The upper

TABLE 1: Cephalometric measurements.

Measurement	Normal	Pretreatment	Posttreatment
SNA (°)	82.0 ± 3.5	88	88
SNB (°)	80.9 ± 3.4	88	88
ANB (°)	1.6 ± 1.5	0	0
IMPA (°)	95.0 ± 7	100	90
U1-NA (mm)	4.3 ± 2.7	16	15
L1-NB (mm)	4 ± 1.8	16	12
Interincisal angle (°)	123.0 ± 6.0	94	106
Upper lip to E-line (mm)	3.0 ± 2.0	0.5	0.5
Lower lip to E-line (mm)	5.0 ± 2.0	9	7
Wits appraisal	−1.0 ± 1.0	−3.5	−2
Occlusal plane-SN (°)	14.4 ± 2.5	8.5	7
SN-MP (°)	33.0 ± 6.0	31	31
FH-MP (°)	26.2 ± 4.5	25	25
U1-SN (°)	108.6 ± 5.5	130	129
U1-NA (°)	22.8 ± 5.7	45	43.5
L1-NB (°)	25.3 ± 6	41	30.5
LFH (ANS-Me/N-Me) (%)	55	59.3	59

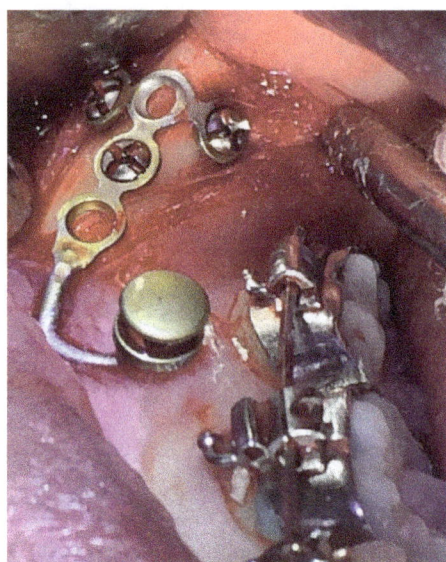

(a)

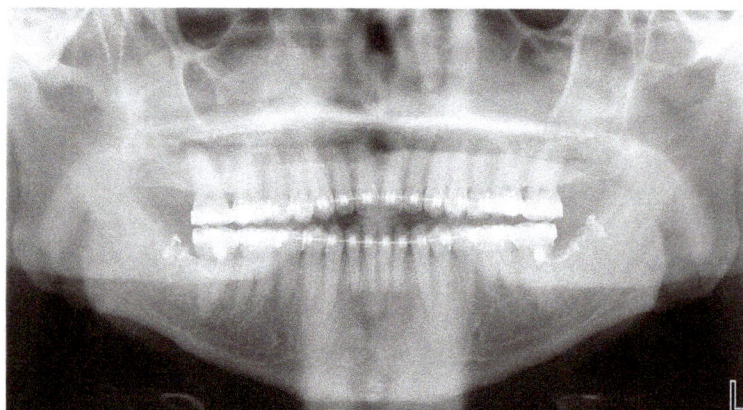

(b)

FIGURE 4: Surgical procedure: (a) intraoral photograph of reflected flap and fixed miniplate; (b) panoramic radiograph after placement of the miniplate.

midline space was closed spontaneously during leveling and alignment.

The patient was referred to an oral surgeon for miniplate placement after the leveling stage. T-plates (Stryker, Kalamazoo, MI, USA) were placed on the external oblique ridge lateral to the third molar area on both sides and fixed by three miniscrews (1.7 mm in diameter and 5 mm in length). The heads of the miniplates were adjusted to the position between the first and second molars (Figure 4). Two weeks after placement of miniplates, two elastomeric chains exerting 250 gm each were applied from the canine and first premolar to the miniplate on both sides to distalize the mandibular arch on a 0.019 × 0.025-inch stainless steel archwire (Figure 5(a)). The distalization was discontinued after 5.5 months when the molars were overcorrected to end-on Class II molar

relationship (Figure 5(b)). Although the molar relationship was overcorrected, the incisal relationship was still edge to edge due to some spacing in the anterior region. A lateral cephalometric film was taken for evaluation, and thin symphysis was noted with the lower incisal roots devoid of labial cortical bone. The patient's mandibular incisors were not suitable for more distal movements because of the thin trabecular bone in the mandibular anterior area that could damage the periodontal tissue. After discussing with patient, the treatment plan was modified to involve only distalization of the mandibular arch instead of both arches.

Thereafter, lower incisor MBT prescription brackets (Opal Orthodontics, USA) were inverted to build up a lingual root torque, and power chain was placed to close the residual anterior spaces. A 0.019 × 0.025-inch stainless steel

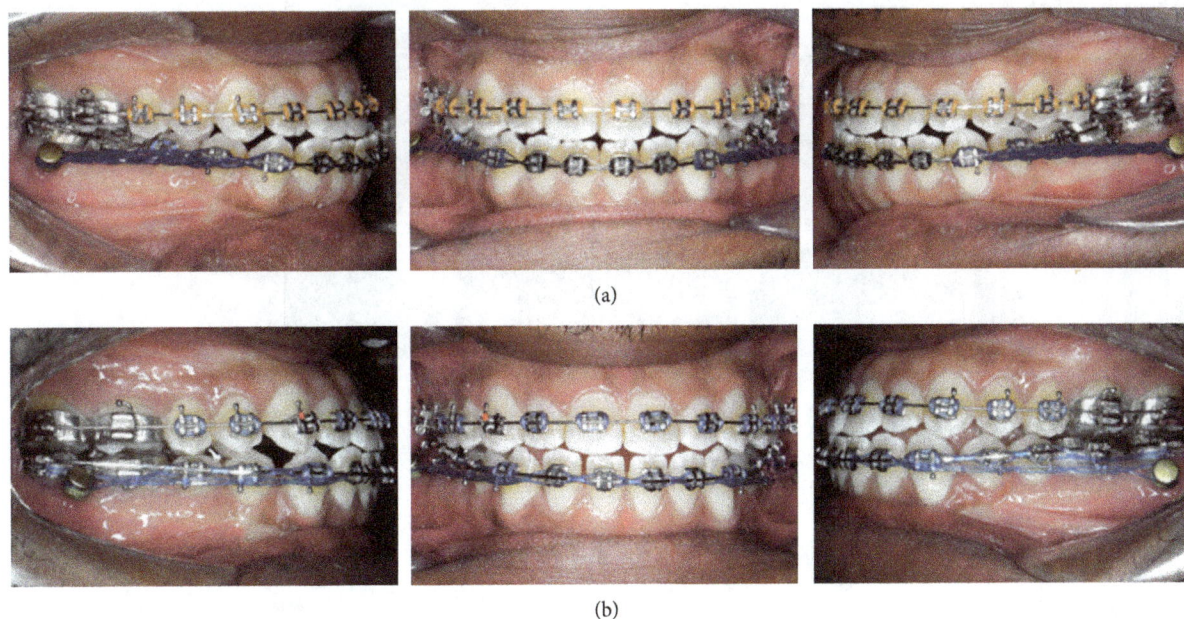

FIGURE 5: Progress intraoral photographs: (a) miniplates are placed on both sides and en masse distalization has just started; (b) the molars are overcorrected to end-on Class II molar relationship.

archwire in the lower arch and a 0.021×0.025-inch TMA archwire in the upper arch were placed for finishing. Due to a Bolton discrepancy, a small amount of interproximal enamel reduction was performed on the lower anterior teeth. The total treatment duration was 23 months. The fixed appliances were removed, and retention was provided by maxillary and mandibular lingual-bonded fixed retainers.

6. Treatment Results

The patient was pleased with the treatment result (Figure 6). The posttreatment records showed improvement of the lower third of the facial profile and retraction of the lower lip with a favorable deepening of the labiomental fold. A Class I canine and molar relationship and normal overjet and overbite were achieved as well as closure of the maxillary midline diastema (Figures 6 and 7).

The transverse dimension was well maintained throughout the treatment. In the maxillary arch, the intercanine width was maintained at 38 mm, whereas the intermolar width was slightly increased from 45 to 45.5 mm. In the mandibular arch, the intercanine width was maintained at 30 mm, and the intermolar width was expanded from 46 to 47 mm (Figures 6 and 7).

The posttreatment panoramic radiograph showed good root parallelism with no significant root resorption (Figure 8(a)). Posttreatment lateral cephalometric analysis and superimposition showed that the ANB angle remained unchanged and the interincisal angle increased as the mandibular incisors uprighted. The patient's facial profile, especially the position of the lower lip, was improved. According to the superimposition, the mandibular anterior teeth were retracted about 4 mm with controlled tipping and the mandibular first molars were distalized 4 mm with bodily movement. The maxillary incisors and molars were slightly uprighted (Figures 8(a) and 9 and Table 1).

7. Discussion

In this patient, very favorable occlusal and esthetic results were achieved despite the large deviation from the norm in some cephalometric numbers. Ideal overjet, overbite, and Class I relationships were achieved. The dentoalveolar compensatory changes contributing most to the correction of his initial dental and skeletal discrepancies were distal en masse movement of the mandibular dentition with counterclockwise rotation of the occlusal plane.

It has always been debatable whether to treat an adult with a skeletal Class III malocclusion by orthognathic surgery or orthodontic camouflage treatment. As Class III patients show complex interactions of skeletal and dentoalveolar components, statistical techniques, including discriminant analysis, have provided differential diagnoses and treatment options for Class III malocclusion patients by allotting them to a treatment modality more objectively [12–15]. In the studies of Stellzig-Eisenhauer et al., the Wits appraisal was described as the best parameter to discriminate between the two groups [15]. According to their developed formula, this patient would have been treated by combined orthodontic-orthognathic therapy. On the other hand, Benyahia et al. proposed using the Holdaway (H) angle—an angle formed by soft-tissue Nasion and soft-tissue Pogonion—tangent to the upper lip, as the decisive parameter between the two treatment groups [14]. According to this philosophy, this patient would have been successfully treated with orthodontics alone. Although ethnic heterogeneity of the sample has been reported in the latter study [14], a possible explanation of this difference could be that the former study was conducted on white Caucasian subjects [15]. Accordingly, their resulting data might not be directly applicable to African American subjects or other ethnicities.

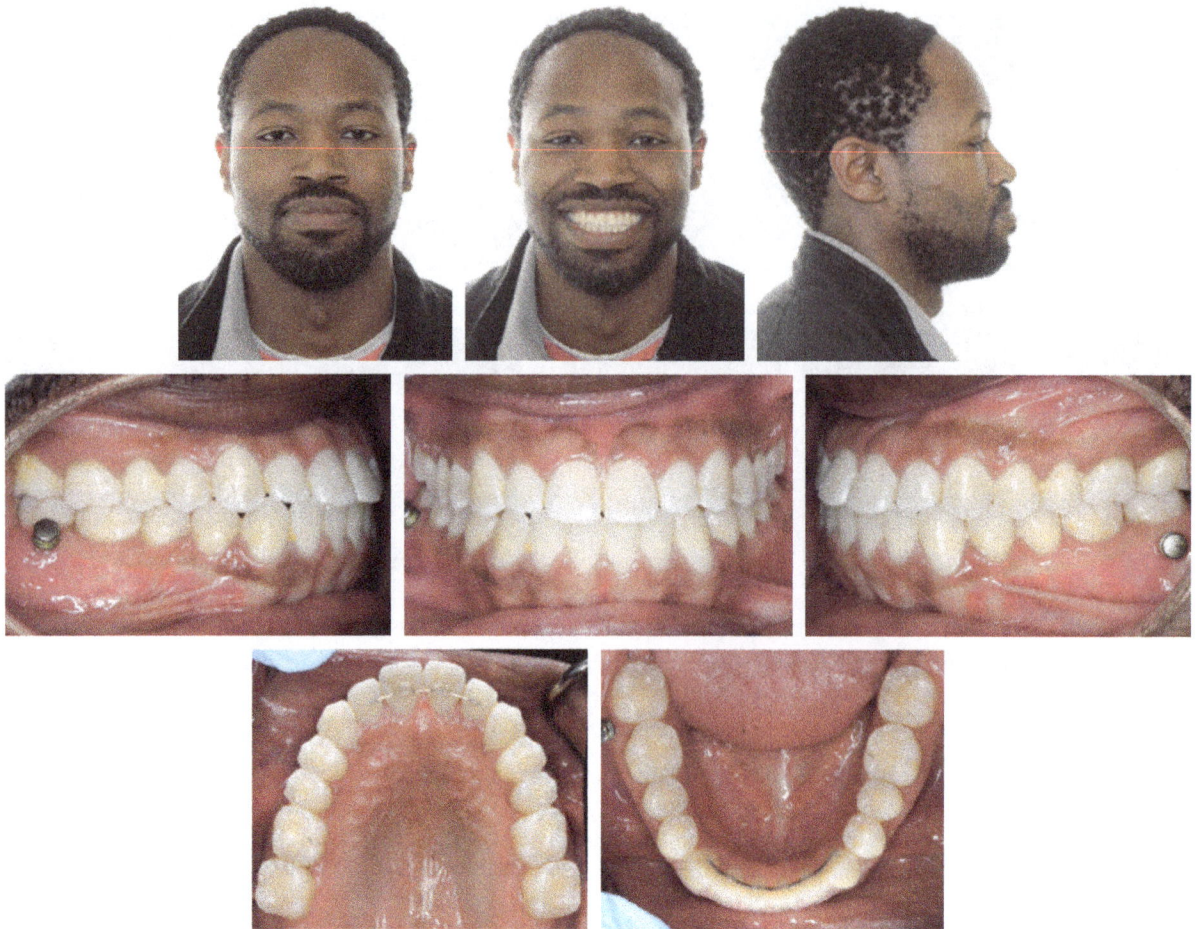

FIGURE 6: Posttreatment facial and intraoral photographs.

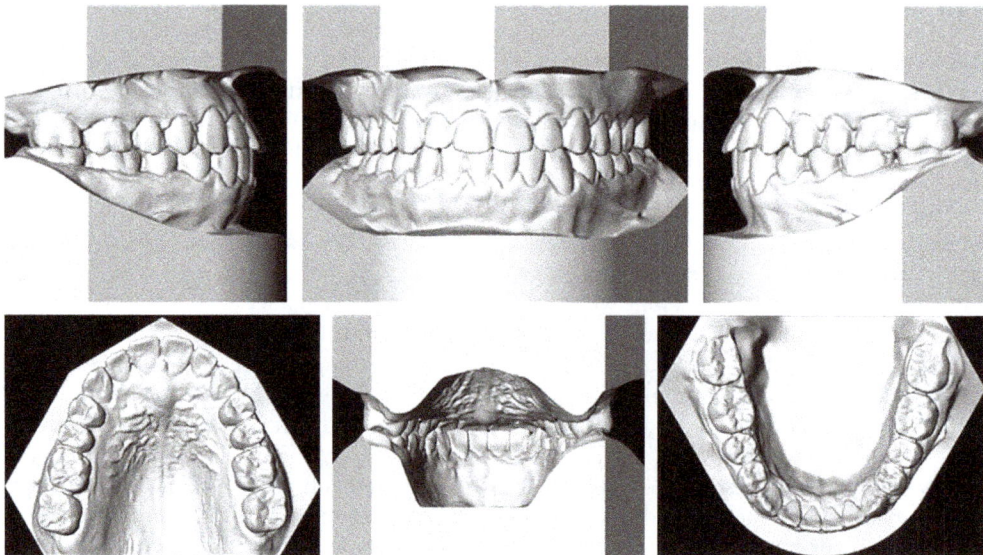

FIGURE 7: Posttreatment dental casts.

In general, tooth movement should be maintained within the boundaries of cortical bone. Since the mandible is a horseshoe-shaped bone, distalization of the mandibular teeth is limited anteriorly by the symphysis and posteriorly by the anterior border of the ramus. Kim et al. suggested that the posterior anatomic limit is the lingual cortex of the mandibular body and not the anterior border of the ramus. Furthermore, they indicated that a root of a mandibular

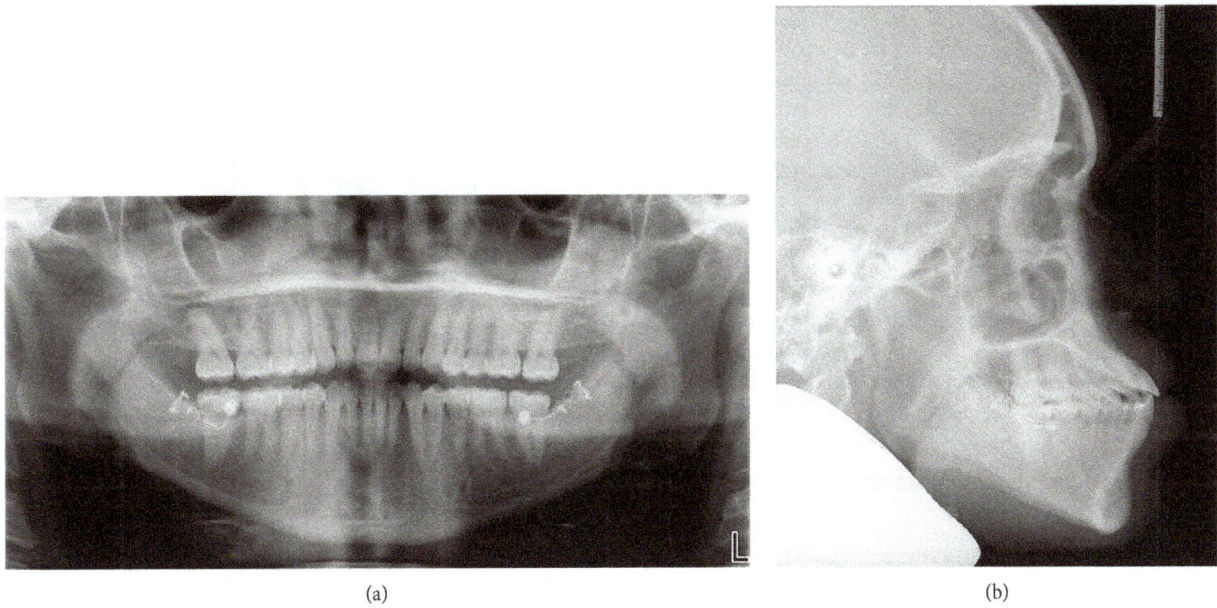

(a)   (b)

FIGURE 8: Posttreatment radiographs: (a) panoramic radiograph; (b) lateral cephalograph.

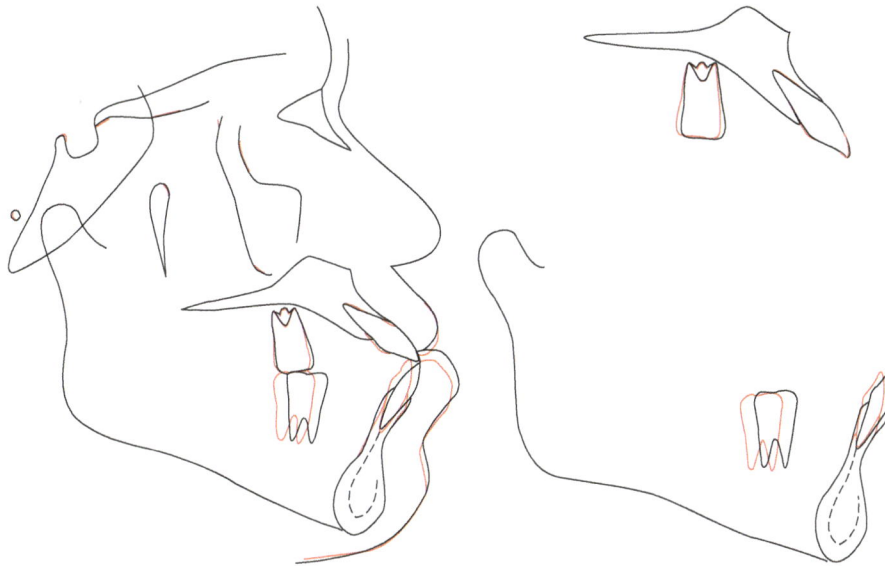

FIGURE 9: Superimpositions of pretreatment (black line) and posttreatment (red line) cephalometrc tracings.

second molar is likely to be contacting the inner lingual cortex of the mandible when the posterior available space in lateral cephalograms is lower than 3.9 mm [16]. This patient had greater than 3.9 mm of posterior space after extraction of his impacted third molars, so significant molar distalization could be performed safely. However, the symphysis of this patient was narrow, thus limiting the amount of incisor retraction because of the risks of dehiscence and loss of bone support [17]. Therefore, we changed the initial treatment plan of en masse distalization in both arches to reduce the bimaxillay proclination to only distalization of the mandibular arch while maintaining the maxillary incisor proclination.

Different amounts of mandibular dentition distalization have been reported using various forms of skeletal anchorage. In general, less than 3.5 mm of mandibular arch distalization using miniscrews placed in different sites has been reported [4, 9]. Ye et al. reported more tipping movement of lower molars retracted by indirect usage of miniscrews in the posterior area of the maxillary compared to direct usage of miniscrews in the retromolar area [9]. Using a miniplate, Sugawara et al. reported 3.5 mm distalization of the first molar at the crown level and 1.8 mm at the root level, with a tipping ratio of 46.3% [5]. Recently, Yu et al. showed that the amount of distalization using a ramal plate, a miniplate inserted in the ramus, was 3.2 mm at the crown level and 2.0 mm at the root level, but with a tipping ratio of 37.5% [18]. Miniplates are relatively invasive, requiring flap elevation and suturing in the placement and removal procedures. Thus, miniscrews are widely accepted by both orthodontists and patients [19].

In our patient, mandibular molars were distalized by 4 mm with near bodily movement. It is possible that this bodily movement is attributable to the force applied near the center of resistance of the lower arch in combination with a large and stiff working archwire that adequately filled the bracket slot. However, as illustrated in Figure 10, the force vector was still above the center of resistance of the mandibular dentition, leading to a slight counterclockwise rotation of the mandibular arch and an alleviation of the negative overbite as documented previously in similar case reports [20]. Moreover, these results are in agreement with a finite element study by Roberts et al., which demonstrated rotation of the mandibular arch resulted in molar intrusion to reduce the vertical dimension of the occlusion and to close the mandibular plane angle in treating Class III patients with anterior open bite [10]. The cephalogram also showed decreased protrusion and 4 mm retraction of the mandibular incisors with controlled tipping, which improved the labiomental fold and retracted the lower lip.

Despite the fact that this patient declined premolar extraction camouflage treatment, various extraction patterns are possible for orthodontic camouflage of Class III malocclusion in adults. Mandibular incisor extraction is most frequently indicated in mild or moderate Class III malocclusions with an edge-to-edge occlusion of the incisors or anterior crossbite and minimal overbite or open bite [21]. Careful diagnosis and thorough treatment planning should be undertaken to consider the amount of overjet, overbite, anterior crowding, and possible Bolton discrepancies [22]. In this patient, lower incisor extraction could have improved the anterior occlusion but also would have compromised the posterior occlusion and buccal segment interdigitation. Alternatively, bilateral mandibular premolar extraction could have been performed. However, a drawback of this option would be that the maxillary second molars would not have an occlusal contact with the opposing dentition after extraction of the impacted third molars.

With regard to the aforementioned contemplations, intermaxillary Class III elastics would also have been a viable camouflage treatment approach. Yet, undesirable side effects including proclination of the maxillary incisors, extrusion of the molars, and unexpected rotation of the mandible are often associated with intermaxillary Class III elastics [23]. This approach would not have been beneficial for our patient because it would have resulted in exacerbating the proclined maxillary incisors. It has also been suggested that excessive use of Class III elastics might be an etiologic factor on temporomandibular disorders because it might exert upward and backward pressures on the mandible [24]. In this case, Class III elastics were not used during the entire treatment period. Therefore, with minimal pressure on the condyle, en masse distalization of the mandibular dentition using miniplates was a quite effective camouflage treatment approach without any further excessive proclination of the maxillary incisors.

Posttreatment stability of orthodontic treatment should always be taken into consideration during treatment planning

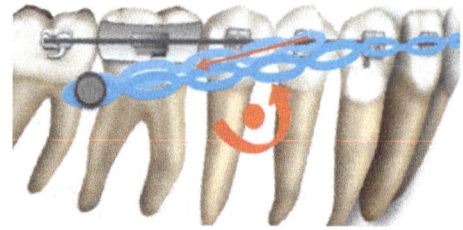

FIGURE 10: Schematic illustration of the en masse mandibular distalization mechanics. Distalization force applied to the miniplate is above the center of the mandibular dentition. This leads to counterclockwise rotation of the mandibular teeth which helps in correcting the anterior open bite.

of Class III patients. It has been suggested that relapse is positively correlated with the amount of tipping or tooth movement in any direction [5, 18]. Sugawara et al. reported 0.3 mm of relapse one year posttreatment for 3.5 mm of distalization. Moreover, they found no significant correlation between the amount of relapse and the tipping ratio and the amount of tooth movement [5]. On the other side, Chung et al. reported a significant relapse after 8 months of retention in a case report of a Class III patient treated with distalization of the mandibular dentition due to severe distal tipping of the mandibular molar [25]. In our patient, mandibular molars were distalized with a translatory type of movement. The mandibular molars were overcorrected to end-on Class II molar relationship and then allowed to relapse gradually over a year during the treatment. Also, the dimensions of both arches were maintained, which is also an important factor in posttreatment stability [5].

8. Conclusion

This case study demonstrates that in mild-to-moderate Class III cases, skeletal anchorage using miniplates is effective in retraction of the whole mandibular dentition leading to correcting the Class III molar relationship and the anterior crossbite without surgery or extraction of premolars. Moreover, this case provides an example that a favorable treatment result, both occlusally and esthetically, can be obtained regardless of a large deviation from the norm in some of the posttreatment cephalometric numbers.

References

[1] I. Egermark-Eriksson, G. E. Carlsson, T. Magnusson, and B. Thilander, "A longitudinal study on malocclusion in relation to signs and symptoms of cranio-mandibular disorders in children and adolescents," European Journal of Orthodontics, vol. 12, no. 4, pp. 399–407, 1990.

[2] W. R. Proffit, H. W. Fields, and D. M. Sarver, Contemporary Orthodontics, pp. 689–693, Mosby, St. Louis, MI, USA, 4th edition, 2007.

[3] K. Chung, S.-H. Kim, and Y. Kook, "C-orthodontic microimplant for distalization of mandibular dentition in Class III correction," Angle Orthodontist, vol. 75, no. 1, pp. 119–128, 2005.

[4] H.-S. Park, S.-K. Lee, and O.-W. Kwon, "Group distal movement of teeth using microscrew implant anchorage," *Angle Orthodontist*, vol. 75, pp. 602–609, 2005.

[5] J. Sugawara, T. Daimaruya, M. Umemori et al., "Distal movement of mandibular molars in adult patients with the skeletal anchorage system," *American Journal of Orthodontics and Dentofacial Orthopedics*, vol. 125, no. 2, pp. 130–138, 2004.

[6] H. Watanabe, T. Deguchi, M. Hasegawa, M. Ito, S. Kim, and T. Takano-Yamamoto, "Orthodontic miniscrew failure rate and root proximity, insertion angle, bone contact length, and bone density," *Orthodontics & Craniofacial Research*, vol. 16, no. 1, pp. 44–55, 2013.

[7] K. Tai, J. H. Park, M. Tatamiya, and Y. Kojima, "Distal movement of the mandibular dentition with temporary skeletal anchorage devices to correct a Class III malocclusion," *American Journal of Orthodontics and Dentofacial Orthopedics*, vol. 144, no. 5, pp. 715–725, 2013.

[8] C. Chang, S. S. Y. Liu, and W. E. Roberts, "Primary failure rate for 1680 extra-alveolar mandibular buccal shelf mini-screws placed in movable mucosa or attached gingiva," *Angle Orthodontist*, vol. 85, no. 6, pp. 905–910, 2015.

[9] C. Ye, Z. Zhihe, Q. Zhao, and J. Ye, "Treatment effects of distal movement of lower arch with miniscrews in the retromolar area compared with miniscrews in the posterior area of the maxillary," *Journal of Craniofacial Surgery*, vol. 24, no. 6, pp. 1974–1979, 2013.

[10] W. E. Roberts, R. F. Viecilli, C. Chang, T. R. Katona, and N. H. Paydar, "Biology of biomechanics: finite element analysis of a statically determinate system to rotate the occlusal plane for correction of a skeletal Class III open-bite malocclusion," *American Journal of Orthodontics and Dentofacial Orthopedics*, vol. 148, no. 6, pp. 943–955, 2015.

[11] M. Schätzle, R. Männchen, M. Zwahlen, and N. P. Lang, "Survival and failure rates of orthodontic temporary anchorage devices: a systematic review," *Clinical Oral Implants Research*, vol. 20, no. 12, pp. 1351–1359, 2009.

[12] W. J. Kerr, S. Miller, and J. E. Dawber, "Class III malocclusion: surgery or orthodontics?," *British Journal of Orthodontics*, vol. 19, no. 1, pp. 21–24, 1992.

[13] W. R. Proffit and J. L. Ackermann, "A systematic approach to orthodontic diagnosis and treatment planning," in *Current Orthodontic Concepts and Techniques*, C. V. Mosby, St. Louis, MI, USA, 3rd edition, 1985.

[14] H. Benyahia, M. F. Azaroual, C. Garcia, E. Hamou, R. Abouqal, and F. Zaoui, "Treatment of skeletal Class III malocclusions: orthognathic surgery or orthodontic camouflage? How to decide," *International Orthodontics*, vol. 9, no. 2, pp. 196–209, 2011.

[15] A. Stellzig-Eisenhauer, C. J. Lux, and G. Schuster, "Treatment decision in adult patients with Class III malocclusion: orthodontic therapy or orthognathic surgery?," *American Journal of Orthodontics and Dentofacial Orthopedics*, vol. 122, no. 1, pp. 27–37, 2002.

[16] S.-J. Kim, T.-H. Choi, H.-S. Baik, Y.-C. Park, and K.-J. Lee, "Mandibular posterior anatomic limit for molar distalization," *American Journal of Orthodontics and Dentofacial Orthopedics*, vol. 146, no. 2, pp. 190–197, 2014.

[17] K. Chen and Y. Cao, "Class III malocclusion treated with distalization of the mandibular dentition with miniscrew anchorage: a 2-year follow-up," *American Journal of Orthodontics and Dentofacial Orthopedics*, vol. 148, no. 6, pp. 1043–1053, 2015.

[18] J. Yu, J. H. Park, M. Bayome et al., "Treatment effects of mandibular total arch distalization using a ramal plate," *Korean Journal of Orthodontics*, vol. 46, no. 4, pp. 212–219, 2016.

[19] M. Suzuki, T. Deguchi, H. Watanabe et al., "Evaluation of optimal length and insertion torque for miniscrews," *American Journal of Orthodontics and Dentofacial Orthopedics*, vol. 144, no. 2, pp. 251–259, 2013.

[20] Y.-A. Kook, J. H. Park, M. Bayome, S. Kim, E. Han, and C. H. Kim, "Distalization of the mandibular dentition with a ramal plate for skeletal Class III malocclusion correction," *American Journal of Orthodontics and Dentofacial Orthopedics*, vol. 150, no. 2, pp. 364–377, 2016.

[21] D. Zhylich and S. Suri, "Mandibular incisor extraction: a systematic review of an uncommon extraction choice in orthodontic treatment," *Journal of Orthodontics*, vol. 38, no. 3, pp. 185–195, 2011.

[22] J. A. Canut, "Mandibular incisor extraction: indications and long-term evaluation," *European Journal of Orthodontics*, vol. 18, no. 5, pp. 485–489, 1996.

[23] J. A. de Alba y Levy, S. J. Chaconas, and A. A. Caputo, "Effects of orthodontic intermaxillary class III mechanics on craniofacial structures. Part II - computerized cephalometrics," *Angle Orthodontist*, vol. 49, no. 1, pp. 29–36, 1979.

[24] W. E. Wyatt, "Preventing adverse effects on the temporomandibular joint through orthodontic treatment," *American Journal of Orthodontics and Dentofacial Orthopedics*, vol. 91, no. 6, pp. 493–499, 1987.

[25] K.-R. Chung, S.-H. Kim, H. Choo, Y.-A. Kook, and J. B. Cope, "Distalization of the mandibular dentition with mini-implants to correct a Class III malocclusion with a midline deviation," *American Journal of Orthodontics and Dentofacial Orthopedics*, vol. 137, no. 1, pp. 135–146, 2010.

14

Fifteen-Year Follow-Up of a Case of Surgical Retreatment of a Single Gingival Recession

Luca Francetti,[1,2] **Silvio Taschieri,**[1,2] **Nicolò Cavalli** (ID),[1,2] **and Stefano Corbella** (ID)[1,2]

[1]*Department of Biomedical, Surgical and Dental Sciences, Università degli Studi di Milano, Milan, Italy*
[2]*IRCCS Istituto Ortopedico Galeazzi, Milan, Italy*

Correspondence should be addressed to Nicolò Cavalli; cavalli.nicolo@gmail.com

Academic Editor: Sonja Pezelj Ribarić

Purpose. The aim of the present case report was to describe the retreatment of the single gingival recession in aesthetic area, in the presence of scar formation and consequent impairment of aesthetic appearance. *Methods.* A young patient with one single recession of 4 mm of 2.1 was treated with coronally advanced flap and subepithelial connective tissue graft, through a microsurgical approach that aimed at the removal of the scarred fibrous tissue. The intervention was performed using a surgical microscope as a magnification device. *Results.* Fifteen years after the surgical treatment, a substantial stable resolution of the gingival recession could be observed. Moreover, a further improvement of the aesthetic appearance could be observed. *Conclusions.* This case report suggests that periodontal microsurgery could be an effective approach for the retreatment of gingival recessions and, in long-term evaluation, to reduce the aesthetic problem due to the presence of scar formation. Further studies with a larger sample size are needed to better evaluate its efficacy.

1. Introduction

Gingival recession is the result of the apical migration of the gingival margin, thus exposing portions of the tooth root that can cause aesthetic impairment when it occurs in anterior regions of the mouth [1, 2]. Moreover, gingival recessions can predispose to root caries development and/or dentinal hypersensitivity [1, 3].

Even though a large debate exists on the etiology of gingival recession, many factors were related to the initiation and development of the apical migration of the gingival margin [4, 5]. In particular, oral piercings, orthodontic forces and appliances, peculiar anatomical conditions in presence of particularly predisposed gingival biotype (thin and scalloped one in particular), and inadequate oral hygiene maneuvers could be related to the presence of recessions [6–10].

Since in most cases gingival recessions remain totally unperceived by patients and asymptomatic, thus limiting the indications to treatment [11], in some cases they could be related to a number of conditions that can cause discomfort to patients or they can be misinterpreted as a sign of periodontitis. Indeed, gingival recessions were recognized as one factor related to dentinal hypersensitivity [3, 12], the formation of carious or noncarious cervical lesions, difficulties in maintaining oral hygiene, and aesthetic impairment [13].

Several surgical techniques were proposed and described in scientific literature for the treatment of gingival recessions [14]. Coronally advanced flap (CAF) with or without connective tissue graft (CTG) is one of the most common surgical techniques in this field, and its application was widely validated by several randomized controlled clinical trials [15–17] and systematic reviews of the literature [18, 19].

One recent review of the literature [14] reported, for cases treated with CAF, only a mean root coverage ranging from 34.0% to 86.7% and a percentage of recessions that resulted complete coverage ranging from 11.0% to 60.0%. As for CAF + CTG, the proportion of recession with complete root coverage ranged from 18.1% to 97.0%, while the mean root coverage ranged from 64.4% to 96.0%.

Since in most cases even partial coverage of the gingival recession could lead to a reduction of symptoms related to dentinal hypersensitivity, an inappropriate technique, in particular regarding the flap management, was related to scar formation and, consequently, an impairment of the aesthetic aspect [14].

The aim of the present paper was to describe the long-term outcomes of a retreatment of one single recession in aesthetic area, treated with a microsurgical approach with the aid of a surgical microscope.

2. Case Presentation

A 21-year-old female patient presented in 2002 with vague symptoms of dentinal hypersensitivity and with a significant dissatisfaction with the aesthetics due to the gingival recession of the tooth 2.1 (left maxillary central incisor) and for the appearance of the surrounding gingival tissues. The patient reported that in 2000 two surgical interventions were already performed to treat the gingival recession after orthodontic treatment and they both resulted in incomplete root coverage and in the formation of scars in the site of surgery which importantly compromised the aesthetics. The exact surgical procedure undergone by the patient was not known. Medical anamnesis was collected before surgery, and the patient was classified as ASA-1 (following the American Academy of Anaesthesiologists classification), having no relative or absolute contraindications to surgical treatment. The subject did not smoke at the time of intervention.

The clinical examination revealed the presence of a Miller I [20] recession of 4 mm on 2.1 and of 1 mm on 2.2. No periodontal pockets deeper than 3.5 mm were found, confirming the absence of active periodontitis. In the region of 2.1, a small band of keratinized tissue (1 mm) was found apical to the gingival margin, and scars extending from the region of 1.1 to 2.2 were found (Figure 1). All teeth were vital and stable, the full-mouth bleeding score was 15%, and the full-mouth plaque score was 15%. From the aesthetic point of view, we evaluated a pink esthetic score (PES) of 4 (on a scale of 10) [21] and a white esthetic score (WES) of 6 (on a scale of 10) [22].

The patient was informed about the clinical conditions and about the treatment alternatives that were, in this particular case, limited. The first proposed option was to perform a surgical retreatment of the gingival recession, aiming to remove the scars through the surgical approach; as an alternative in order to treat the dentinal hypersensitivity, a topical desensitizing treatment was proposed, in case the patient preferred to avoid a surgical approach. After complete explanation of the procedures that could be adopted, the patient decided to undergo a surgical retreatment and signed an inform consent form, approving also the publication of clinical pictures.

2.1. Surgical Procedure. The surgical procedure was performed in 2003 by one oral surgeon with more than ten years of experience in periodontal plastic surgery and a specific training for the use of surgical microscope (LF). The surgery was performed under magnification obtained by a surgical microscope (Universa 300, MÖLLER-WEDEL GmbH & Co. KG, Wedel, Germany).

Local anesthesia with articaine 4% + epinephrine 1 : 100,000. was performed buccally in the site of the intervention

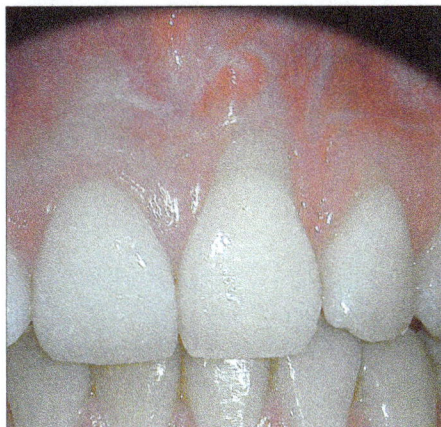

FIGURE 1: Clinical conditions at baseline. It was noticeable the scar tissue in the region of the intervention and the persistence of a gingival recession of 2.1.

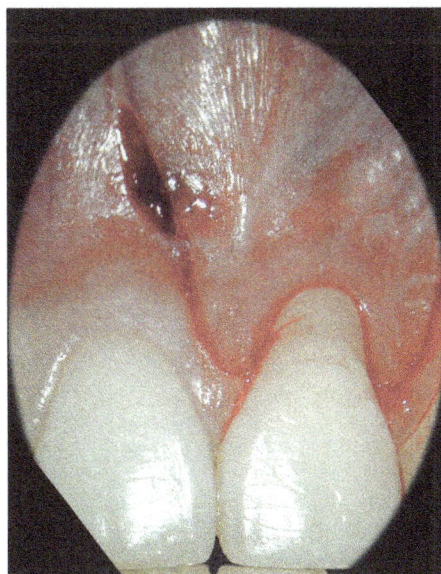

FIGURE 2: Trapezoidal flap was prepared. The vertical incisions extended significantly beyond the mucogingival junction and were beveled.

A trapezoidal flap, made of two beveled and slightly divergent vertical incisions extending beyond the mucogingival junction, was elevated using microsurgical blades. The vertical incisions were connected by one sulcular, which was performed in the gingival sulcus of the affected tooth (Figure 2). A split-thickness flap was carefully elevated, extending beyond the mucogingival junction, leaving the periosteum attached to the bone surface and untouched. In the region of the mesial and distal papilla of the treated tooth, the epithelium was removed, leaving the vascular connective tissue in site. The exposed root surface was accurately debrided through sharp curette (Figure 3).

Afterwards, a connective tissue graft (1-2 mm thick) was harvested from the palate in the region extending from the second premolar to the second molar using the trap door approach [23] and trimmed as necessary to remove

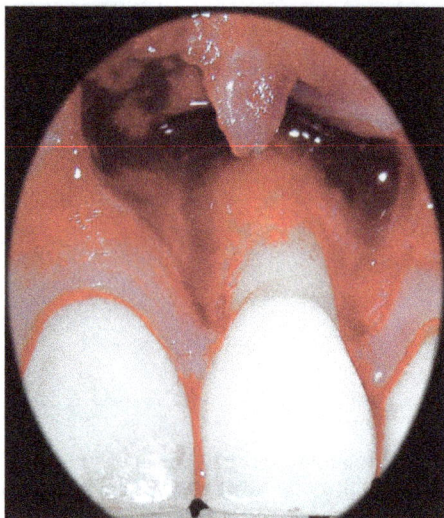

FIGURE 3: After the dissection of the scar tissues that limited the mobility of the flap, it can be repositioned coronally without tensions.

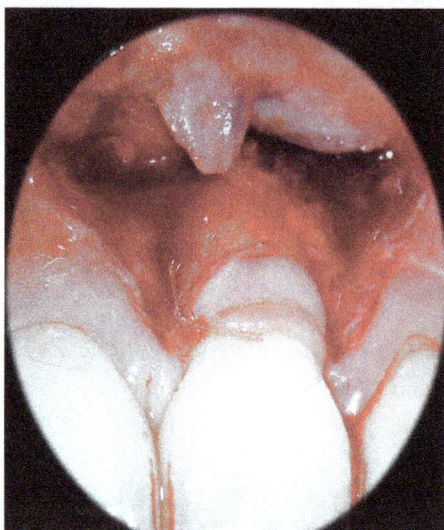

FIGURE 4: A connective tissue graft was placed in the site of the recession and stabilized by the use of resorbable sutures.

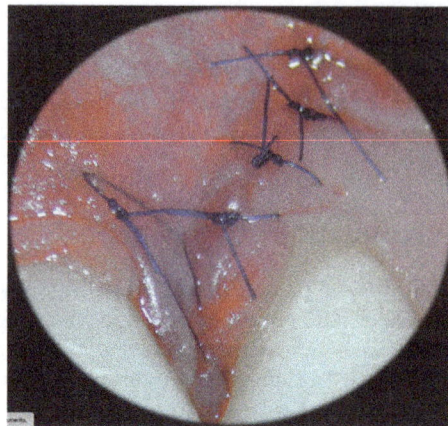

FIGURE 5: Detail of the sutures placed for vertical incisions.

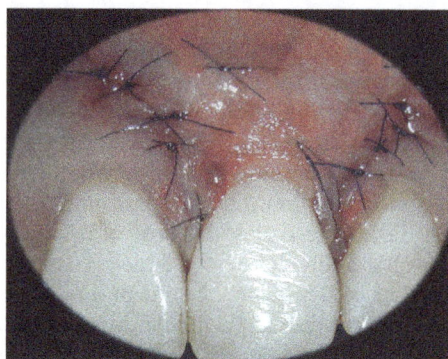

FIGURE 6: The flap was sutured in a more coronal position, and the connective tissue graft was partially covered.

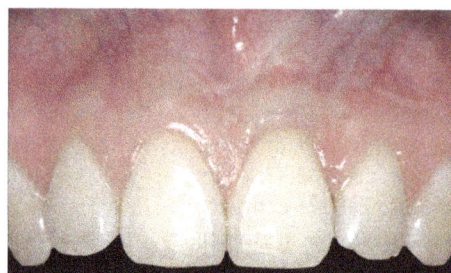

FIGURE 7: Clinical conditions one year after surgical intervention. If compared to baseline, a significant reduction of gingival recession could be observed.

visible epithelium. The graft was then placed to cover the recession defect, at the level of the CEJ, and stabilized using resorbable sutures (Monocryl® 5-0, Ethicon, Inc., Johnson & Johnson, Piscataway, NJ, USA) anchored to the periosteum (Figure 4).

In order to obtain a coronal repositioning of the flap, excluding tensions deriving from muscles, the elevated flap was released through partial-thickness incisions of muscular insertions to the periosteum deep apically. Then, the flap was sutured with interrupted sutures on the vertical release incisions (Deknalon® 6-0 Deknatel, Genzyme GmbH, Lübeck, Germany) and one sling suture (Deknalon 6-0 Deknatel, Genzyme GmbH, Lübeck, Germany) (Figures 5 and 6).

The patient was advised to avoid any trauma in the region of surgery and not to consume hard food during the first three days. Ketoprofen and lysine salt 80 mg was prescribed twice a day for two days for inflammation and pain control. Toothbrushing in the region of surgery was avoided for three weeks, and plaque control was obtained using 0.5% chlorhexidine digluconate spray, applied twice a day. After this period, the patient was instructed to resume toothbrushing using ultrasoft bristles for three more weeks. Subsequently, standard oral hygiene procedures were reintroduced.

The patient was recalled 3, 6, and 12 months after surgery and annually after. Professional oral hygiene was performed in each follow-up visit up to 15 years. After one year, a significant reduction of the gingival recession was observed with an almost complete root coverage (Figure 7). This clinical

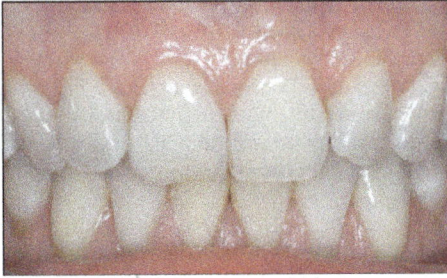

FIGURE 8: Clinical conditions 15 years after the surgical intervention.

condition remained stable also after 15 years (Figure 8). The PES was 8, and WES was 8 highlighting an improvement also in aesthetic appearance.

3. Discussion

The case report described above shows the long-term follow-up of one case of surgical retreatment of one gingival recession in the aesthetic area in a young patient.

As a result of the surgical retreatment, the aspect of the gingival tissues improved, with a complete root coverage and the removal of the scars from the failure of a prior surgical intervention. Fifteen years after the surgical intervention, the result remained unchanged.

As it was observed, scars occurred less frequently at the level of the oral mucosa than skin, probably due to the faster healing of the epithelial tissues of the oral cavity or to the presence of saliva [24]. The presence or persistence of inflammation during the healing process could be recognized as one factor related to scar formation [24, 25].

Some authors have related the formation of scars to a trauma that occurred during surgery to the periosteum that could lead to the formation of fibrous tissues during the healing period [17]. This could occur during surgery when vertical incisions were performed [26]. One study performed investigating scar formation after apical surgery evaluated the outcomes after 1 year of 57 apical surgeries [27]. In the study on scar formation after apical surgery, the outcomes of 57 cases were evaluated after one year follow-up. Authors failed to demonstrate a correlation between some of the tested variables (age, gender, jaw, region, duration of surgery, and time of suture removal) but stressed out the importance of an adequate surgical protocol to avoid the formation of scars [27].

Moreover, the presence of scar tissue could impair importantly the aesthetic outcome of the treatment even in cases when complete root coverage was obtained [28].

To our knowledge, there are no studies (either prospective or retrospective) in the literature on the number of retreatments after failure of the surgical intervention for gingival recession coverage. However, from the technical point of view, the procedure that was performed can be supported by sound scientific evidence.

A few randomized controlled clinical trials compared CAF and CAF + CTG for the treatment of the single gingival recession defects showing short-term (6 months) results [15, 29]. In 2004, Da Silva and coworkers reported that the application of a CTG as an adjunct to CAF could significantly improve the treatment compared to CAF alone [29]. More recently, the results of a multicentric randomized controlled clinical trial were published by Cortellini and coworkers in 2009 [15]. The authors reported better clinical results of CAF + CTG compared to CAF.

Even though some authors found that short-term results after CAF procedures could be a reliable predictor of the medium-term results (3 years), just few studies presented long-term results.

One randomized clinical trial published in 2013 presented the 5-year clinical results of CAF or CAF + CTG for the treatment of single gingival recession [30]. Considering the 5-year residual recession, the CAF + CTG group showed superior results (0.19 ± 0.44 mm) than the CAF group (0.46 ± 0.60 mm). Furthermore, 5 years after surgery, in the CAF + CTG group, 82.5% of sites presented complete root coverage (CRC), while 59.6% of sites treated with CAF alone showed CRC. The authors concluded that CAF + CTG could be considered more effective than CAF alone for the treatment of single gingival recession.

As for the choice of the treatment approach, the existing literature provided a valid support for using CAF + CTG technique in the presented case, hence allowing to augment the width of the gingival tissue to correct the aesthetic appearance.

Even though in the present case report the substantial stability of the gingival tissue level was evaluated, it cannot be predicted how it will evolve over the time in a longer period.

Considering the long-term outcomes of the described case report, it can be affirmed that the treatment of the single gingival recession can be successfully performed, even in the presence of scar formation, using the micro-surgical technique, and stable results could be maintained long term.

Further research performed on the large sample could help in better understanding of the efficacy of surgical retreatment of gingival recessions.

Ethical Approval

All procedures performed in studies involving human participants were in accordance with the ethical standards of the institutional and/or national research committee and with the 1964 Helsinki declaration and its later amendments or comparable ethical standards.

Consent

Informed consent was obtained from all individual participants included in the study.

References

[1] G. K. Merijohn, "Management and prevention of gingival recession," *Periodontology 2000*, vol. 71, no. 1, pp. 228–242, 2016.

[2] D. M. Kim and R. Neiva, "Periodontal soft tissue non-root coverage procedures: a systematic review from the AAP regeneration workshop," *Journal of Periodontology*, vol. 86, no. 2, pp. S56–S72, 2015.

[3] N. X. West, M. Sanz, A. Lussi, D. Bartlett, P. Bouchard, and D. Bourgeois, "Prevalence of dentine hypersensitivity and study of associated factors: a European population-based cross-sectional study," *Journal of Dentistry*, vol. 41, no. 10, pp. 841–851, 2013.

[4] P. Cortellini and G. Pini Prato, "Coronally advanced flap and combination therapy for root coverage. Clinical strategies based on scientific evidence and clinical experience," *Periodontology 2000*, vol. 59, no. 1, pp. 158–184, 2012.

[5] P. S. Rajapakse, G. I. McCracken, E. Gwynnett, N. D. Steen, A. Guentsch, and P. A. Heasman, "Does tooth brushing influence the development and progression of non-inflammatory gingival recession? A systematic review," *Journal of Clinical Periodontology*, vol. 34, no. 12, pp. 1046–1061, 2007.

[6] G. Sangnes and P. Gjermo, "Prevalence of oral soft and hard tissue lesions related to mechanical toothcleansing procedures," *Community Dentistry and Oral Epidemiology*, vol. 4, no. 2, pp. 77–83, 1976.

[7] L. A. Litonjua, S. Andreana, P. J. Bush, and R. E. Cohen, "Toothbrushing and gingival recession," *International Dental Journal*, vol. 53, no. 2, pp. 67–72, 2003.

[8] I. Joss-Vassalli, C. Grebenstein, N. Topouzelis, A. Sculean, and C. Katsaros, "Orthodontic therapy and gingival recession: a systematic review," *Orthodontics & Craniofacial Research*, vol. 13, no. 3, pp. 127–141, 2010.

[9] P. Mehta and L. P. Lim, "The width of the attached gingiva—much ado about nothing?," *Journal of Dentistry*, vol. 38, no. 7, pp. 517–525, 2010.

[10] N. L. Hennequin-Hoenderdos, D. E. Slot, and G. A. Van der Weijden, "Complications of oral and peri-oral piercings: a summary of case reports," *International Journal of Dental Hygiene*, vol. 9, no. 2, pp. 101–109, 2011.

[11] M. Nieri, G. P. Pini Prato, M. Giani, N. Magnani, U. Pagliaro, and R. Rotundo, "Patient perceptions of buccal gingival recessions and requests for treatment," *Journal of Clinical Periodontology*, vol. 40, no. 7, pp. 707–712, 2013.

[12] M. M. Kassab and R. E. Cohen, "The etiology and prevalence of gingival recession," *Journal of the American Dental Association*, vol. 134, no. 2, pp. 220–225, 2003.

[13] M. S. Tonetti, S. Jepsen, and Working Group 2 of the European Workshop on P, "Clinical efficacy of periodontal plastic surgery procedures: consensus report of Group 2 of the 10th European Workshop on Periodontology," *Journal of Clinical Periodontology*, vol. 41, no. 15, pp. S36–S43, 2014.

[14] G. Zucchelli and I. Mounssif, "Periodontal plastic surgery," *Periodontology 2000*, vol. 68, no. 1, pp. 333–368, 2015.

[15] P. Cortellini, M. Tonetti, C. Baldi et al., "Does placement of a connective tissue graft improve the outcomes of coronally advanced flap for coverage of single gingival recessions in upper anterior teeth? A multi-centre, randomized, double-blind, clinical trial," *Journal of Clinical Periodontology*, vol. 36, no. 1, pp. 68–79, 2009.

[16] F. Cairo, P. Cortellini, A. Pilloni et al., "Clinical efficacy of coronally advanced flap with or without connective tissue graft for the treatment of multiple adjacent gingival recessions in the aesthetic area: a randomized controlled clinical trial," *Journal of Clinical Periodontology*, vol. 43, no. 10, pp. 849–856, 2016.

[17] G. Zucchelli, M. Stefanini, S. Ganz, C. Mazzotti, I. Mounssif, and M. Marzadori, "Coronally advanced flap with different designs in the treatment of gingival recession: a comparative controlled randomized clinical trial," *International Journal of Periodontics & Restorative Dentistry*, vol. 36, no. 3, pp. 319–327, 2016.

[18] L. Chambrone and D. N. Tatakis, "Periodontal soft tissue root coverage procedures: a systematic review from the AAP regeneration workshop," *Journal of Periodontology*, vol. 86, no. 2, pp. S8–S51, 2015.

[19] L. Chambrone, F. Sukekava, M. G. Araujo, F. E. Pustiglioni, L. A. Chambrone, and L. A. Lima, "Root-coverage procedures for the treatment of localized recession-type defects: a Cochrane systematic review," *Journal of Periodontology*, vol. 81, no. 4, pp. 452–478, 2010.

[20] P. D. Miller, "A classification of marginal tissue recession," *International Journal of Periodontics & Restorative Dentistry*, vol. 5, no. 2, pp. 8–13, 1985.

[21] R. Furhauser, D. Florescu, T. Benesch, R. Haas, G. Mailath, and G. Watzek, "Evaluation of soft tissue around single-tooth implant crowns: the pink esthetic score," *Clinical Oral Implants Research*, vol. 16, no. 6, pp. 639–644, 2005.

[22] U. C. Belser, L. Grutter, F. Vailati, M. M. Bornstein, H. P. Weber, and D. Buser, "Outcome evaluation of early placed maxillary anterior single-tooth implants using objective esthetic criteria: a cross-sectional, retrospective study in 45 patients with a 2- to 4-year follow-up using pink and white esthetic scores," *Journal of Periodontology*, vol. 80, no. 1, pp. 140–151, 2009.

[23] B. Langer and L. Langer, "Subepithelial connective tissue graft technique for root coverage," *Journal of Periodontology*, vol. 56, no. 12, pp. 715–720, 1985.

[24] A. Sculean, R. Gruber, and D. D. Bosshardt, "Soft tissue wound healing around teeth and dental implants," *Journal of Clinical Periodontology*, vol. 41, no. 15, pp. S6–S22, 2014.

[25] P. Martin and S. J. Leibovich, "Inflammatory cells during wound repair: the good, the bad and the ugly," *Trends in Cell Biology*, vol. 15, no. 11, pp. 599–607, 2005.

[26] G. Zucchelli, M. Mele, C. Mazzotti, M. Marzadori, L. Montebugnoli, and M. De Sanctis, "Coronally advanced flap with and without vertical releasing incisions for the treatment of multiple gingival recessions: a comparative controlled randomized clinical trial," *Journal of Periodontology*, vol. 80, no. 7, pp. 1083–1094, 2009.

[27] T. von Arx, S. F. Janner, S. Hanni, and M. M. Bornstein, "Scarring of soft tissues following apical surgery: visual assessment of outcomes one year after intervention using the Bern and Manchester scores," *International Journal of Periodontics & Restorative Dentistry*, vol. 36, no. 6, pp. 817–823, 2016.

[28] F. Cairo, R. Rotundo, P. D. Miller, and G. P. Pini Prato, "Root coverage esthetic score: a system to evaluate the esthetic outcome of the treatment of gingival recession through evaluation of clinical cases," *Journal of Periodontology*, vol. 80, no. 4, pp. 705–710, 2009.

[29] R. C. da Silva, J. C. Joly, A. F. de Lima, and D. N. Tatakis, "Root coverage using the coronally positioned flap with or without a subepithelial connective tissue graft," *Journal of Periodontology*, vol. 75, no. 3, pp. 413–419, 2004.

[30] D. Kuis, I. Sciran, V. Lajnert et al., "Coronally advanced flap alone or with connective tissue graft in the treatment of single gingival recession defects: a long-term randomized clinical trial," *Journal of Periodontology*, vol. 84, no. 11, pp. 1576–1585, 2013.

15

Implant-Supported PMMA Monolithic Full-Arch Rehabilitation with Surgical Computer-Planned Guide and Immediate Provisional: A Case Report with One Year Follow-Up

Vincenzo Luca Zizzari [1,2] and Gianmarco Tacconelli[2]

[1]Private Practice, Via Benedetto Croce, 85/D, Foggia 71122, Italy
[2]Department of Medical, Oral and Biotechnological Sciences, University "G. d'Annunzio", Chieti-Pescara, Italy

Correspondence should be addressed to Vincenzo Luca Zizzari; vincenzoluca.zizzari@unich.it

Academic Editor: Gerardo Gómez-Moreno

The aim of this case report is to describe the surgical and prosthetic procedures to achieve maxillary and mandibular implant-supported PMMA monolithic full-arch rehabilitation (PMFR) with surgical computer-planned guide and immediate provisional. In such cases, the correct planning of dental implants' position, length, and diameter and the prosthetic phases via computer-aided design are very important to achieve good aesthetic and functional long-lasting results.

1. Introduction

Edentulism is prevalent worldwide among elderly people, and it is mainly attributed to dental caries and periodontal diseases. However, there is an association between sociodemographic factors, age, gender, low family-income, lifestyle, and tooth loss. In addition, earlier studies have shown edentulism to be a global issue, and it seems to be associated with systemic disorders [1].

When a condition of full-arch edentulism or pre-edentulism occurs, different rehabilitative options may be chosen: a complete removable denture, an implant-retained removable denture, and an implant-supported fixed prosthesis, either fixed or hybrid [1–4]. The increase in functional demand and social confidence, is leading more and more patients towards the fixed implant-supported options [5].

As regards implant fixtures inserted in edentulous areas, traditional Branemark's protocols recommend 4 or 6 months of submerged and unloaded healing period, respectively, in the mandible and maxilla, after which it is possible to proceed to prosthetic loading, being the process of osseointegration completed [6, 7].

However, in the last few years, the chance to rehabilitate totally edentulous arches through immediately loaded implant-supported prosthesis was found to be a significant opportunity [6–8] due to good success rates and technical simplification introduced by such procedure as widely reported in previous studies [9–12].

Immediate loading is defined as a restoration placed in occlusion with the opposing dentition within 48 h of implant placement [13]. Integration between dental implants and host tissue is strictly dependent upon control of micromovement at the bone/implant interface during the first healing period, and it could be critical in case of immediate implant loading [9, 14, 15]. With full-arch immediate-loading prostheses, the control of micromovement could be achieved only when respecting some conditions: implants should have adequate primary stability at the time of placement, they should be subjected to rigid interimplant splinting, and occlusal forces should be appropriately controlled during the osseointegration period [16, 17].

Computer-aided design/computer-aided manufacturing (CAD/CAM) guided flapless surgery for implant placement using stereolithographic templates is gaining popularity among clinicians and patients [18, 19]. Its advantages are visualization of anatomical hard and soft tissue structures, virtual prototype of definitive prosthesis, accuracy of implant placement, minimally invasive surgical procedures,

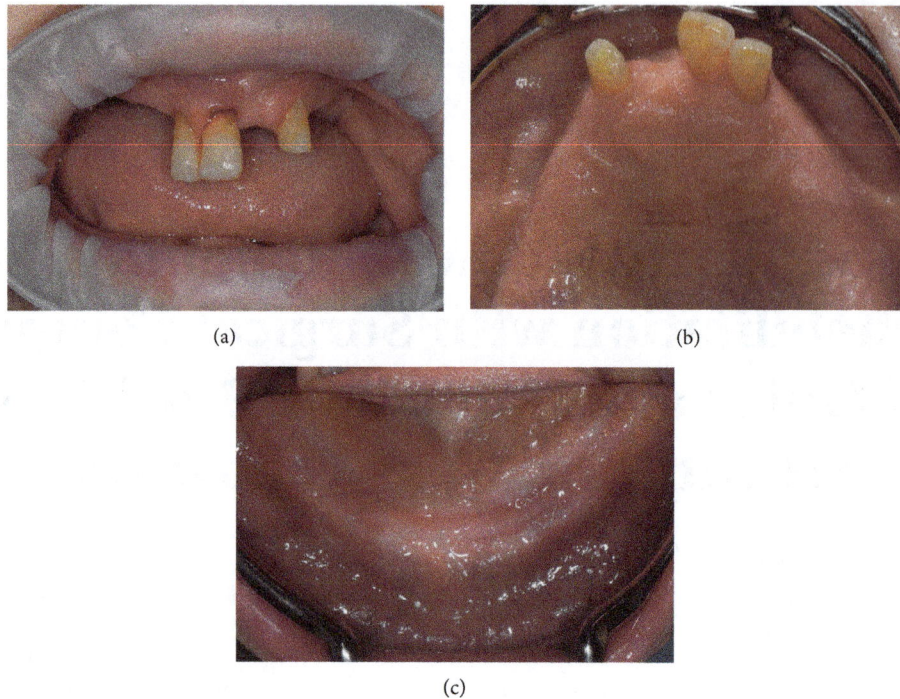

(a)   (b)

(c)

FIGURE 1: Preliminary clinical evaluation of the patient: (a) maxilla intraoral frontal view; (b) maxilla intraoral occlusal view; (c) mandible intraoral occlusal view.

more predictability, and decreasing time required for definitive rehabilitation. Also, it allows the optimization of implants' position and their parallelism because of the high precision of planning, thus preventing damage to anatomical structures and helping to produce a suitable immediate provisional rehabilitation before surgery [18–20].

The surgical and prosthetic procedures to achieve maxillary and mandibular implant-supported PMMA monolithic full-arch rehabilitation (PMFR) with surgical computer-planned guide and immediate provisional are described below.

2. Case Presentation

A 58-year-old man presented few natural teeth in the upper jaw (dental elements 1.2, 1.1, and 2.2) and long-term complete mandibular edentulism (Figure 1). Due to scarce retention of the removable dentures, the patient had not worn them for several years and reported difficulties in eating and speaking, besides aesthetic problems. The patient presented mild hypertension under treatment and antiaggregant therapy and was not a smoker. The primary patient request was a nonremovable rehabilitation. The remaining superior teeth appeared not to be suitable for supporting a fixed rehabilitation, both for their position and for the periodontal attachment loss, and were considered hopeless.

In order to plan an implant-supported oral rehabilitation, a preliminary cone beam computed tomography (CBCT) was prescribed to better evaluate the bone volume of both jaws.

Preliminary radiographic examination through CBCT revealed the presence of sufficient bone volume in the anterior maxilla and poor bone volume in the lower jaw except for the

interforaminal area; no periapical radiolucency was discovered in correspondence of the remaining teeth (Figure 2).

The treatment planned consisted in a fixed full-arch rehabilitation of maxilla supported by 5 implants after the extraction of remaining teeth, and a fixed full-arch rehabilitation on 4 implants in the mandible. Both interventions were scheduled to be conducted through a flapless approach after computer-aided planning in order to reduce intraoperative and postoperative morbidity. The strong request of the patient to try everything possible to avoid a provisional mobile restoration led to carefully planning not only implant insertion but also prosthetic rehabilitation. Thus, the patient was informed about the possibility of applying immediate fixed provisional prosthesis if at the time of implant insertions; most of the implants had showed an insertion torque higher than 45 N·cm, as reported by Cannizzaro et al. [21].

The patient was informed about the treatment and a written consensus was obtained according to local legislation.

Initially, a biphasic impression in vinyl polyether silicone (EXA'lence Putty and EXA'lence Light Body, GC Europe) of both arches was obtained to have initial stone models. After having simulated maxillary teeth extraction on the upper working model, both stone models were put in a medium-values articulator to realize the diagnostic wax-up in order to previsualize the aesthetic result, also considering the extraction of the residual teeth (Figure 3).

As the remaining teeth showed no pathological mobility and their position could not affect the insertion of sufficient number of implants, they could be used for supporting the surgical guide. However, their extraction would be performed

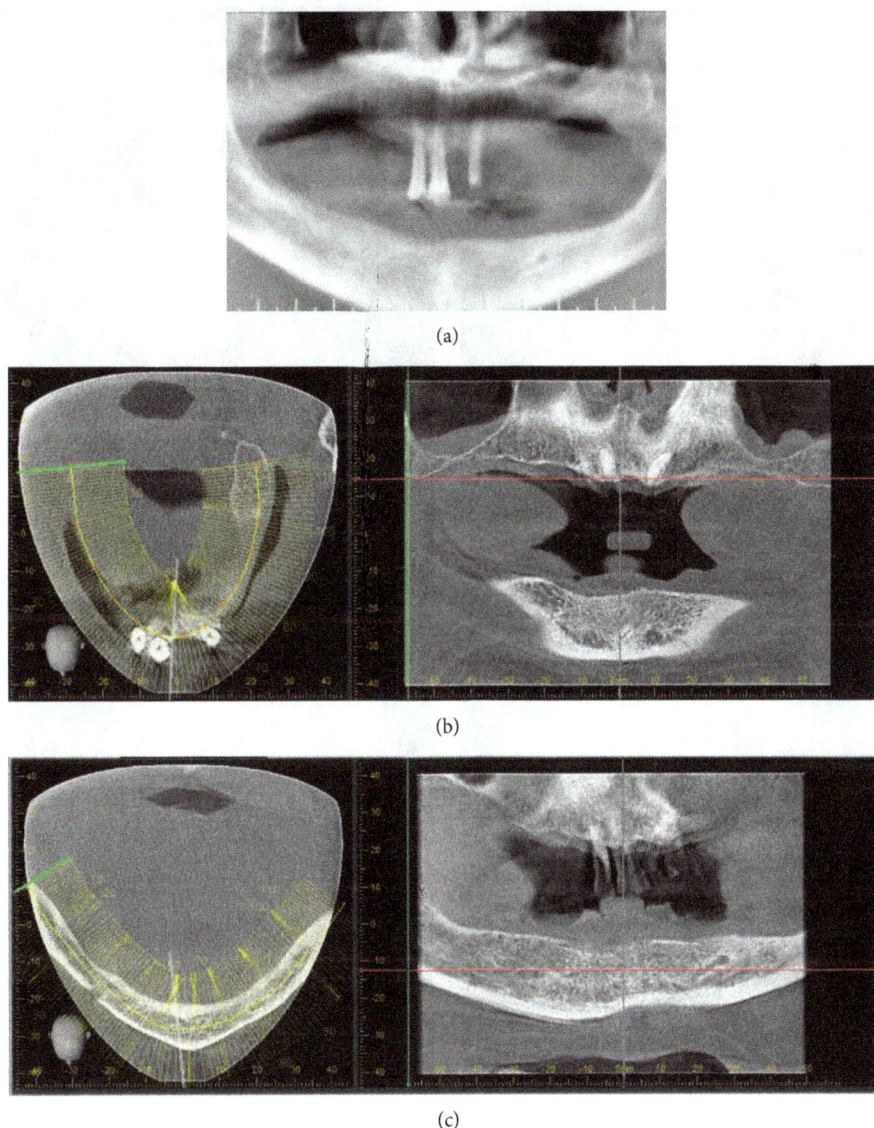

(a)

(b)

(c)

FIGURE 2: Views of preliminary CBCT evidencing sufficient bone volume in the anterior maxilla and poor bone in the lower jaw except for the interforaminal area: (a) panorex reconstruction; (b) maxilla view; (c) mandible view.

on the same day of implant insertion, as they were not necessary for the definitive restoration.

The stone model of the upper jaw was sent to the laboratory, where it was scanned through a model scanner equipped with a computer (7 Series, Dental Wings, Montreal, Canada) to generate STL (STereo Lithography interface format) files. Then, DICOM (Digital Imaging and Communications in Medicine) files derived from preliminary CBCT of the maxilla and STL files from maxilla model scanning were coupled using 3Dyagnosis software (3Diagnosys 4.2, 3DIEMME srl, Italy) so as to be perfectly superimposed, thus obtaining the 3D image that allows the implementation of the intervention planning. Thanks to the presence of the remaining teeth, it was possible to directly couple STL files from the model scan and DICOM files from CBCT using the teeth themselves as reference points, thus avoiding the production of an acrylic guide with radiopaque markers.

Then, a virtual simulation of the rehabilitation was performed. Once having digitally reproduced the diagnostic wax-up, the position of the implants was planned, considering the bone availability and in a prosthetically driven approach in order to have a favourable emergence of the prosthetic screws (Figure 4). Once the implant position was planned, the project was sent to a CAM center (3DIEMME srl, Italy), and the guided surgical template, being supported by the remaining teeth, was printed by stereolithography in biocompatible material (class I CE). Together with the template, a model with implant analogue holes was provided. In laboratory, the implant analogues were inserted into the model, and a metal-reinforced acrylic provisional prosthesis—1.5 mm diameter steel bar reinforcement—(Acry Pol LL, Ruthinium Group, Badia Polesine, Italy) to be relined on the abutments in the patient's mouth after the implant positioning was produced based on the diagnostic wax-up (Figure 5).

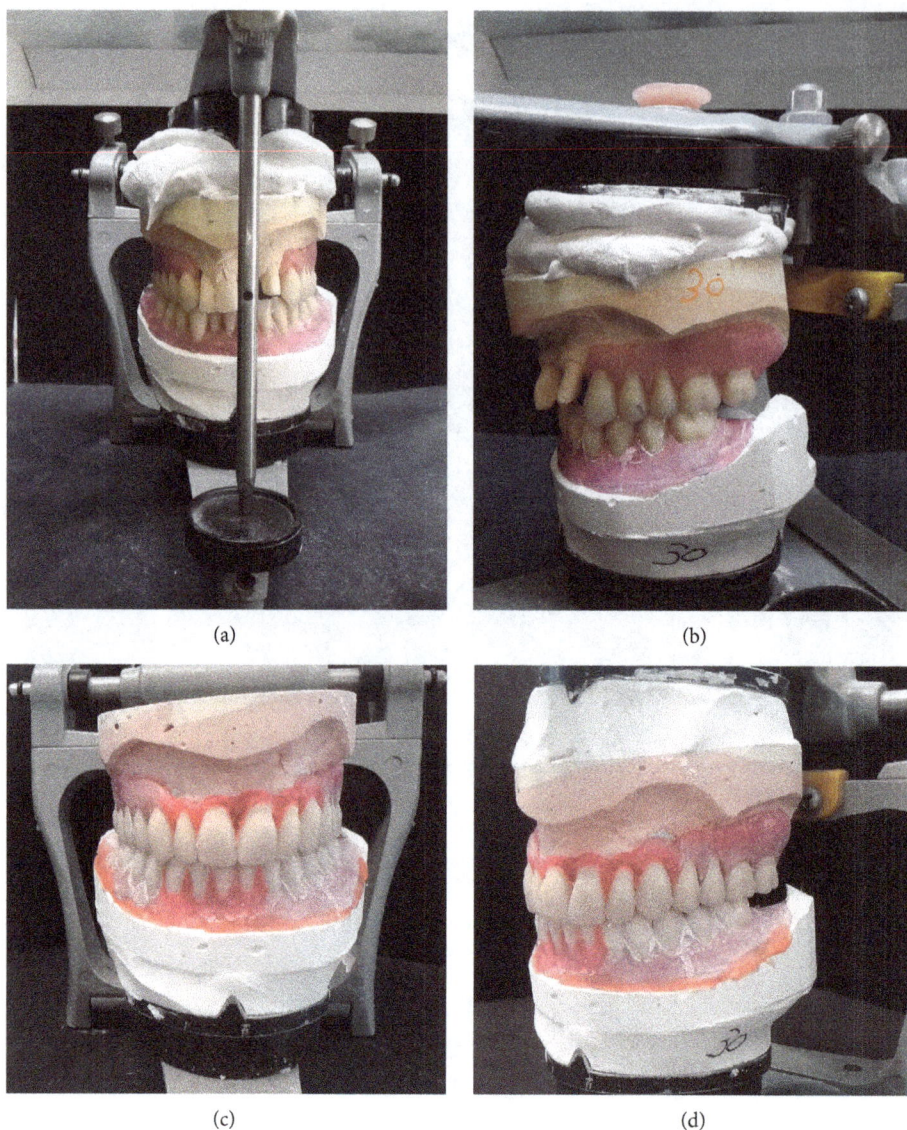

(a)

(b)

(c)

(d)

FIGURE 3: Diagnostic wax-up realized on stone models put in medium-values articulator prior (a, b) and after (c, d) simulating teeth extraction.

The following preintervention drug therapy was prescribed:

(i) Antibiotic prophylaxis with amoxicillin 2 g 1 hour before surgery

(ii) Rinse with chlorhexidine 0.20% for 1 minute before surgery

At the time of surgery, local anesthesia was administered through articaine with epinephrine 1 : 100000, and implant insertion was performed through a flapless approach. After checking the correct seating of the teeth-supported surgical template, soft tissue plugs in correspondence of the sites of implant insertion were removed with the help of a soft tissue punch through the surgical guide. Then, a sequence of calibrated drills with increasing diameters (RealGUIDE surgical kit, 3DIEMME srl) was used to prepare the implant sites under abundant irrigation with refrigerated physiological solution using an implant motor (i-Surge+, Satelec

Acteon, France) at a speed of 800 rpm, while implants were inserted mechanically at 25 rpm with no irrigation and under torque measurement control. The implants inserted had external hexagon connection, diameter of 4.2 mm, and length of 11 or 13 mm (MIS Lance Standard Platform; MIS Implant Technologies Ltd., Karmiel, Israel). All the implants showed an insertion torque higher than 45 N·cm, so the remaining teeth could be removed (Figure 6), postextractive alveoli were filled with collagen sponges, and screwed provisional prosthesis was delivered.

In brief, five temporary abutments (Temporary Cylinder Standard Platform, MIS Implant Technologies Ltd.), which height had been previously studied in laboratory in order not to protrude occlusally from the provisional prosthesis, were screwed on the implants, and metal-reinforced resin provisional prosthesis was directly relined and fixed on the abutments with resin (Splintline, Lang Dental Mfg. Co. Inc., Wheeling, IL) and then refined and

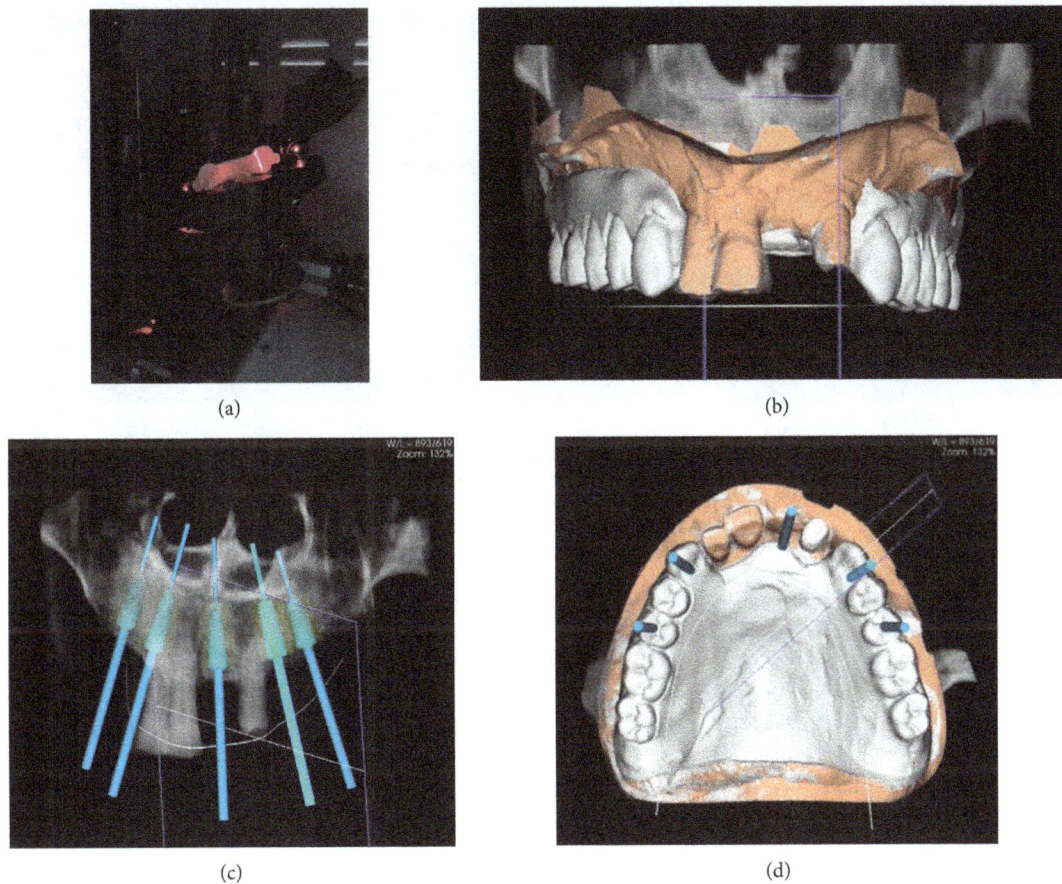

FIGURE 4: (a) Stone model scanning; (b) coupling DICOM files from CBCT with STL files from model scan; (c, d) computer planning of implant position.

polished in the dental laboratory and finally placed in the mouth (Figure 7). The provisional prosthesis was screwed on the implants and tightened at 25 N·cm, and then the holes for screws were filled with light-curing resin. Resorbable 4.0 sutures were necessary only at the sites of teeth extraction.

Final orthopantomography (OPG) was performed to control implant insertion and prosthesis fitting (Figure 8). Postintervention drug therapy consisted in

(i) amoxicillin 1 g twice a day for 5 days,

(ii) ibuprofen 400 mg 2–4 times a day to be taken where necessary,

(iii) rinses with chlorhexidine 0.2% for 1 minute 3 times a day for 2 weeks.

About one month later, impressions of the edentulous mandible and of the maxillary provisional rehabilitation were collected, and a radiological acrylic template with five radiopaque markers reproducing the lower diagnostic wax-up and in occlusion with the maxillary provisional prosthesis was produced. The patient underwent a CBCT of the mandible wearing the radiological template, biting into the established position of centric occlusion. DICOM data from CBCT were processed with the 3Dyagnosis software together with STL files derived from stone model and template scans. The

implant insertion was virtually planned as previously described (Figure 9).

Moreover, the insertion of three anchor pins for the rigid stabilization of the mucosa-supported guide into its appropriate position during the surgical drilling phase was also planned. Files deriving from the project were processed, and the surgical template, the acrylic model, and the provisional prostheses were produced as described above (Figure 10).

In order to provide the correct positioning of the surgical template in the patient's mouth, a silicon index (Occlufast Rock, Zhermack, Badia Polesine, Italy) was realized after seating the surgical guide on the mandible model and putting it in the appropriate three-dimensional relationship to the maxillary model, according to the centric occlusion registered previously (Figure 11).

On the day of surgery, after local anesthesia was administered, the correct seating of the surgical template was checked in mouth and, asking the patient to bite the previously obtained silicon index, it was stabilized in its correct intermaxillary relationship through three anchor pins: a 1.2 mm diameter drill was passed through the three vestibular pin holes of the surgical template under irrigation with refrigerated physiological solution using the implant motor at 1000 rpm and the anchor pins inserted. Once the surgical template was stabilized, the silicon index was

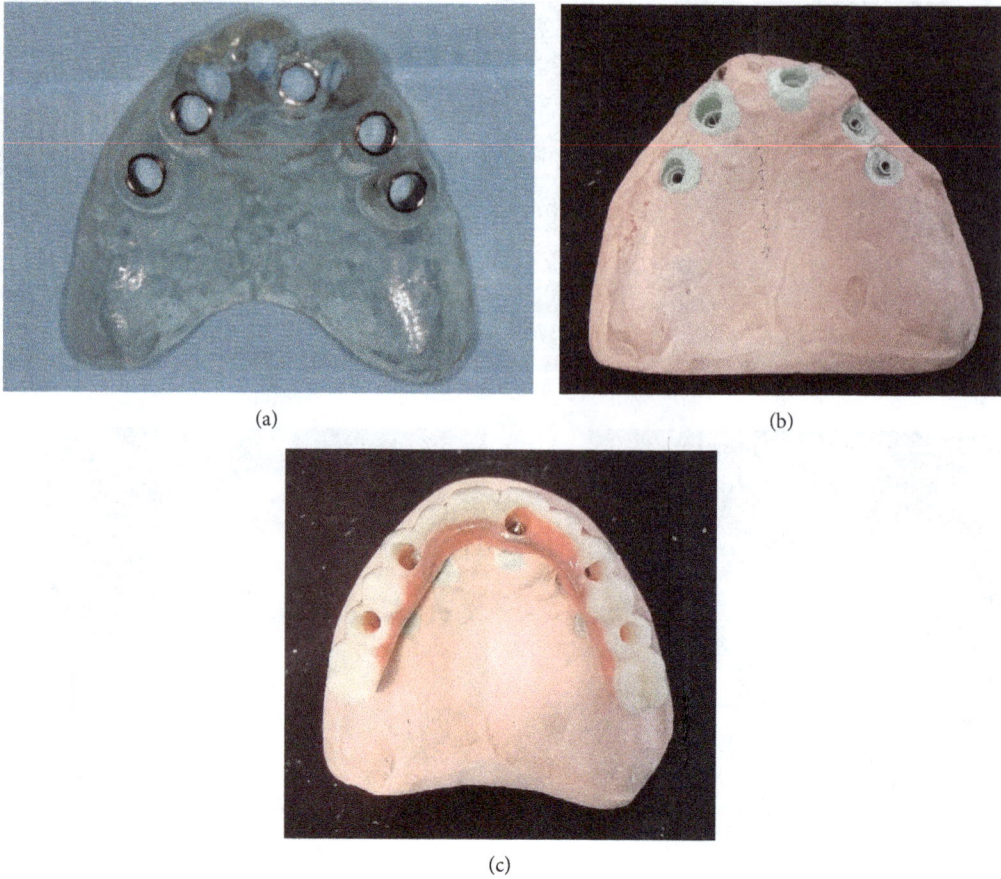

(a)

(b)

(c)

FIGURE 5: (a) Occlusal view of the teeth-supported maxillary-guided surgical template; (b) maxillary model with analogues inserted in correspondence of planned implant position; (c) maxillary metal-reinforced acrylic provisional prosthesis.

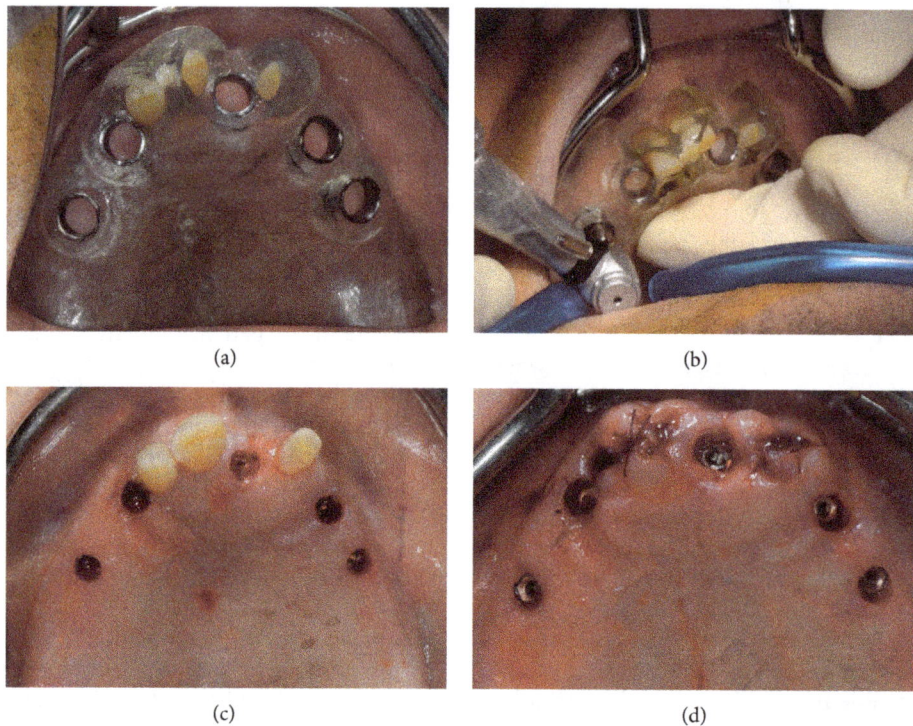

(a)

(b)

(c)

(d)

FIGURE 6: (a) In-mouth try-in of the maxillary teeth-supported surgical template; (b) positioning of the superior dental implants with the aid of the surgical guide; (c) five dental implants positioned in the maxilla before teeth extraction; (d) clinical aspect after teeth extraction.

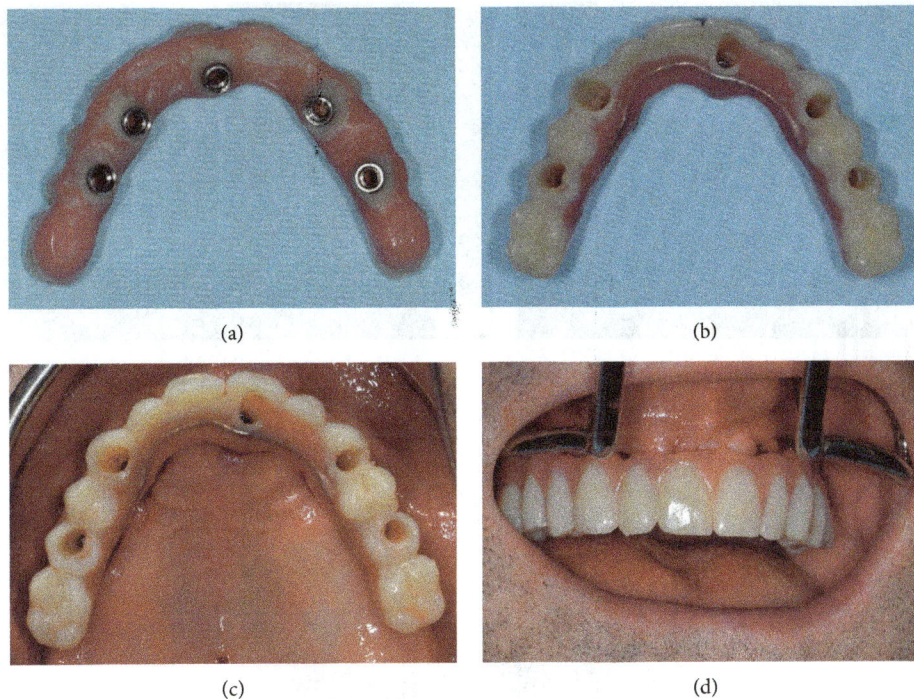

(a)   (b)

(c)   (d)

FIGURE 7: (a, b) View of the provisional upper prosthesis after in-mouth direct abutment fixing; (c) occlusal view of the prosthesis after screwing; (d) frontal view.

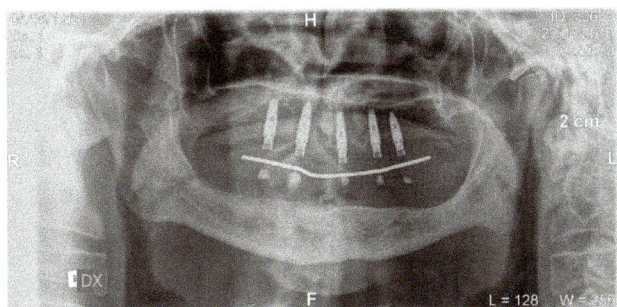

FIGURE 8: OPG performed after maxillary rehabilitation.

removed and four external hexagon dental implants, diameter of 4.2 mm and length of 11 or 13 mm (MIS Lance Standard Platform), were inserted following the same procedure as above. No sutures were necessary. As all implants showed an insertion torque higher than 45 N·cm, the patient could receive provisional prosthesis at the same time of surgery, following the same protocol as for the maxilla (Figure 12). Minor occlusal adjustments were performed as required, and the access holes were filled. Preintervention and postintervention drug therapy was administered as described above, and the patient was advised to chew only lightly during the first six to eight weeks after intervention. The patient underwent periodical controls to evaluate mucosal healing and to perform occlusal adjustments to the provisional prosthesis. About four months after the second intervention, biphasic impressions in vinyl polyether silicone (EXA'lence Putty and EXA'lence Light Body) were obtained through individual trays and using the provisional prosthesis as implant

transfer, according to the pick-up technique. Moreover, bite registration of the provisional prosthesis was also obtained through a silicon base material (Occlufast Rock).

Impressions were immediately poured to obtain stone models, which were fixed in a medium-values articulator and put in their correct intermaxillary relationship by means of the provisional prosthesis and of the bite registration obtained. Then, articulated stone models were scanned (7Series, Dental Wings), the definitive prostheses virtually designed by the use of a planning software (DWOS, Dental Wings), and related files were transferred to the milling machine.

Definitive PMMA monolithic prosthesis was realized from 98 × 20 mm three-layered PMMA blocks (VIPI BLOCK TRILUX®, VIPI Industria, Pirassununga, SP, Brazil) through a 3D milling machine (DWX-50, Roland DG Mid Europe S.R.L., Acquaviva Picena, Italy), according to the manufacturer's instruction. After milling, the milled pieces were removed from the block by sectioning with a diamond disc, the connection peduncles, and mechanically finished and polished using rubbers and gloss, respectively.

After checking the prosthesis adaptation to the stone models, they were delivered to the patients and connection screws tightened at 25 N·cm; screw accesses were filled with light-curing restoration material (Figure 13).

The patient was instructed about oral hygiene behaviors to follow at home, and periodic controls for in-office hygiene were scheduled every four months. After one year follow-up, the patient was satisfied with the result, with good functional and aesthetical integration of the rehabilitation. Only a few accumulations of bacterial plaque were found on the prosthesis between one control visit and another. Good clinical

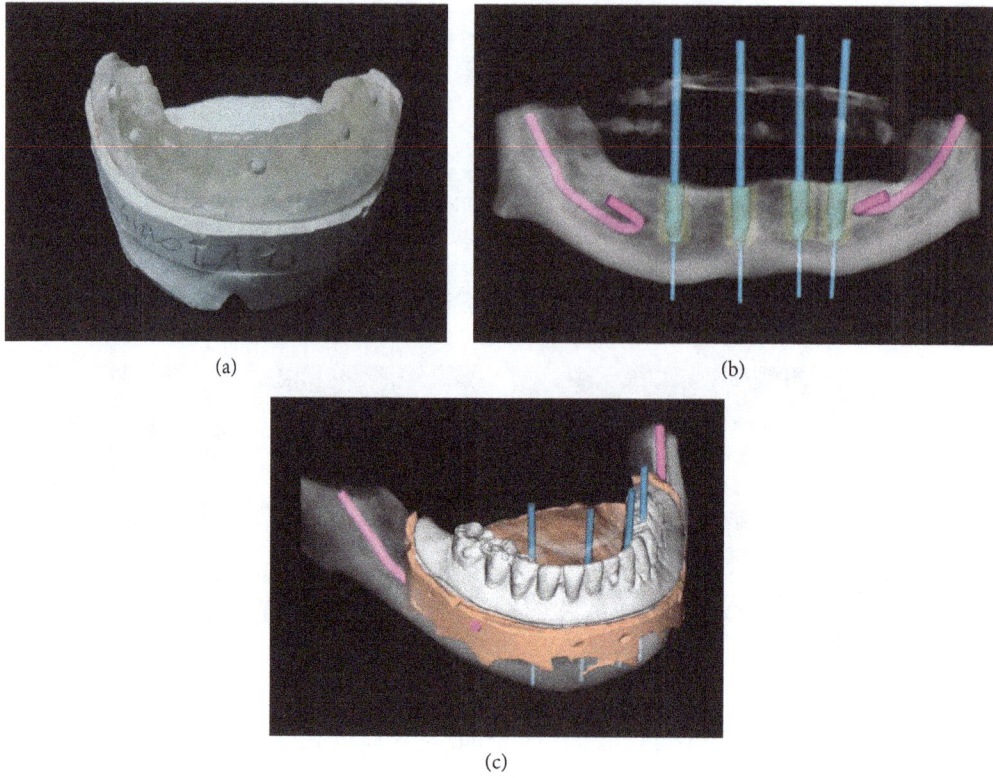

FIGURE 9: Planning of lower intervention: (a) radiological acrylic template with radiopaque markers; (b, c) virtual planning of implant insertion.

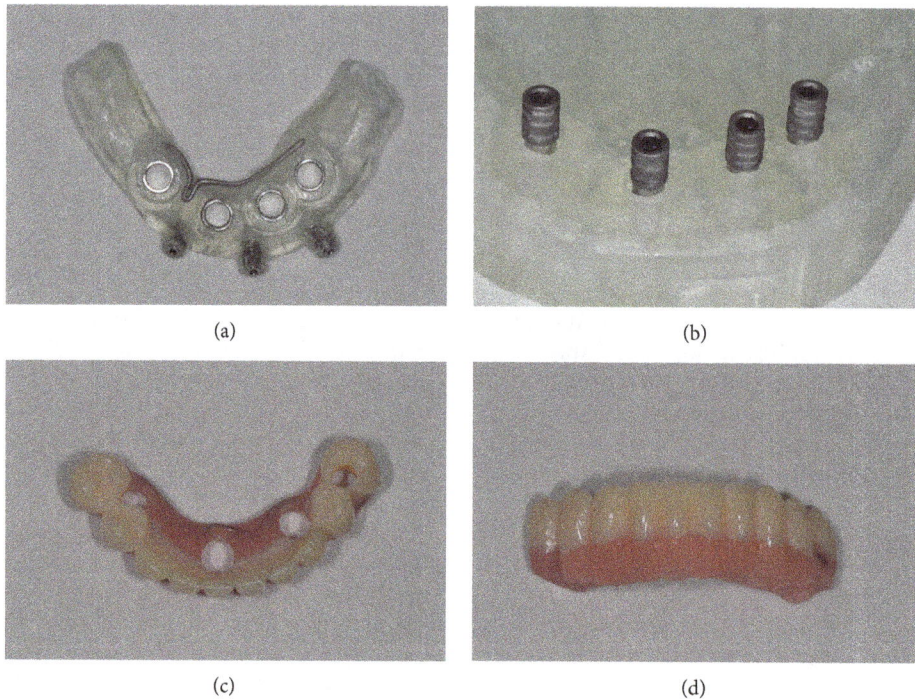

FIGURE 10: (a) Coronal view of the mandibular guided surgical template; (b) a particular of the mandible model with temporary abutments screwed on the analogues inserted in correspondence of planned implant position; (c) occlusal and (d) frontal views of mandible metal-reinforced acrylic provisional prosthesis.

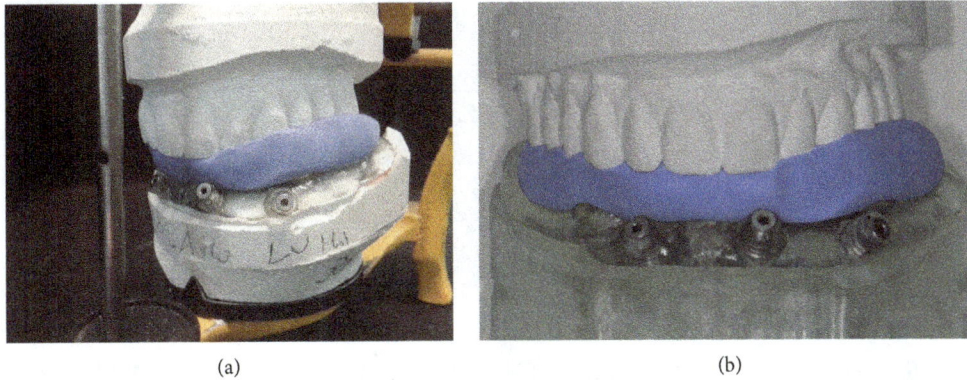

FIGURE 11: (a) Surgical template seated on the mandible model and put in medium-values articulator for the realization of the silicon index; (b) detail of the three-dimensional relationship between maxilla and mandible models.

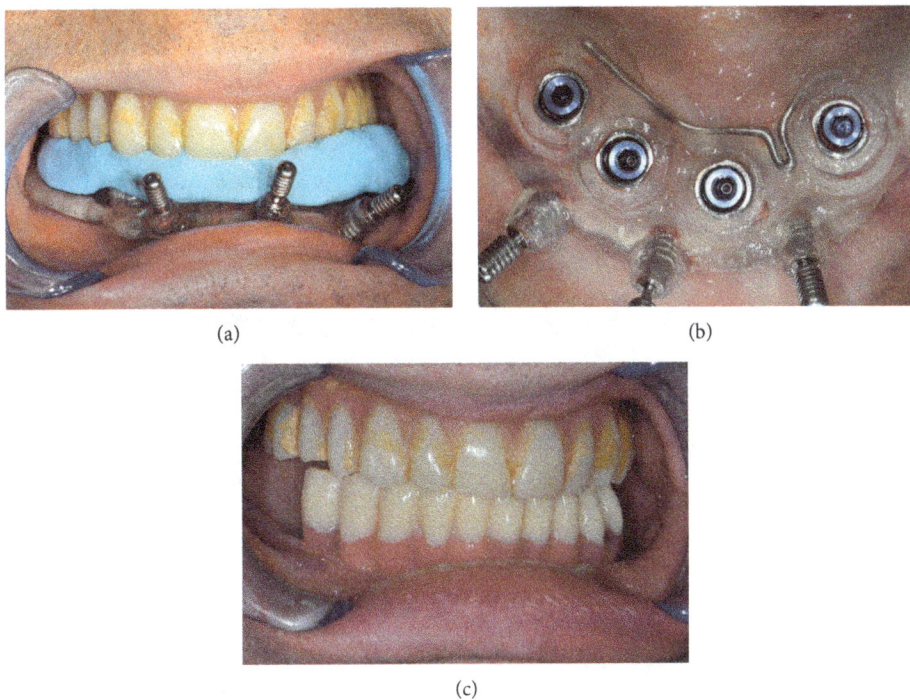

FIGURE 12: (a) Clinical setting of the template through the silicon index; (b) occlusal view of the inferior implant inserted before removing the surgical template; (c) provisional restorations.

and radiographic results could be reported, with no sign of soft tissue inflammation and limited bone resorption around the implant necks (Figure 14).

3. Discussion

Computer-aided planning of dental implant position is of crucial importance when approaching patients with severe bone atrophy as it allows inserting implants, taking advantage of residual bone and optimizing the prosthetic procedures, as established in previous studies [22–25]. In fact, when the bone volume is really scarce, the only alternative to removable denture could be appealing to more invasive, more time-consuming and sometimes less predictable surgical options, such as guided bone regeneration and maxillary sinus augmentation prior to implant insertion, or the use of zygomatic implants [26–28].

Even if several studies focused on the degree of offset between computer planning and the real position of dental implants [29, 30], other studies confirm the high predictability of more recent 3D planning software and the high level of precision between what is accomplished by the surgeon in respect to what is planned [31].

The use of precise and stable surgical templates also allows clinicians to insert dental implants with a flapless approach [32]. It has already been described how bone tissue exposure during oral surgery causes anoxia damage to the outer bone tissue, resulting in a peri-implant bone resorption [33]. Moreover, a flapless approach is doubtless associated with minor postoperative edema and pain [34], so

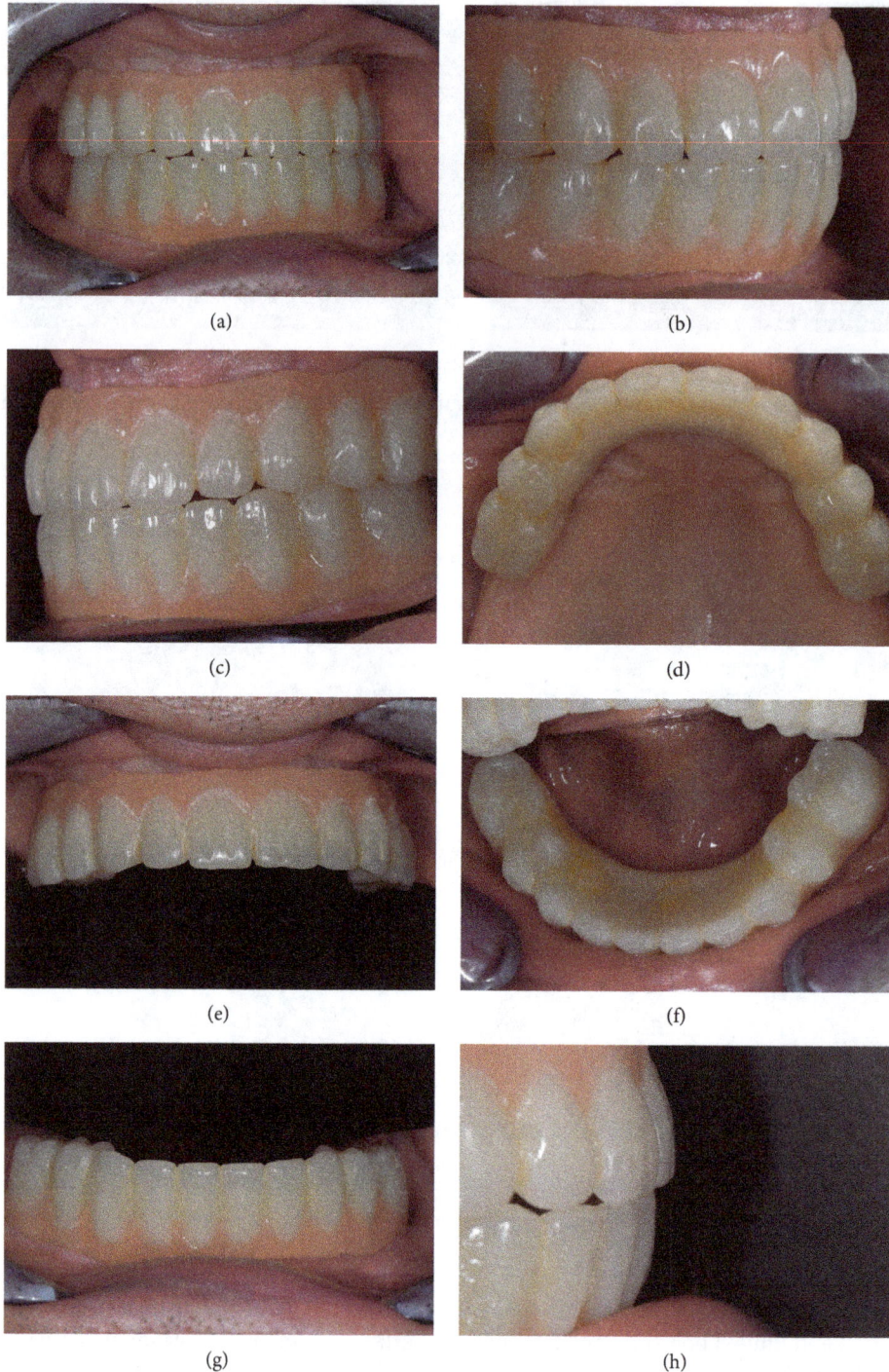

FIGURE 13: Definitive PMMA monolithic restoration: (a) frontal view; (b) right-side view; (c) left-side view; (d) occlusal view of the maxillary arch; (e) frontal view of the maxillary arch; (f) occlusal view of the mandibular arch; (g) frontal view of the mandibular arch; (h) detail of the frontal bite.

that it could be considered a preferable approach to treating patients with systemic diseases [35].

The utilization of milling CAD/CAM resins in the fabrication of the definitive prostheses offers many advantages over the use of the traditional acrylic resin. The use of milled PMMA ensures better mechanical properties than using autopolymerizing acrylic resin, due to the lack of polymerization shrinkage

[36]. Moreover, the content of residual monomer is significantly reduced, due to the method of polymerization under high pressure that PMMA blocks experience before milling, thus enhancing hardness and wear resistance, decreasing surface worsening and the adhesion of bacterial plaque [37].

A further advantage of using CAD/CAM manufacturing is the data storage and reproducibility of prosthetic device in

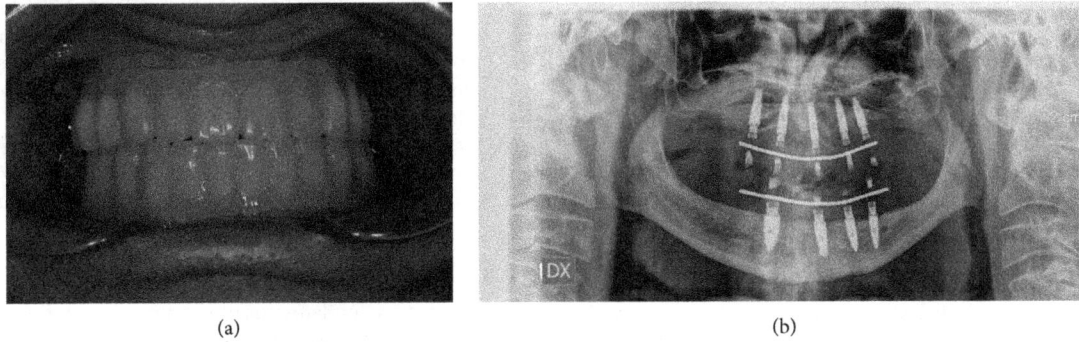

(a)　　　　　　　　　　　　　　　　　　　　　(b)

FIGURE 14: (a) Clinical and (b) radiographical aspect of the definitive restoration after 1 year follow-up.

case of its breaking in short time and with minor discomfort for the patients.

4. Conclusion

Even if the described procedure requires a considerable amount of pretreatment planning and the need to attend for CBCT scanning, it could be considered as a valuable and predictable approach to provide full-arch immediate fixed rehabilitation, with many aesthetical and functional advantages especially in cases of severe bone atrophy, where the alternative would be conventional removable denture or more invasive interventions, and in patients with coagulation disorders, who could take advantage from the flapless approach.

Acknowledgments

The authors wish to thank the CAD/CAM center and dental laboratory "Dental Division s.a.s. di Nicola Corso e Teofilo Ferrandino" for the production of the radiographical and surgical templates and for provisional and definitive prostheses.

References

[1] D. A. Felton, "Edentulism and comorbid factors," *Journal of Prosthodontics*, vol. 18, no. 2, pp. 88–96, 2009.

[2] G. C. Boven, J. W. A. Slot, G. M. Raghoebar, A. Vissink, and H. J. A. Mejer, "Maxillary implant-supported overdentures opposed by (partial) natural dentitions: a 5-year prospective case series study," *Journal of Oral Rehabilitation*, vol. 44, no. 12, pp. 988–995, 2017.

[3] E. Agliardi, M. Clericò, P. Ciancio, and D. Massironi, "Immediate loading of full-arch fixed prostheses supported by axial and tilted implants for the treatment of edentulous atrophic mandibles," *Quintessence International*, vol. 41, no. 4, pp. 285–293, 2010.

[4] P. Malò, M. de Araùjo Nobre, A. Lopes, C. Francischone, and M. Rigolizzo, ""All-on-4" immediate-function concept for completely edentulous maxillae: a clinical report on the medium (3 years) and long-term (5 years) outcomes," *Clinical*

Implant Dentistry and Related Research, vol. 14, no. 1, pp. e139–e150, 2012.

[5] E. Emami and J. M. Thomason, "In individuals with complete tooth loss, the mandibular implant-retained overdenture increases patient satisfaction and oral health related quality of life compared to conventional dentures," *Journal of Evidence Based Dental Practice*, vol. 13, no. 3, pp. 94–96, 2013.

[6] P. I. Branemark, "Osseointegration and its experimental background," *Journal of Prosthetic Dentistry*, vol. 50, no. 3, pp. 399–410, 1983.

[7] T. Albrektsson, F. Dahl, and L. Enbom, "Osseointegrated oral implants: a Swedish multicenter study of 8139 consecutively inserted Nobelpharma implants," *Journal of Periodontology*, vol. 59, no. 5, pp. 287–296, 1988.

[8] H. De Bruyn, S. Raes, P. O. Ostman, and J. Cosyn, "Immediate loading in partially and completely edentolous jaws: a review of the literature with clincal guidelines," *Periodontology 2000*, vol. 66, no. 1, pp. 153–187, 2014.

[9] C. E. Misch, H. L. Wang, and C. M. Misch, "Rationale for the application of immediate load in implant dentistry: part I," *Implant Dentistry*, vol. 13, no. 3, pp. 207–217, 2004.

[10] D. P. Tarnow, S. Emtiaz, and A. Classi, "Immediate loading of threaded implants at stage I surgery in edentulous arches: ten consecutive case reports with 1 to 5 year data," *International Journal of Oral & Maxillofacial Implants*, vol. 12, no. 3, pp. 319–324, 1997.

[11] U. Grunder, "Immediate functional loading of immediate implants in edentulous arches: two-year results," *International Journal of Periodontics & Restorative Dentistry*, vol. 21, no. 6, pp. 545–551, 2001.

[12] T. Testori, S. Szmukler-Moncler, and L. Francetti, "Immediate loading of osseotite implants: a case report and histologic analysis after 4 months of occlusal loading," *International Journal of Periodontics & Restorative Dentistry*, vol. 21, no. 5, pp. 451–459, 2001.

[13] D. L. Cochran, D. Morton, and H. P. Weber, "Consensus statements and recommended clinical procedures regarding loading protocols for endosseous dental implants," *International Journal of Oral & Maxillofacial Implants*, vol. 19, pp. 109–113, 2004.

[14] M. Esposito, M. G. Grusovin, H. Maghaireh, and H. V. Worthington, "Interventions for replacing missing teeth: different times for loading dental implants," *Cochrane Database of Systematic Reviews*, vol. 3, p. CD003878, 2013.

[15] L. Sennerby and J. Gottlow, "Clinical outcomes of immediate/early loading of dental implants: a literature review of recent controlled prospective clinical studies," *Australian Dental Journal*, vol. 53, no. 1, pp. S82–S88, 2008.

[16] S. Szmulkler-Monkler, A. Piattelli, G. A. Favero, and J. H. Dubruille, "Considerations preliminary to the application of early and immediate loading protocols in dental implantology," *Clinical Oral Implants Research*, vol. 11, no. 1, pp. 12–25, 2000.

[17] C. E. Misch, J. Hahn, K. W. Judy, J. E. Lemons, and L. I. Linkow, "Immediate Function Consensus Conference: workshop guidelines on immediate loading in implant dentistry," *Journal of Oral Implantology*, vol. 30, no. 5, pp. 283–288, 2004.

[18] S. Chandran and N. Sakkir, "Implant-supported full mouth rehabilitation: a guided surgical and prosthetic protocol," *Journal of Clinical and Diagnostic Research*, vol. 10, no. 2, pp. ZJ05–ZJ06, 2016.

[19] M. Cassetta, L. V. Stefanelli, M. Giansanti, and S. Calasso, "Accuracy of implant placement with a stereolithographic surgical template," *International Journal of Oral & Maxillofacial Implants*, vol. 27, no. 3, pp. 655–663, 2012.

[20] C. B. Marchack and P. K. Moy, "Computed tomography-based, template-guided implant placement and immediate loading: an 8-year clinical report," *Journal of Prosthetic Dentistry*, vol. 112, no. 6, pp. 1319–1323, 2014.

[21] G. Cannizzaro, M. Leone, and M. Esposito, "Immediate functional loading of implants placed with flapless surgery in the edentulous maxilla: 1-year follow-up of a single cohort study," *International Journal of Oral & Maxillofacial Implants*, vol. 22, no. 1, pp. 87–95, 2007.

[22] O. Ozan, E. Seker, S. Kurtulmus-Yilmaz, and A. E. Ersoy, "Clinical application of stereolithographic surgical guide with a handpiece guidance apparatus: a case report," *Journal of Oral Implantology*, vol. 38, no. 5, pp. 603–609, 2012.

[23] L. Amorfini, F. Storelli, and R. Romeo, "Rehabilitation of a dentate mandible requiring a full arch rehabilitation, immediate loading of a fixed complete denture on 8 implants placed with a bone-supported surgical computer-planned guide: a case report," *Journal of Oral Implantology*, vol. 37, pp. 106–113, 2011.

[24] P. Papaspyridakos, N. Rajput, Y. Kudara, and H. P. Weber, "Digital workflow for fixed implant rehabilitation of an extremely atrophic edentulous mandible in three appointments," *Journal of Esthetic and Restorative Dentistry*, vol. 29, no. 3, pp. 178–188, 2017.

[25] V. Arisan, C. Z. Karabuda, E. Mumcu, and T. Özdemir, "Implant positioning errors in freehand and computer-aided placement methods: a single-blind clinical comparative study," *International Journal of Oral & Maxillofacial Implants*, vol. 28, no. 1, pp. 190–204, 2013.

[26] C. Aparicio, W. Ouazzani, and N. Hatano, "The use of zygomatic implants for prosthetic rehabilitation of severely resorbed maxilla," *Periodontology 2000*, vol. 47, no. 1, pp. 162–171, 2008.

[27] P. Malo, M. De Araùjo Nobre, and I. Lopes, "A new approach to rehabilitate the severely atrophic maxilla using extra-maxillary anchored implants in immediate function: a pilot study," *Journal of Prosthetic Dentistry*, vol. 100, no. 5, pp. 354–366, 2008.

[28] P. Malo, M. De Araùjo Nobre, and A. Lopes, "Immediate loading of "All-on-4" maxillary prostheses using trans-sinus tilted implants without sinus bone grafting: a retrospective study reporting the 3-year outcome," *European Journal of Oral Implantology*, vol. 6, no. 3, pp. 273–283, 2013.

[29] G. Windmann and R. J. Bale, "Accuracy in computer aided implant surgery-a review," *International Journal of Oral & Maxillofacial Implants*, vol. 21, no. 2, pp. 305–313, 2006.

[30] O. Ozan, I. Turkyilmaz, A. Ersoy, E. A. Mc Glumphy, and S. F. Rosenstiel, "Clinical accuracy of 3 different types of computed tomography derived stereolithographic surgical guides in implant placement," *Journal of Oral and Maxillofacial Surgery*, vol. 67, no. 2, pp. 394–401, 2009.

[31] D. P. Sarment, P. Sukovic, and N. Clinthorne, "Accuracy of implant placement with a stereolithographic surgical guide," *International Journal of Oral & Maxillofacial Implants*, vol. 18, no. 4, pp. 571–577, 2003.

[32] R. Marra, A. Accoccella, R. Alessandra, S. D. Ganz, and A. Blasi, "Rehabilitation of full-mouth edentulism: immediate loading of implants inserted with computer-guided flapless surgery versus conventional dentures: a 5-year multicenter retrospective analysis and OHIP questionnaire," *Implant Dentistry*, vol. 26, no. 1, pp. 54–58, 2017.

[33] Z. Vlahovic, A. Markòvic, Z. Lazìc, M. Scepanovic, A. Dinìc, and M. Kalanovic, "Histopathological comparative analysis of periimplant bone inflammatory response after dental implant insertion using flap and flapless surgical technique: an experimental study in pigs," *Clinical Oral Implants Research*, vol. 28, no. 9, pp. 1067–1073, 2017.

[34] I. Lalemn, L. Bernard, M. Vercruyssen, R. Jacobs, M. M. Bornstein, and M. Quirynen, "Guided implant surgery in the edentulous maxilla: a systematic review," *International Journal of Oral & Maxillofacial Implants*, vol. 31, pp. s103–s117, 2016.

[35] K. K. Agrawal, J. Rao, M. Anwar, K. Singh, and D. Himanshu, "Flapless vs. flapped implant insertion in patients with controlled type 2 diabetes subjected to delayed loading: 1-year follow-up results from a randomised controlled trial," *European Journal of Oral Implantology*, vol. 10, no. 4, pp. 403–413, 2017.

[36] A. AlHelal, H. S. AlRumaih, M. T. Kattadiyil, N. Z. Baba, and C. J. Goodacre, "Comparison of retention between maxillary milled and conventional denture bases: a clinical study," *Journal of Prosthetic Dentistry*, vol. 117, no. 2, pp. 233–238, 2017.

[37] A. D. Ayman, "The residual monomer content and mechanical properties of CAD\CAM resins used in the fabrication of complete dentures as compared to heat cured resins," *Electron Physician*, vol. 9, no. 7, pp. 4766–4772, 2017.

16

Conservative Vertical Groove Technique for Tooth Rehabilitation: 3-Year Follow-Up

Dhanalaxmi Karre [ID],[1] Mahesh Kumar duddu [ID],[2] Silla Swarna Swathi [ID],[1] Abdul Habeeb Bin Mohsin [ID],[3] Bhogavaram Bharadwaj [ID],[4] and Sheraz Barshaik [ID][5]

[1]Department of Pedodontics, Sri Sai College of Dental Surgery, Vikarabad, India
[2]Department of Pedodontics, G Pulla Reddy Dental College, Kurnool, India
[3]Department of Prosthodontics, Sri Sai College of Dental Surgery, Vikarabad, India
[4]Department of Oral and Maxillofacial Surgery, Sri Sai College of Dental Surgery, Vikarabad, India
[5]Department of Oral and Maxillofacial Surgery, MNR Dental College & Hospital, Sangareddy, India

Correspondence should be addressed to Dhanalaxmi Karre; dr.dhana87@gmail.com

Academic Editor: Michelle A. Chinelatti

Reattachment of tooth fragment is a simple, conservative, and noninvasive procedure, and it is the most currently acceptable treatment option. This article presents management of two accidentally damaged maxillary incisors using direct composite resin restoration and fractured tooth fragment. With the advancements in adhesive dentistry, tooth fragment reattachment procedure has become simpler and clinically reliable. The present paper is a report of 3-year follow-up of coronally fractured tooth treated with a very conservative technique of tooth fragment reattachment using vertical groove preparation and reinforcement with fiber post.

1. Introduction

Coronal fractures are the most common frequent form of traumatic dental injuries commonly involving maxillary incisors. This can be explained by their anterior placement and protrusion due to eruption pattern. Factors such as age, gender, race, and overjet predispose dental trauma in maxillary anterior teeth with higher prevalence in the age groups between 2-3 years and 8–12 years [1, 2]. Based on involvement of tooth structure, coronal fractures are broadly categorized as complicated and uncomplicated fractures [3]. Reconstruction of coronal fractures immediately is important for the positive psychological status and to maintain esthetics [4]. Although direct composite restoration has expanded over the past decade, fragment reattachment is increasingly opted due to its minimal invasion, promising esthetics, and a natural form of restoration [5]. In the present case, there was Ellis class II fracture of maxillary left central

and lateral incisors. Tooth fragment for maxillary left central incisor was not available; hence, it was reconstructed with direct composite restoration. Maxillary left lateral incisor was managed with fragment reattachment using vertical groove technique followed by fiber post placement in the vertical groove thus offering higher esthetics and improved function.

2. Case Report

A 12-year-old boy reported to the Department of Pedodontics with fractured maxillary incisors due to sudden strike on the wooden bench. There was no history of loss of consciousness and vomiting. His parent brought intact tooth fragment in a water filled container. Clinical examination revealed fracture of maxillary left central and lateral incisors involving enamel and dentin with no pulp exposure (Figure 1). There was a lacerated labial gingiva in

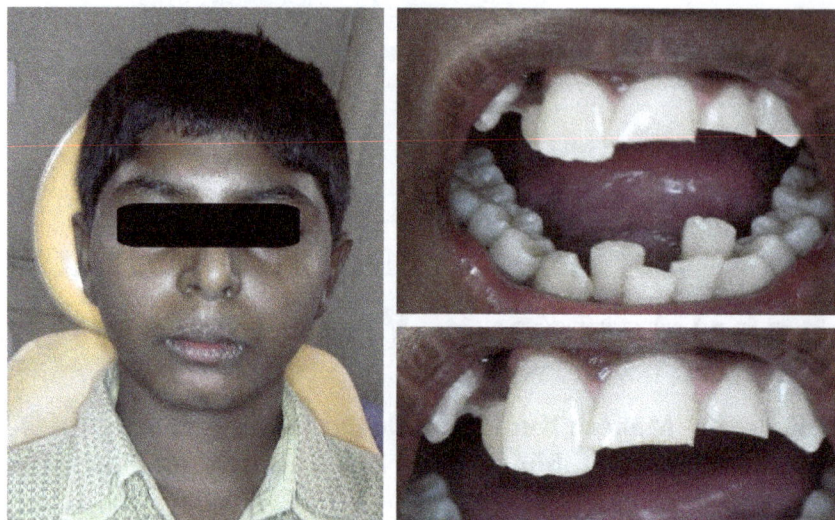

FIGURE 1: Preoperative view showing psychologically disturbed boy due to Ellis class II fractured teeth 21 and 22.

the mandibular incisors region. Periapical radiograph of maxillary left central and lateral incisors showed absence of alveolar fracture with intact roots and closed apices with no periapical pathology. Considering various treatment options available, reattachment of tooth fragment of maxillary left lateral incisor and direct composite restoration of maxillary left central incisor was planned. The chosen treatment was a less invasive technique which promotes an immediate repair of the esthetics and function of fractured tooth. Treatment was explained to parents, and an informed consent was taken.

Under strict asepsis condition, bilateral mental nerve block was administered using 2 percent lidocaine with 1 : 80000 adrenaline, and lacerated labial gingiva was sutured. Composite reconstruction of maxillary left central incisor was performed with total etch multilayered technique. The fractured component and tooth structure of maxillary left lateral incisor were cleaned and acid etched with 37% orthophosphoric acid gel for 20 seconds. After thorough rinsing and drying, adhesive was placed on both tooth fragment (Figure 2(a)) and tooth structure and air thinned and light cured for 10 seconds. Tooth fragment was reattached using low-viscosity flowable resin cement and light cured. After reattachment, two vertical grooves of depth and width 2 mm were placed along the fracture line on the labial surface using depth orientation bur (Figure 2 (b)). Fiber-reinforced composite posts (quartz no. 1) were cut of the same size and placed in the prepared grooves (Figure 2(c) and 2(d)). Posts were attached to tooth using resin cement and light cured. Excess composite material was removed, finished, and polished (Figure 3(a)). The patient was advised dietary, oral hygiene instructions and recalled after one week for the suture removal. One-year follow-up showed successfully retained fragment of maxillary left lateral incisor while composite restoration of maxillary left central incisor was dislodged; hence, reconstruction of dislodged composite restoration was done again. 2-year and 3-year follow-up showed successfully

retained fragment and composite restoration serving their function, and the patient was asymptomatic throughout the period (Figure 3(b)).

3. Discussion

Preservation of healthy tissue, longevity, esthetics, and function of restored tooth structure represented major objective of restorative dentistry [6]. Traumatized teeth with coronal fractures can be managed by various techniques such as resin crowns, ceramic crowns, orthodontic bands, and composite restoration with or without posts [7]. With the development of adhesive dentistry, reattachment of tooth fragment is considered as the best alternative for restoring coronal fractures in anterior teeth. Tooth fragment reattachment is far superior to direct composite restoration as enamel is maintained thus restoring natural color, contour of the fractured tooth, and it is considered as a viable treatment alternative. Conceição reported fragment reattachment as a simple, safer, and extremely conservative technique offering excellent esthetics and maintaining occlusal function [8]. Crucial aspects in the fragment reattachment technique are the location of the fracture, adaptation of the fragment to the remaining tooth structure, size of the fragment, and its hydration [9, 10]. In the present case, availability of tooth fragment with satisfactory surface area and size indicated fragment reattachment technique for maxillary left lateral incisor.

Various factors play a vital role in longevity and function of reattached fragment. These factors include storage media used for tooth fragment, material, and technique used for fragment reattachment. According to the recent literature, there is no effect on fracture strength when a different resin material was used. Many techniques are proposed for fragment reattachment which include simple reattachment, chamfering, over contour, and internal dentin groove. In simple reattachment technique, only bonding is done without any additional wearing of

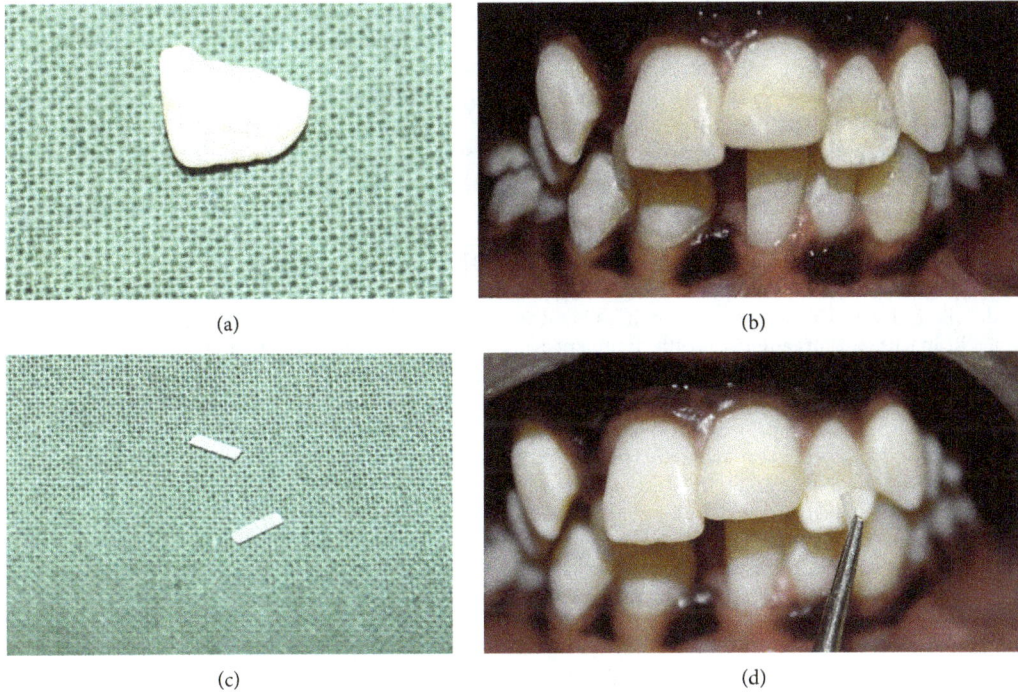

FIGURE 2: Intact tooth fragment of tooth 22 (a). Composite reconstruction of tooth 21 and fragment reattachment with vertical groove placement of tooth 22 (b). Fiber post sectioned and placed in prepared vertical grooves (c, d).

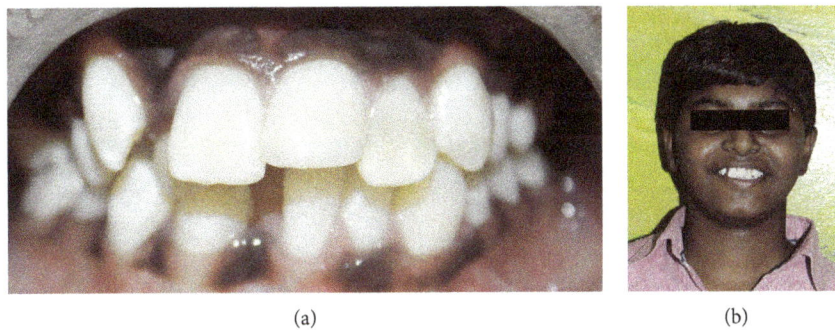

FIGURE 3: Immediate postoperative picture (a). 3-year follow-up picture showing intact tooth fragment (b).

tooth fragment or remaining tooth structure [11, 12]. External chamfer, over contour, and internal dentin groove techniques help in obtaining adequate function, retention, and esthetics.

In this case, vertical groove technique was used in which two vertical grooves were prepared along the fracture line creating space for fiber post placement thus increasing the fracture strength of retained tooth fragment. Low-viscosity resin was used for reattachment of tooth fragment to obtain minimum thickness along cementation line. Fiber post was used extracoronally as it was an uncomplicated crown fracture. Studies have reported that fragment reattachment is superior to direct composite restoration as higher fracture strength can be attained [13]. In the present case, over 1-year follow-up, there was dislodged composite restoration while tooth restored with fragment reattachment was intact and functional. Fragment reattachment should be attempted in priority in young children as it showed higher retention rate and better esthetics and boosts psychological confidence when compared to other treatment options [14].

4. Conclusion

Fragment reattachment is an esthetically acceptable and a conservative approach in the management of traumatic dental injuries. This procedure of vertical groove preparation and fiber post showed excellent stabilization even after a 3-year follow-up, and it was esthetically pleasing with no color change.

References

[1] J. Traebert, D. D. Bittencourt, K. G. Peres, M. A. Peres, J. T. de Lacerda, and W. Marcenes, "Aetiology and rates of treatment

of traumatic dental injuries among 12-year-old school children in a town in southern Brazil," *Dental Traumatology*, vol. 22, no. 4, pp. 173–178, 2006.

[2] E. B. Bastone, T. J. Freer, and J. R. McNamara, "Epidemiology of dental trauma: a review of literature," *Australian Dental Journal*, vol. 45, no. 1, pp. 2–9, 2000.

[3] K. P. Bharath, R. U. Patil, H. V. Kambalimath, and A. Alexander, "Autologous reattachment of complicated crown fractures using intra canal anchorage: report of two cases," *Journal of Indian Society of Pedodontics and Preventive Dentistry*, vol. 33, no. 2, pp. 147–151, 2015.

[4] G. V. Macedo, P. I. Diaz, C. A. De O Fernandes, and A. V. Ritter, "Reattachment of anterior teeth fragments: a conservative approach," *Journal of Esthetic and Restorative Dentistry*, vol. 20, no. 1, pp. 5–18, 2008.

[5] U. Iseri, Z. Ozkurt, and E. Kazazoglu, "Clinical management of a fractured anterior tooth with reattachment technique: a case report with an 8-year follow up," *Dental Traumatology*, vol. 27, no. 5, pp. 399–403, 2011.

[6] M. Szmidt, M. Górski, K. Barczak, and J. Buczkowska-Radlińska, "Direct resin composite restoration of maxillary central incisors with fractured tooth fragment reattachment: case report," *International Journal of Periodontics & Restorative Dentistry*, vol. 37, no. 2, pp. 249–253, 2017.

[7] R. B. Anchieta, E. P. Rocha, M. U. Watanabe et al., "Recovering the function and esthetics of fractured teeth using several restorative cosmetic approaches. Three clinical cases," *Dental Traumatology*, vol. 28, no. 2, pp. 166–172, 2012.

[8] E. N. Conceição, *Colagem de Fragmento Dental*, pp. 209–226, ArtMed, Yerevan, Armenia, 2000.

[9] A. Reis and A. D Loguercio, "Tooth fragment reattachment: current treatment concepts," *Practical Procedures and Aesthetic Dentistry*, vol. 16, no. 10, pp. 739–740, 2004.

[10] A. Rajput, I. Ataide, and M. Fernandes, "Uncomplicated crown fracture, complicated crown-root fracture, and horizontal root fracture simultaneously treated in a patient during emergency visit: a case report," *Oral Surgery, Oral Medicine, Oral Pathology, Oral Radiology, and Endodontology*, vol. 107, no. 2, pp. e48–e52, 2009.

[11] L. Venugopal, M. N. Lakshmi, D. A. Babu, and V. R. Kiran, "Comparative evaluation of impact strength of fragment bonded teeth and intact teeth: an in vitro study," *Journal of International Oral Health*, vol. 6, no. 3, pp. 73–76, 2014.

[12] V. K. Kulkarni, C. P. Bhusari, D. S. Sharma, P. Bhusari, A. V. Bansal, and J. Deshmukh, "Autogenous tooth fragment reattachment: a multidisciplinary management for complicated crown-root fracture with biologic width violation," *Journal of Indian Society of Pedodontics and Preventive Dentistry*, vol. 32, no. 2, pp. 190–194, 2014.

[13] V. L. Deepa, S. N. Reddy, V. C. Garapati, S. R. Sudhamashetty, and P. Yadla, "Fracture fragment reattachment using projectors and anatomic everStick post™: An ultraconservative approach," *Journal of International Society of Preventive and Community Dentistry*, vol. 7, no. 7, pp. 52–54, 2017.

[14] R. Arora, B. Shivakumar, H. Murali Rao, and R. Vijay, "Rehabilitation of complicated crown root fracture by fragment reattachment and intraradicular splinting: case reports," *Journal of International Oral Health*, vol. 5, no. 5, pp. 129–138, 2013.

17

Desmoplastic Fibroma Recurrence Associated with Tuberous Sclerosis in a Young Patient

A. M. Espinoza-Coronado,[1] **J. P. Loyola-Rodríguez ⓘ,**[2] **J. H. Olvera-Delgado,**[1]
J. O. García-Cortes ⓘ,[1] **and J. F. Reyes-Macías**[1]

[1]*Advanced Education in General Dentistry, Master Degree Program at San Luis Potosi University,*
 Faculty of Dentistry of San Luis Potosi, Universidad Autónoma de San Luis Potosí, San Luis Potosi, SLP, Mexico
[2]*Escuela Superior de Odontología y Doctorado en Ciencias Biomédicas, Universidad Autónoma de Guerrero, Acapulco, GRO, Mexico*

Correspondence should be addressed to J. O. García-Cortes; obedslp@hotmail.com

Academic Editor: Jose López-López

Case Report. A nine-year-old patient with a diagnosis of tuberous sclerosis (with no pathological record) that showed calcifications at the brain level. Besides, the case showed the Vogt triad (epilepsy, mental retardation, and sebaceous adenoma). The patient clinically showed a volume increase of hard consistency, without suppuration and no sessile that included the following teeth 73, 74, and 75. Cone beam computed tomography (CBCT) was obtained, and it displayed a delimited unilocular lesion. After surgical excision, the histopathological report was desmoplastic fibroma (DF). It was observed that the patient had an aggressive recurrence of DF at four months after surgery treatment. Due to these clinical findings, resective osseous surgery and curettage were carried out. It is uncommon to find these two pathologies together (DF and tuberous sclerosis). Since DF is a benign pathology but very invasive and destructive, it is necessary a constant follow-up examination due to a high recurrence frequency.

1. Introduction

Tuberous sclerosis (TS) is a rare disease described by Von Recklinghausen of neurocutaneous autosomal dominant origin, which is characterized by the development of benign tumors. This disease exhibits a triad known as the Vogt triad, the full triad that includes seizures, mental retardation, and cutaneous angiofibroma occuring in only 30% of reported cases. It is described by the presence of hamartomatous benign tumors, neurofibromas, and angiofibroma, which can be developed in the eyes, kidneys, heart, skin, brain, lungs, and progressive intracranial calcifications. There is a family history of the disease in 50% of all affected subjects, and the birth prevalence is as high as 1 in 6000 birth cases [1–3].

Oral manifestations of TS occur in 11% of affected subjects, and oral abnormalities include the presence of delayed eruption, bifid uvula, enamel hypoplasia, cystic hyperostosis, hyperplasia, enamel pitting, haemangioma, multiple osteomas, cleft lip and palate, and desmoplastic fibromas (DF) [2, 4]. The combination of desmoplastic fibroma and tuberous sclerosis is uncommon; there is little information about its clinical features. However, 84% of cases appear between the third and fourth decades of life, involving the mandible and maxillary area, having a predilection of 86% for the mandible and 14% in the maxilla. This tumor has a high percentage of relapse after surgical removal that usually occurs in 20%–40% of cases in which enucleation or excision of the fibroma occurs; while in cases with curettage, the relapse has a recurrence of 70%. Radiographically, a radiolucent area of a trabecular shape is seen, which is linked to soft tissue. The treatment is carried out using surgery, pharmacotherapy, or radiotherapy [5–10].

2. Case Presentation

A nine-year-old patient with tuberous sclerosis, who was diagnosed at five months of age, presented the Vogt triad (sebaceous adenomas, epilepsy, and mental retardation).

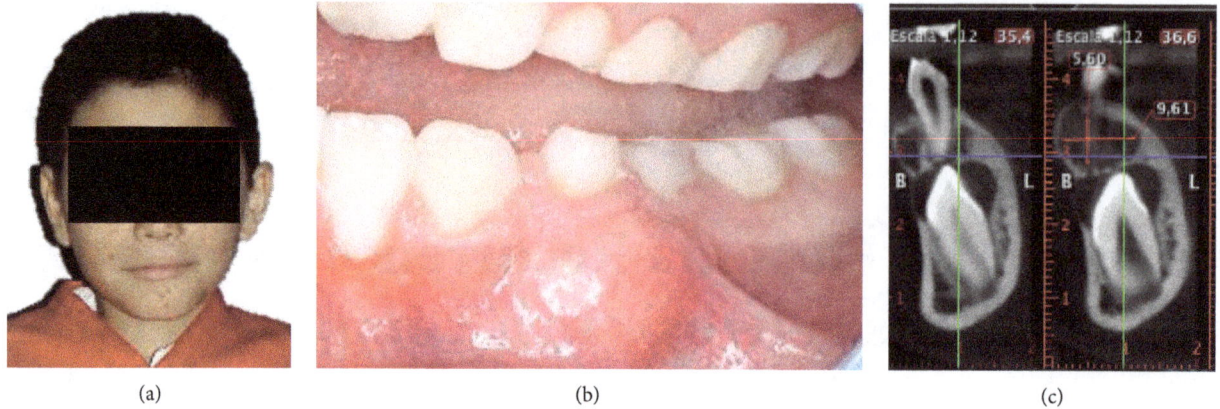

FIGURE 1: (a) Patient with sebaceous adenoma. (b) Oral examination revealed a facial asymmetry with a nonmovable mass about 8 mm in diameter 873 (74 and 75). (c) The tumor size is measured in the tomography, which is $5.6 \times 9.6 \times 8.3$ mm in the left mandible site.

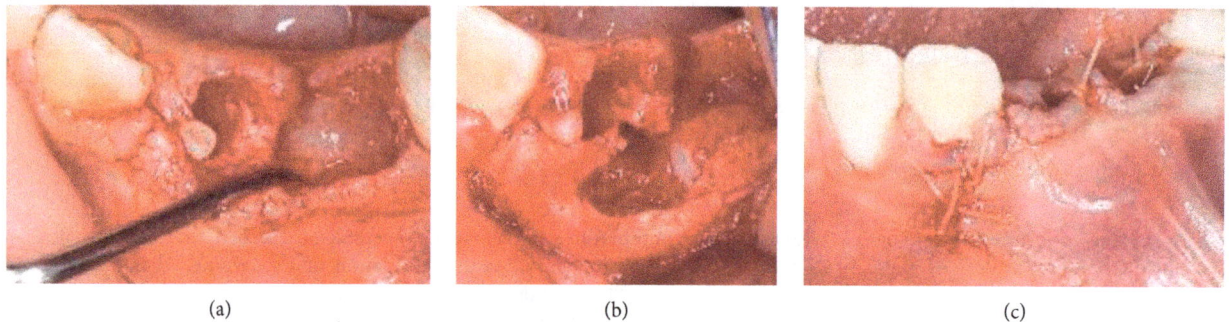

FIGURE 2: (a) The deciduous teeth 73 and 74 were removed. (b) A surgical enucleation was carried out. (c) The flap was repositioned and sutured with Vicryl 4-0.

There was not a family history of tuberous sclerosis, epilepsy, nor mental retardation. However, cone beam computed tomography (CBCT) showed multiple radioopacities throughout the brain, which were diagnosed by the neuropediatrician (Figure 1(a)).

In March (2016), the patient attended to the dental clinic at San Luis Potosi University, oral examination revealed a facial asymmetry, and this increase of volume has no movement with a measure of about 8 mm in diameter overlying the left mandible from the canine to the second molar of the primary dentition. In addition, the enamel of permanent anterior teeth showed pitting or irregularities. Radiographs (panoramic and periapical) and a cone beam computed tomography (CBCT, Software Planmeca Romexis Viewer, Finland) were taken. The tomography shows the presence of a lesion of approximately $5.6 \times 9.6 \times 8.3$ mm, and the cortical bone was covered with an incomplete fibrous capsule. Radiographic examination of the mandible revealed a large, round, radiolucent lesion with edges well circumscribed (Figures 1(b) and 1(c)). Therefore, it was decided to remove the lesion and perform a histopathological study.

3. Surgical Procedure

Before the clinical procedure, the caregivers received an informed consent form where ethical principles were taken into consideration based on the Declaration of Helsinki on Ethical Principles for Medical Research Involving Human Subjects (version 2013). After the acceptance of the treatment by their parents, asepsis with iodopovidone was performed in the patient in the intervention site; local infiltration of lidocaine containing 2% of epinephrine (Zeyco FD, Mexico) was carried out. Deciduous teeth 73 and 74 were removed, and then a full-thickness flap technique was performed; debridement and surgical enucleation of the lesion ($10 \times 15 \times 13$ mm) were carried out, ensuring that no fibrous tissue was left in the area. Subsequently, the flap was repositioned and sutured with Vicryl 4-0 (Ethicon, Polyglactin 910, USA). The biopsy was sent to the pathology department, and the following week, the patient attended to his follow-up appointment for stitches removal (Figures 2(a)–2(c)).

The histopathological showed a DF, constituted by a proliferation of connective tissue with the presence of fusiform fibroblasts deposited between dense hyalinized collagen bundles (Figure 3(a)). Once the diagnosis was established, the patient was referred for monthly follow-ups (clinical and radiographic evaluation) to assess the eruption of permanent teeth (33 and 34). Also, the patient was referred to the pediatric dentist for placement of a space maintainer.

In the clinical follow-ups, radiographically was observed that the first premolar (34) during the first three months, and there was no visible lesion (Figure 3(b)). However, in fourth-month

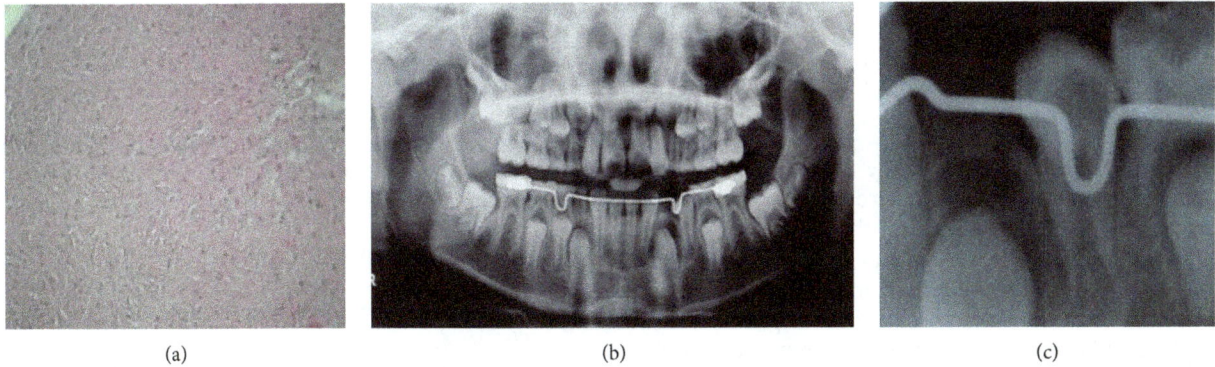

FIGURE 3: (a) The histopathological result was desmoplastic fibroma, which was constituted by a proliferation of connective tissue with the presence of fusiform fibroblasts. (b) Radiographic control after first surgery. (c) At the fourth month follow-up, it was observed in the radiograph a radiolucent area apically around the left mandibular canine (33).

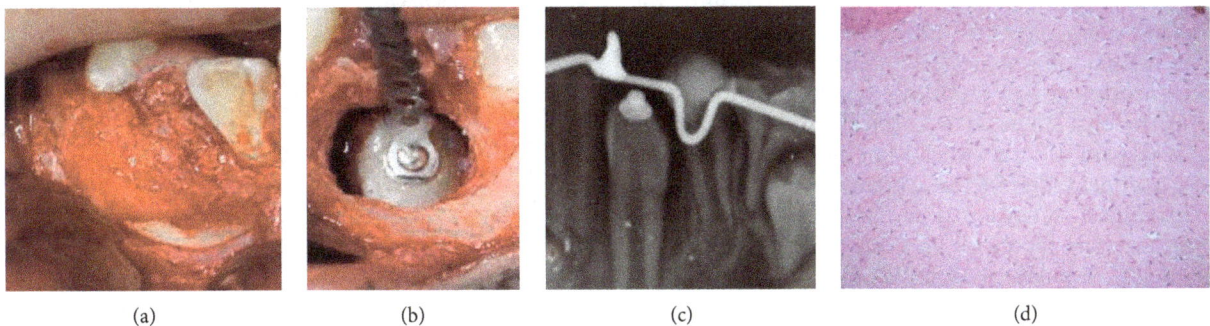

FIGURE 4: (a) At the fourth month, a surgical excision was performed, and the lesion was observed delimited and adhered to adjacent tissues. (b) The lesion was removed, and an osteotomy was performed. (c) A button was placed on the left mandibular canine, and a close orthodontic chain without traction was placed. (d) Histopathological result of 4 months of desmoplastic fibroma relapse.

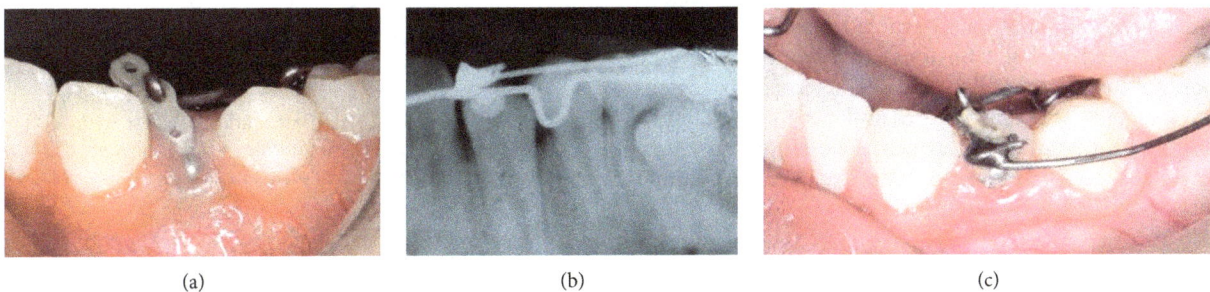

FIGURE 5: (a) Two months after the last surgery. (b) The eruption of canine. (c) Five months follow-up.

control appointment, the presence of tissue adjacent to the erupting teeth was observed radiographically, as well as an asymmetry in the left mandible, so a second intervention was decided (Figure 3(c)). An asepsis technique was performed with iodopovidone and infiltration with lidocaine 2% with epinephrine (Zeyco FD, Mexico). A full-thickness flap technique was made for accessing to the lesion by the vestibular site, especially to have a clean access for the left-lower permanent canine. During the surgery procedure, multiple fragments of both soft and hard tissues were removed; the fragments were sent to the pathology department with a diagnosis of a presumption of recurrent desmoplastic fibroma.

An osseous resective surgery with safe margins and curettage of the surgical site was performed with a subsequent use of the orthodontic button onto the left mandible canine. It was placed a closed chain without traction (Figure 4(a)). Finally, the flap was repositioned by using Vicryl Suture 4-0 (Ethicon, Polyglactin 910, USA), leaving the orthodontic chain free (Figure 4(b)). Eight days later, the patient had an appointment for suture removal and then referred to his pediatric dentist for the space maintainer placement. The Department of Oral Pathology reported the presence of desmoplastic fibroma recurrence with bundles of spindle-shaped, fibroblast-like cells in a collagen matrix

(Figure 5(a)). The canine was erupted after 5 months (Figures 5(b) and 5(c)).

4. Discussion

There is little information about the combination of desmoplastic fibroma and tuberous sclerosis; this combination is uncommon [8, 10, 11]. Likewise, there are no epidemiologic studies due to its low frequency, and the features are not well-known. In the world, there are few cases reported; however, some authors described a higher prevalence of desmoplastic fibroma in the mandible compared to the maxilla, as occurred in this case report [8, 12, 13].

It has been observed radiographically that relapsing lesions are unilocular or multilocular; the patient showed a unilocular radiolucent area at four months of the first surgery, coronal to the erupting dental organ 33 [5, 11]. DF is a collagenous lesion that lacks odontogenic epithelium; for maxillofacial surgeons, this information is crucial since a wider margin of resection is required when provided definitive treatment and probably it could be the cause of relapsing lesions. There is a controversy related to the presence of pain; the patient did not show pain prior the surgical treatment, despite the aggressive growth of the lesion. This clinical finding is in accordance with other reports; however, there are reports of pain due to the growth of the lesion [8, 14]. The removed DF showed lower size than previous reports, where the lesions had variable sizes of 2 to 7 cm [7, 14, 15].

Establishing a diagnosis of DF is difficult by imaging studies alone, since many tumors resemble DF. The differential diagnosis includes a wide range of lesion from benign lesions (fibrous dysplasia, bone cysts ossifying fibroma, and eosinophilic granuloma) to malignant lesions (osteosarcoma). In addition, DF includes pathologies from soft tissues (desmoplastic fibroma) to bone tissues (bone desmoid tumor). Besides, due to its high recurrence, osseus resective surgery with safe margins and curettage should be considered as the optimal treatment. The follow-up examination is an important issue to detect recurrence; it should be done monthly for the first year.

5. Conclusion

In the present case report, it was observed that the patient had an aggressive recurrence of DF at four months after the first surgical resection; it was necessary a second surgery that included safe margins and curettage. However, most reported cases did not mention the relapse time, just a high rate of recurrence. Besides, it is uncommon to find these two pathologies together (DF and tuberous sclerosis). Furthermore, it is necessary an excellent follow-up control due to a high recurrence frequency. The DF is benign pathology but is very invasive and destructive.

References

[1] R. Radhakrishnan and S. Verma, "Clinically relevant imaging in tuberous sclerosis," *Journal of Clinical Imaging Science*, vol. 1, no. 1, p. 39, 2011.

[2] S. Sodhi, R. S. Dang, and G. Brar, "Tuberous sclerosis with oral manifestations : a rare case report," *International Journal of Applied and Basic Medical Research*, vol. 6, no. 1, pp. 60–63, 2016.

[3] F. E. Jansen, O. van Nieuwenhuizen, and A. C. van Huffelen, "Tuberous sclerosis complex and its founders," *Journal of Neurology, Neurosurgery and Psychiatry*, vol. 75, no. 5, p. 770, 2004.

[4] S. U. Mbibi, S. L. Segelnick, and M. A. Weinberg, "Epithelial and fibrous hyperplasia : an oral manifestation of tuberous sclerosis complex. A case study," *New York State Dental Journal*, vol. 81, no. 5, pp. 37–41, 2015.

[5] A. M. Taylor, "Fibroma desmoplásico, reporte de un caso y revisión de la literatura," *Revista Española de Cirugía Oral y Maxilofacial*, vol. 32, no. 1, pp. 21–24, 2010.

[6] M. Schneider, A. C. Zimmermann, R. A. Depprich et al., "Desmoplastic fibroma of the mandible–review of the literature and presentation of a rare case," *Head and Face Medicine*, vol. 5, no. 1, p. 25, 2009.

[7] S. Tandon and R. K. Garg, "Intraoral desmoplastic fibroma : a manifestation," *Fetal and Pediatric Pathology*, vol. 31, no. 4, pp. 195–201, 2012.

[8] R. Vargas-gonzalez, W. S. Martin-Brieke, C. Gil-Orduna, and F. Lara-hernandez, "Desmoplastic fibroma-like tumor of maxillofacial region associated with tuberous sclerosis," *Pathology and Oncology Research*, vol. 10, no. 4, pp. 237–239, 2004.

[9] A. Ferri, M. Leporati, D. Corradi, T. Ferri, and E. Sesenna, "Huge desmoplastic fibroma of the paediatric mandible: surgical considerations and follow-up in three cases," *Journal of Cranio-Maxillofacial Surgery*, vol. 41, no. 5, pp. 367–370, 2013.

[10] T. R. Woods, D. M. Cohen, M. N. Islam, Y. Rawal, and I. Bhattacharyya, "Desmoplastic fibroma of the mandible : a series of three cases and review of literature," *Head and Neck Pathology*, vol. 9, no. 2, pp. 196–204, 2015.

[11] H. V. Talla, R. K. Alaparthi, and S. Yelamanchili, "Desmoplastic fibroma of the mandible : a rare case report," *Journal of Indian Academy of Oral Medicine and Radiology*, vol. 26, no. 2, pp. 222–224, 2014.

[12] N. J. Cross, M. Rcps, and D. E. Fung, "Tuberous sclerosis : a case report," *Special Care in Dentistry*, vol. 30, no. 4, pp. 157–159, 2010.

[13] S. Nithya, S. Sundaravel, D. Uppala, and K. Rao, "Desmoplastic fibroma-a rare case report," *Journal of Oral and Maxillofacial Pathology*, vol. 19, no. 2, p. 270, 2015.

[14] Y. Miyamoto, K. Satomura, K. Rikimaru, and Y. Hayashi, "Desmoplastic fibroma of the mandible associated with tuberous sclerosis," *Journal of Oral Pathology and Medicine*, vol. 24, no. 2, pp. 93–96, 1995.

[15] M. A. Feria and A. C. Carranza, "Desmoplastic fibroma of the jaw associated with tuberous sclerosis," *Revista Española de Cirugía Oral y Maxilofacial*, vol. 2, pp. 107–114, 2008.

18

A Combined Approach for the Aesthetic Management of Stained Enamel Opacities: External Bleaching Followed by Resin Infiltration

O. Marouane ⓘⅅ, N. Douki, and F. Chtioui

Restorative Dentistry, Dental Surgery Department, Sahloul University Hospital, Sousse, Tunisia

Correspondence should be addressed to O. Marouane; marouane.omar@yahoo.com

Academic Editor: Muawia A. Qudeimat

Stained enamel opacities are frequently encountered in dental practice. However, due to the risk of unaesthetic outcome, managing such lesions by resin infiltration techniques alone is not advised. Therefore, performing external bleaching before resin infiltration procedure is mandatory to eliminate stains from the hypomineralized lesions in order to aesthetically infiltrate them. In this work, we describe clinical cases in which external bleaching and resin infiltration techniques were used for managing stained enamel hypomineralized lesions related to traumatic dental injuries and molar incisor hypomineralization. Despite the fact that this approach has some limitations, it could be concluded that external bleaching associated with the resin infiltration technique shows promising results to aesthetically manage stained enamel opacities when the stain is totally removed after bleaching.

1. Introduction

Stained enamel opacities (SEO) are frequently observed in our dental practice. They can be defined as aberrations of the quality of dental enamel which ranges clinically from yellow to brown due to its pigmentation while it appears to be histologically hypomineralized. SEO differs from unstained enamel opacities as they show a bright opaqueness in the absence of pigments in the hypomineralized enamel [1, 2].

The underlying aetiologies are multiple, but the categories are mainly twofold: posteruptive and preeruptive damages. A preeruptive damage is a consequence of a dysfunction in the enamel organ due to a variety of agents and leading to various pathological conditions such as fluorosis, traumatic hypomineralisation, and molar-incisor hypomineralization (MIH) [3–5]. Posteruptive damage of the enamel is, however, a result of the early manifestation of the carious process leading to lesion called brown spot [6, 7].

From an aesthetic point of view, treating SEO conservatively using the resin infiltration procedure is very complex. Indeed, it has been shown that performing resin infiltration on SEO is not effective. It induces a stain reemergence with

an unpleasant aesthetic outcome [2]. For this reason, aesthetic management of SEO using resin infiltration technique alone is avoided and more invasive treatment options such as composite restorations, veneers, or crowns are used to correct the aesthetic defect [7–9]. Biologically, resin infiltration technique is a therapeutic of choice to aesthetically manage SEO. Indeed, resin infiltration allows to correct the aesthetic defect in a microinvasive way with improving the mechanical properties of such lesions [5, 7, 10, 11].

To date, there are only few papers reporting the aesthetic management of SEO using the resin infiltration technique.

In the aim of improving the aesthetic appearance of three patients, we describe in this paper the aesthetic management of cases presenting SEO using external bleaching followed by resin infiltration.

2. Case Report

Three patients between 12 and 23 years of age, with SEO located in their maxillary incisors, were referred to the Dental Medicine Department at Sahloul University Hospital, Sousse, Tunisia. All patients reported the discomfort caused by the

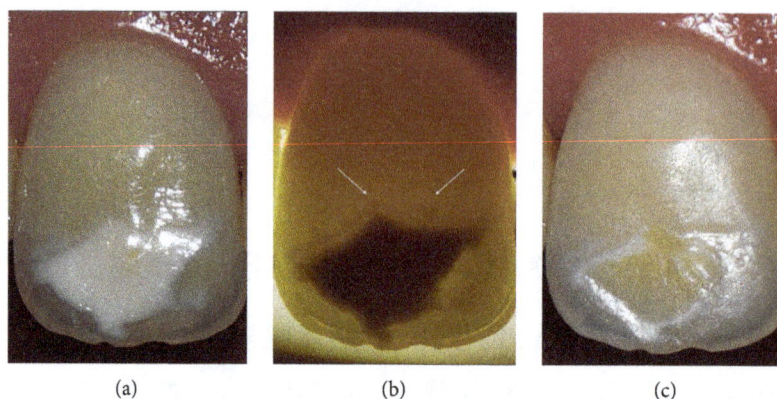

(a)   (b)   (c)

FIGURE 1: Stained enamel opacity related to traumatic dental injuries (a). The underestimation of the presence of stain into the lesion have led to unaesthetic outcomes after performing resin infiltration (c). Note the presence of enamel cracks (white arrow), observed under transillumination, which could constitute a possible pathway for chromatogenic substances (b). This case is considered a failure.

presence of opacities on their anterior teeth as they affected their self-esteem and social lives.

Meticulous clinical examination helped us to properly set the aetiology for each lesion. In the first case, SEO related to traumatic dental injury (TDI) (Figure 1(a)), and in the remaining cases, SEO related to molar incisor hypomineralization (MIH) (Figures 2(a) and 3(a)).

In order to aesthetically manage these SEO, the treatment consisted on external bleaching followed by resin infiltration. The idea behind this approach is to, first of all, remove the stain then perform resin infiltration. However, for the first patient (Figure 1(a)), due to the lack of evidence of staining, solely, resin infiltration procedure was adopted.

After obtaining a full written consent, each patient received an external bleaching procedure which was performed as follows:

(i) The second patient applied in-office bleaching gel (38% H_2O_2 Opalescence Xtra Boost; Ultradent) according to the manufacturer's instructions for 15 min selectively on the stained enamel opacity on a single session (Figure 2(b)).

(ii) The third patient was instructed to use a whitening gel which contained 10% carbamide peroxide 10% (Philips Zoom NiteWhite, Discus Dental, Stamford, USA) (Figures 3(b) and 3(c)) delivered via a custom-fitting mouth tray for 21 nights.

Two weeks after completing the whitening treatment, resin infiltration procedure was performed. The surface layer was etched at first by applying of a 15% hydrochloric acid gel (Icon-etch) for 120 seconds followed by a water rinse for 30 seconds.

Then, the lesion was dried out with ethanol solution for 30 seconds (Icon-dry). After this step, the resin (Icon-infiltrant) was applied gently in a circular motion for 3 minutes then light-cured for 40 seconds. Finally, the excess was removed and the enamel surface was polished.

Except for the first patient, where the infiltration technique produced unsatisfactory and unaesthetic results, a considerable esthetic improvement was achieved in the other cases.

3. Discussion

As presented in these cases, enamel opacities may be discoloured with an appearance ranging from stain hardly distinguishable (Figure 1(a)) to yellow (Figure 2(a)) or brown (Figure 3(a)).

The histological structure of MIH or enamel opacity related to TDI has been described in the literature in a number of papers. On a microscopic scale, these lesions exhibit disorganised enamel prisms, separated with gaps containing a protein-rich matrix [1, 12–14]. Moreover, these lesions present a lower hardness and higher porosity than sound enamel [15, 16]. This histological structure implicates their weak mechanical properties and explains why these lesions often crack (Figure 1(b)) [14–16].

As presented, in the first case (Figures 1(a)–1(c)), performing resin infiltration on SEO must be avoided. In fact, the infiltration itself is probably not altered, but since the colour masking effect is related to the refractive index of the low viscosity resin, it has no effect on the brownish staining that still remained at the end of the treatment. Therefore, even if the stain is hardly distinguishable or questionable, it may reemerge following the infiltration procedure leading to an unaesthetic outcome [2].

The latter however once observed at the first patient cannot be attributed solely to the discolouring agents trapped within the enamel. In fact, the camphorquinone (CQ) used as a photoinitiator in the resin presents a yellowish colour. Yet during light curing, the CQ loses this colour as it infiltrates the lesion. In case of incomplete consumption of CQ, the resin may remain yellowish which may indicate the presence of unconsumed CQ [17, 18].

As illustrated in the second and third cases, removing stains from enamel opacities using external bleaching provides an essential pretreatment step to aesthetically manage SEO before proceeding with the resin infiltration. The aim of the bleaching procedure is to remove the stains within and acquire the desired esthetic outcome. Despite the fact that no differences in treatment efficacy were detected between at-home bleaching and in-office bleaching, other considerations must be, yet, taken before choosing one or the other [19].

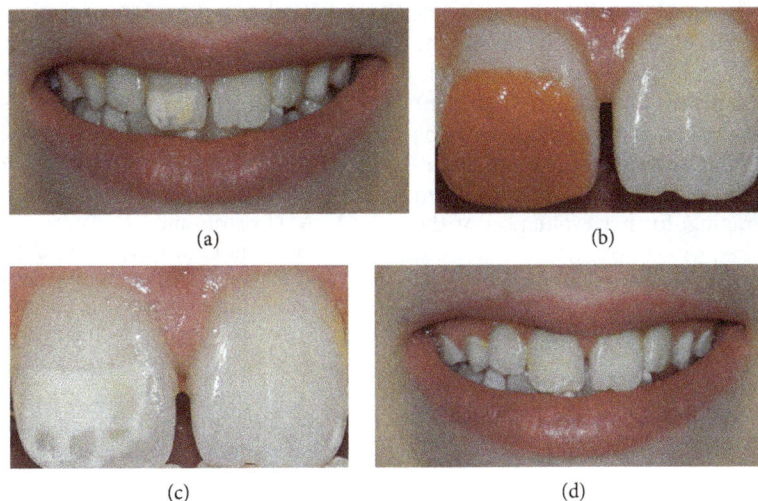

FIGURE 2: Yellowish lesion related to molar incisor hypomineralization (a). The combination of in-office bleaching (38% H_2O_2) (b) applied on a single visit for 15 min (c) and resin infiltration procedure were sufficient to end up with an esthetically satisfying result. By the end of the infiltration step, the incisal part of the lesion was not completely infiltrated probably due to excessive depth of the lesion at this area (d).

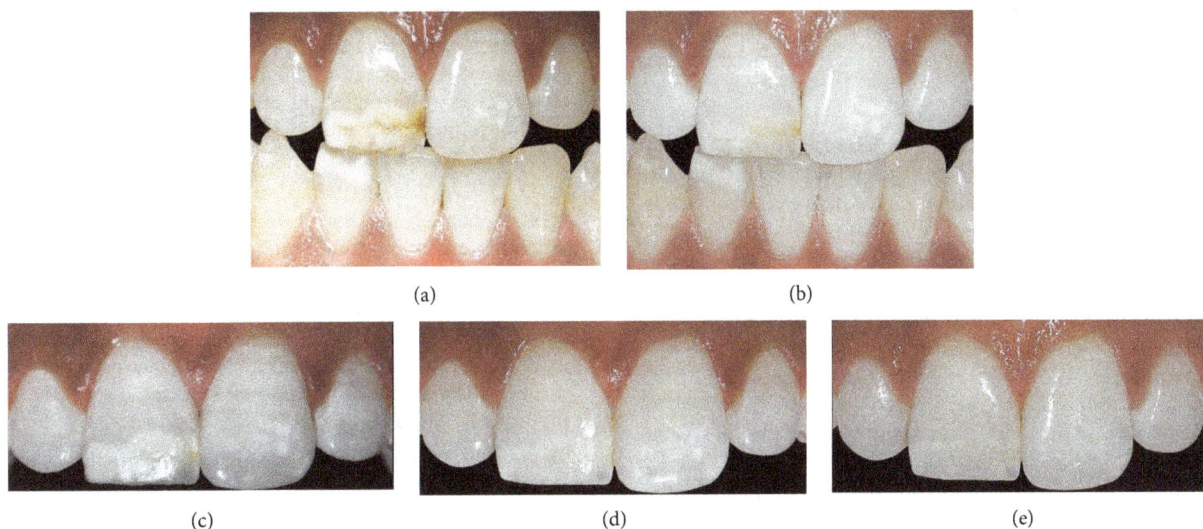

FIGURE 3: Brownish lesion related to molar incisor hypomineralization (a). After one week of at-home whitening using 10% carbamide peroxide gel (b), the stain was partially removed and has disappeared completely by the end of the bleaching treatment (c). Immediate result after performing resin infiltration (d). 3 months after treatment (e). Significant improvement in the aesthetic appearance of this patient's teeth was achieved, and the case was thus considered to be a success.

In the second case, we performed a focal in-office bleaching for several reasons: firstly, due to the young age of the patient and, secondly, due to the mild colouration (yellow) of the opacity in association with correct brightness of the remaining teeth (Figures 2(a) and 2(b)) [20].

Otherwise, as was performed on the third patient, at-home whitening treatment containing 10% carbamide peroxide may also be effective to completely remove stains from the enamel opacity.

In addition to masking enamel opacities, resin infiltration technique also produces a positive side effect. It genuinely leads to an increase in the enamel surface hardness reinforcing its weakened histological structure that was additionally affected by the external bleaching [21].

After performing external bleaching, the adhesion of resin to the enamel becomes compromised for up to 14 days, and so a two- to three-week waiting period is necessary. Moreover, it was recently demonstrated that performing resin infiltration, directly after a bleaching procedure, affects negatively the penetration depth of the infiltrant [21].

4. Conclusion

To aesthetically manage stained enamel opacities, the stain must be totally removed by performing an external bleaching. Once the latter is successfully achieved, resin infiltration technique may subsequently allow a significant improvement in the appearance of teeth in a relatively short working time.

Although the results in the cases described in this work showed a partial disappearance of the stained lesions, the treatment outcome may be, all in all, considered successful.

However, the suggested treatment protocol might present some limitations. A correct inspection of these lesions remains essential to make a proper diagnosis and to propose a correct treatment plan. Although the final results flowing from the present cases are encouraging, further evaluation of the proposed procedure is required.

Acknowledgments

The authors acknowledge the Research Laboratory of Oral Health and Orofacial Rehabilitation, LR12 ES11, Faculty of Dental Medicine, Monastir University, Tunisia.

References

[1] M. Denis, A. Atlan, E. Vennat, G. Tirlet, and J. P. Attal, "White defects on enamel: diagnosis and anatomopathology: two essential factors for proper treatment (part 1)," *International Orthodontics*, vol. 11, no. 2, pp. 139–165, 2013.

[2] J. P. Attal, A. Atlan, M. Denis, E. Vennat, and G. Tirlet, "White spots on enamel: treatment protocol by superficial or deep infiltration (part 2)," *International Orthodontics*, vol. 12, no. 1, pp. 1–31, 2014.

[3] A. Leppaniemi, P. L. Lukinmaa, and S. Alaluusua, "Nonfluoride hypomineralizations in the permanent first molars and their impact on the treatment need," *Caries Research*, vol. 35, no. 1, pp. 36–40, 2001.

[4] N. Chawla, L. B. Messer, and M. Silva, "Clinical studies on molar-incisor- hypomineralisation part 1: distribution and putative associations," *European Archives of Paediatric Dentistry*, vol. 9, no. 4, pp. 180–190, 2008.

[5] A. B. Borges, T. M. F. Caneppele, D. Masterson, and L. C. Maia, "Is resin infiltration an effective esthetic treatment for enamel development defects and white spot lesions? A systematic review," *Journal of Dentistry*, vol. 56, pp. 11–18, 2017.

[6] A. Watts and M. Addy, "Tooth discolouration and staining: tooth discolouration and staining: a review of the literature," *British Dental Journal*, vol. 190, no. 6, pp. 309–316, 2001.

[7] S. Paris and H. Meyer-Lueckel, "Masking of labial enamel white spot lesions by resin infiltration—a clinical report," *Quintessence International*, vol. 40, no. 9, pp. 713–718, 2009.

[8] L. D. Carvalho, J. K. Bernardon, G. Bruzi, M. A. C. Andrada, and L. C. C. Vieira, "Hypoplastic enamel treatment in permanent anterior teeth of a child," *Operative Dentistry*, vol. 38, no. 4, pp. 363–368, 2013.

[9] M. A. Muñoz, L. A. Arana-Gordillo, G. M. Gomes et al., "Alternative esthetic management of fluorosis and hypoplasia stains: blending effect obtained with resin infiltration techniques," *Journal of Esthetic and Restorative Dentistry*, vol. 25, no. 1, pp. 32–39, 2013.

[10] A. M. Kielbassa, I. Ulrich, L. Treven, and J. Mueller, "An updated review on the resin infiltration technique of incipient proximal enamel lesions," *Medicine in Evolution*, vol. 16, no. 4, pp. 3–15, 2010.

[11] S. Paris, F. Schwendicke, J. Keltsch, C. Dörfer, and H. Meyer-Lueckel, "Masking of white spot lesions by resin infiltration in vitro," *Journal of Dentistry*, vol. 41, pp. e28–e34, 2013.

[12] J. O. Andreasen, B. Sundström, and J. J. Ravn, "The effect of traumatic injuries to primary teeth on their permanent successors," *European Journal of Oral Sciences*, vol. 79, no. 3, pp. 219–284, 1971.

[13] A. Thylstrup and J. O. Andreasen, "The influence of traumatic intrusion of primary teeth on their permanent successors in monkeys a macroscopic, polarized light and scanning electron microscopic study," *Journal of Oral Pathology & Medicine*, vol. 6, no. 5, pp. 296–306, 1977.

[14] B. Jälevik and J. G. Norén, "Enamel hypomineralization of permanent first molars: a morphological study and survey of possible aetiological factors," *International Journal of Paediatric Dentistry*, vol. 10, no. 4, pp. 278–289, 2000.

[15] T. G. Fagrell, W. Dietz, B. Jälevik, and J. G. Norén, "Chemical, mechanical and morphological properties of hypomineralized enamel of permanent first molars," *Acta Odontologica Scandinavica*, vol. 68, no. 4, pp. 215–222, 2010.

[16] T. G. Fagrell, P. Salmon, L. Melin, and J. G. Norén, "Onset of molar incisor hypomineralization (MIH)," *Swedish Dental Journal*, vol. 37, no. 2, pp. 61–70, 2013.

[17] L. F. J. Schneider, L. M. Cavalcante, S. Consani, and J. L. Ferracane, "Effect of co-initiator ratio on the polymer properties of experimental resin composites formulated with camphorquinone and phenyl-propanedione," *Dental Materials*, vol. 25, no. 3, pp. 369–375, 2009.

[18] D. D. S. A. Maciel, A. B. Caires-Filho, M. Fernandez-Garcia, C. Anauate-Netto, and R. C. B. Alonso, "Effect of camphorquinone concentration in physical-mechanical properties of experimental flowable resin composites," *BioMed Research International*, vol. 2018, Article ID 7921247, 10 pages, 2018.

[19] J. L. De Geus, L. M. Wambier, S. Kossatz, A. D. Loguercio, and A. Reis, "At-home vs in-office bleaching: a systematic review and meta-analysis," *Operative Dentistry*, vol. 41, no. 4, pp. 341–356, 2016.

[20] H. H. Hamama, "FOCAL bleaching technique," *Journal of Cosmetic Dentistry*, vol. 29, no. 2, 2013.

[21] S. A. Horuztepe and M. Baseren, "Effect of resin infiltration on the color and microhardness of bleached white-spot lesions in bovine enamel (an in vitro study)," *Journal of Esthetic and Restorative Dentistry*, vol. 29, no. 5, pp. 378–385, 2017.

19

Successful Management of Teeth with Different Types of Endodontic-Periodontal Lesions

Hind Alquthami ⓘ,[1] Abdulaziz M. Almalik,[2] Faisal F. Alzahrani,[3] and Lana Badawi[4]

[1]*Department of Dentistry, Division of Endodontics, Prince Sultan Military Medical City, P.O. Box 7897, Riyadh 11159, Saudi Arabia*
[2]*Department of Dentistry, Division of Periodontics, Prince Sultan Military Medical City, Riyadh, Saudi Arabia*
[3]*Department of Dentistry, Division of Orthodontics, Prince Sultan Military Medical City, Riyadh, Saudi Arabia*
[4]*Department of Dentistry, Division of Endodontics, Prince Sultan Military Medical City, Riyadh, Saudi Arabia*

Correspondence should be addressed to Hind Alquthami; halqathami@pscc.med.sa

Academic Editor: Samir Nammour

Endodontic-periodontal diseases often present great challenges to the clinician in their diagnosis, management, and prognosis. Understanding the disease process through cause-and-effect relationships between the pulp and supporting periodontal tissues with the aid of rational classifications leads to successful treatment outcomes. In this report, we present several treatment modalities in patients with different endodontic-periodontal lesions. A modification to the new endodontic-periodontic classification, Al-Fouzan's classification, was also added. The first case was classified as retrograde periodontal disease (i.e., primary endodontic lesion with drainage through the periodontal ligament). The second case was diagnosed as an iatrogenic periodontal lesion caused by root perforation. The third case was diagnosed as an iatrogenic periodontal lesion caused by tooth trauma due to orthodontic treatment. The first two cases were managed with a nonsurgical approach, whereas the third case was managed with nonsurgical and surgical approaches. All patients showed complete healing of soft and hard tissue lesions. A thorough understanding of the disease history and the patient's signs and symptoms, complete examination with full investigation, and the use of a systematic step-by-step approach in the management of such challenging endodontic-periodontal lesions with regular recall visits were very useful and successful.

1. Introduction

An endodontic-periodontal lesion consists of concurrent pulpal and periodontal disease in the same tooth. The spread of infection between the dental pulp and the periodontal ligament can occur through the apical foramen, lateral canals, dentinal tubules, and palatogingival grooves. Moreover, nonanatomic factors can have a role in this communication such as iatrogenic root canal perforations or a vertical root fracture. These pathways cause the spread of infection and bone destruction in a coronal-to-apical direction in the case of periodontal infection or in an apical-to-coronal direction in the case of endodontic infection [1].

In 1964, Simring and Goldberg [2] were the first to describe the relationship between pulpal and periodontal disease and referred to it as an "endo-perio lesion." The most common classifications of endodontic-periodontal lesions were primary endodontic disease, primary periodontal disease, and combined disease, depending on the cause of the lesion [3]. In 2014, Al-Fouzan [4] suggested a new endodontic-periodontal interrelationship classification, based on the primary disease and its secondary effect. The classification is as follows.

(1) Retrograde periodontal disease

    (a) Primary endodontic lesion with drainage through the periodontal ligament

    (b) Primary endodontic lesion with secondary periodontal involvement

(2) Primary periodontal lesion

(3) Primary periodontal lesion with secondary endodontic involvement

(4) Combined endodontic-periodontal lesion

(5) Iatrogenic periodontal lesion

This rational classification increases the understanding of the disease process and its origin. This understanding is essential in determining the correct diagnosis and providing treatment with predictable success. The success rate of joined endodontic-periodontal lesions without a regenerative procedure is between 27% and 37% [5]. These rates are much lower than the success rate of 95% with conventional nonsurgical root canal therapy [6]. The use of barrier membranes and/or bone-grafting materials during treatment encourages the growth of surrounding lost tissues such as the periodontal ligament, bone cementum, and connective tissue while preventing unwanted cell types such as epithelial cells [7]. The aim of this paper was to present the diagnosis and management of different endodontic-periodontal disease conditions with or without the use of regenerative bone techniques.

2. Case Presentations

2.1. Case 1: Retrograde Periodontal Disease: A Primary Endodontic Lesion with Drainage through the Periodontal Ligament. A 55-year-old woman with a noncontributory medical history was referred to the endodontic specialist clinic at Prince Sultan Military Medical City (PSMMC; Riyadh, Saudi Arabia) complaining of intraoral sinus with pus drainage in the right mandibular molar area. Clinical and radiographic examinations revealed a large amalgam restoration with recurrent caries and periapical and furcal radiolucency related to tooth #46. There was localized swelling in the gingival sulcus and the sinus in the gingival area. Tooth mobility was grade II. A midbuccal area with a narrow periodontal pocket > 10 mm was noted. The tooth had a negative response to the thermal vitality test (Endo-Ice; Hygenic Corp., Akron, OH, USA). The diagnosis was a necrotic pulp and chronic apical abscess.

Endodontic treatment was accomplished in two visits with calcium hydroxide [Ca(OH)2] medication between appointments. Local anesthesia (1.8 mL of lidocaine with epinephrine 1 : 100,000) was administered, and the tooth was isolated with a rubber dam. An access opening was created and four canals were located. During the second visit, the localized swelling and sinus opening were thoroughly resolved, and the root canal treatment was completed with RaCe NiTi rotary files (FKG Dentaire, La Chaux-de-Fonds, Switzerland) and 5.25% sodium hypochlorite irrigation. The tooth was obturated with lateral condensation of guttapercha and AH Plus sealer (AH Plus; Dentsply Maillefer, Tulsa, OK, USA). No periodontal treatment was administered. Follow-up X-ray images were obtained from 1 year to 6 years, which showed complete healing of the bone in the periapical and furcation areas (Figure 1).

2.2. Case 2: Iatrogenic Periodontal Lesion: Root Perforation. A 30-year-old woman with a noncontributory medical history

was referred to the endodontic specialist clinic at PSMMC complaining of pain and localized intraoral swelling in the left first mandibular molar. One year earlier, the tooth had undergone root canal treatment with cementation of the post and core and placement of a permanent crown. The clinical examination revealed localized swelling in the gingival sulcus. Periodontal probing through the furcation showed increased probing values with a grade II defect [2] (Figure 2). The radiographic examination revealed a large post in the distal canal and a large furcal lesion related to the distal root opposite the post placement. Iatrogenic root perforation was suspected.

After the administration of local anesthesia (1.8 mL of lidocaine with 1 : 100,000 epinephrine), the crown was removed with a crown removal instrument, and the post was removed with an ultrasonic instrument using a light brush and cutting motion to break up the cement around the post. A paper point was used to check for the presence of blood spots to determine the location and size of the perforation. The perforation site was irrigated with 2.5% sodium hypochlorite followed by drying of the canal and sealing of the perforation with mineral trioxide aggregate (MTA; Dentsply Tulsa Dental) mixed with saline and placed with a microapical placement system (Dentsply Tulsa Dental) and condensed with a paper point (Figure 2). A wet cotton pellet was then placed on the MTA material. The tooth was temporized with glass-ionomer cement and cementation of the crown. At the second visit, the cotton pellet was removed and the MTA setting was checked.

The patient was referred to the prosthodontics department for permanent crown placement. Follow-up appointments at 3 months, 6 months, 9 months, and up to 4 years showed complete healing of the soft tissue and bone lesions and a normal pocket depth of 3 mm.

2.3. Case 3: Iatrogenic Periodontal Lesions: Dental Injury/ Trauma. A 27-year-old woman with a noncontributory medical history was referred from the orthodontic department at PSMMC complaining of pus discharge from the gingival sulcus and slight gingival swelling on the palatal side opposite tooth #22 (i.e., maxillary left lateral incisor) after orthodontic treatment. Clinical and radiographic examinations revealed a sound tooth #22 with a mobility of grade II and a deep periodontal pocket > 10 mm mesial to tooth #22 with pus discharge from the pocket (Figure 3(a)). The thermal vitality test demonstrated a negative response. Moreover, the area was tender to percussion and palpation. Methylene blue stain was applied to exclude the presence of a crack or root fracture. It showed a negative result. The radiographic examination showed advanced bone resorption extending from the mesial bone crest toward the apex of tooth #22 (Figure 3(b)).

The diagnosis was necrotic pulp due to trauma during orthodontic treatment with symptomatic apical periodontitis. The first stage of the treatment plan was endodontic treatment, which was performed during two visits with calcium hydroxide medication between appointments (Figure 3(b)). Chemicomechanical debridement was administered with the ProFile.04 and ProFile.06 Taper Series 29 rotary

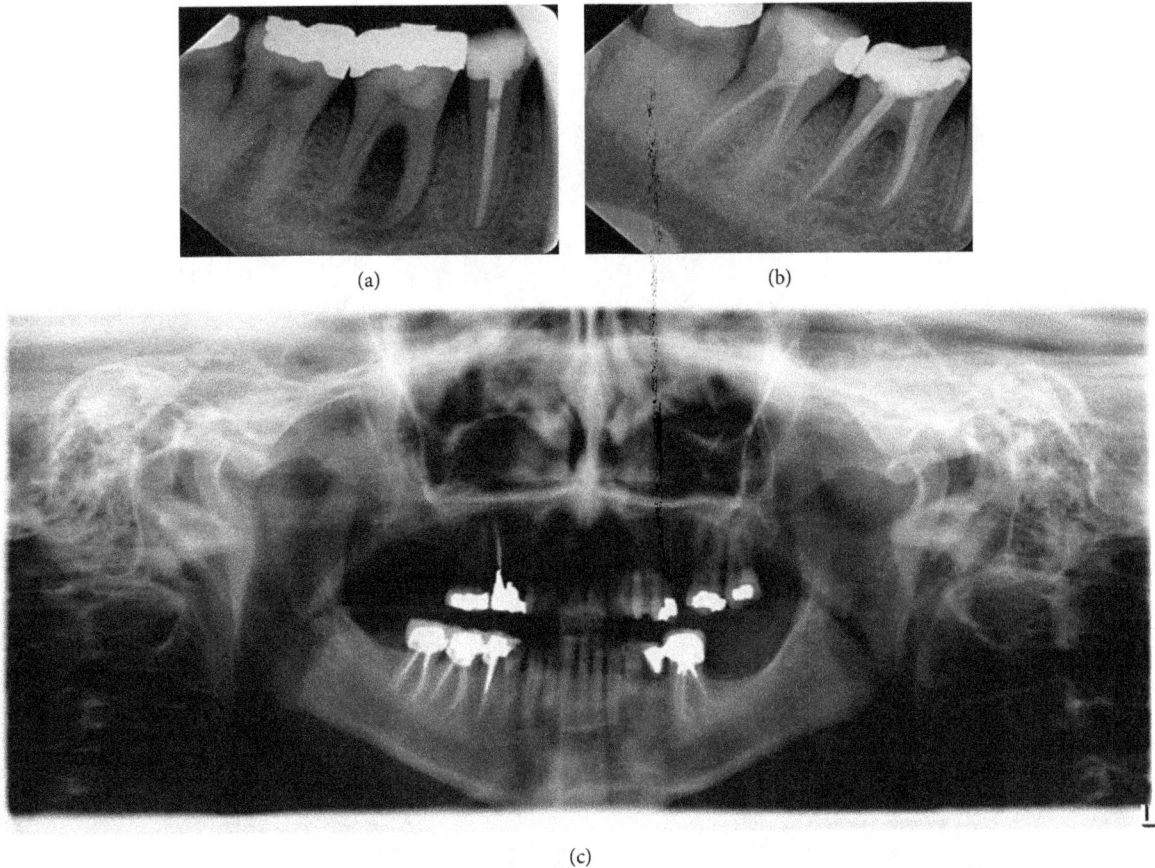

FIGURE 1: Case 1. (a) The initial radiograph of tooth #46 shows periapical and furcation bone resorption. (b) The 1-year recall radiograph shows healing of the bone lesion. (c) The 6-year follow-up radiograph shows tooth #46 with a permanent crown.

instruments (Tulsa Dental Products) and sodium hypochlorite. The canal was obturated with lateral condensation of gutta-percha and AH Plus sealer (Dentsply Maillefer, Tulsa, OK, USA) (Figure 3(b)). The second stage of the treatment plan, which was a surgical procedure, was performed after the permanent composite restoration and a follow-up period of 3 months. Before surgery, the patient signed a consent form.

Local anesthesia (two 1.8 mL carpules of 2% lidocaine with 1 : 100,000 epinephrine) was then administered labially and palatally. A mucoperiosteal flap was raised mesially to the upper left canine tooth, and two vertical releasing incisions were formed in the anterior palatal area opposite teeth #21 and #23. A horizontal incision was formed from the left maxillary central incisor to the left maxillary canine. After flap reflection, a sling suture was placed in the tissue flap to secure it with the premolar tooth on the opposite side of the maxillary arch to aid the surgeon in improving visual and operative access by eliminating the need to manually retract the flap in the palatal area (Figure 3(c)) [8]. Cortical bone was absent on the mesial side of tooth #22. The root surface was covered with black calculus and the area was obliterated with granulation tissues. After removing the granulation tissues and calculus from the root surface with ultrasonic tips (Figures 3(c) and 3(d)), bone graft material (Puros Particulate Allograft; Zimmer Biomet Dental) mixed

with saline was placed into the bony defect with a plastic instrument, and a resorbable barrier membrane (CopiOs membrane, Zimmer Biomet Dental) was placed above the bone graft. The flap was then repositioned and sutured with 4-0 Vicryl thread (Ethicon Inc., Somerville, NJ, USA). The patient was prescribed Augmentin (amoxicillin (875 mg) and clavulanic acid (125 mg)) (GlaxoSmithKline (Ireland) Ltd.) 1 g twice daily for 5 days and ibuprofen (600 mg) orally every 6 h for 2 days. Follow-up of the patient showed no tooth mobility, a reduced pocket depth of 4 mm, and healing of the soft and hard tissues (Figure 3(e)).

3. Discussion

The management of endodontic-periodontal lesions is a true challenge for the dentist because of the deleterious effects on the tooth structure and the supporting periapical structures (i.e., bone and periodontal membrane). The key to success in treating these cases depends on taking a correct history to determine the cause and reach an exact diagnosis of the case development. In addition, a clinician's ability to classify a lesion makes the treatment strategy or protocol very clear and precise. In this report, several successful endodontic-periodontal lesion cases were presented with different treatment modalities and classified according to the new classification system reported by Al-Fouzan in 2014 [4].

(a) Post removal

(b) Preoperative, postoperative, and 9-month recall

(c) Four-year recall

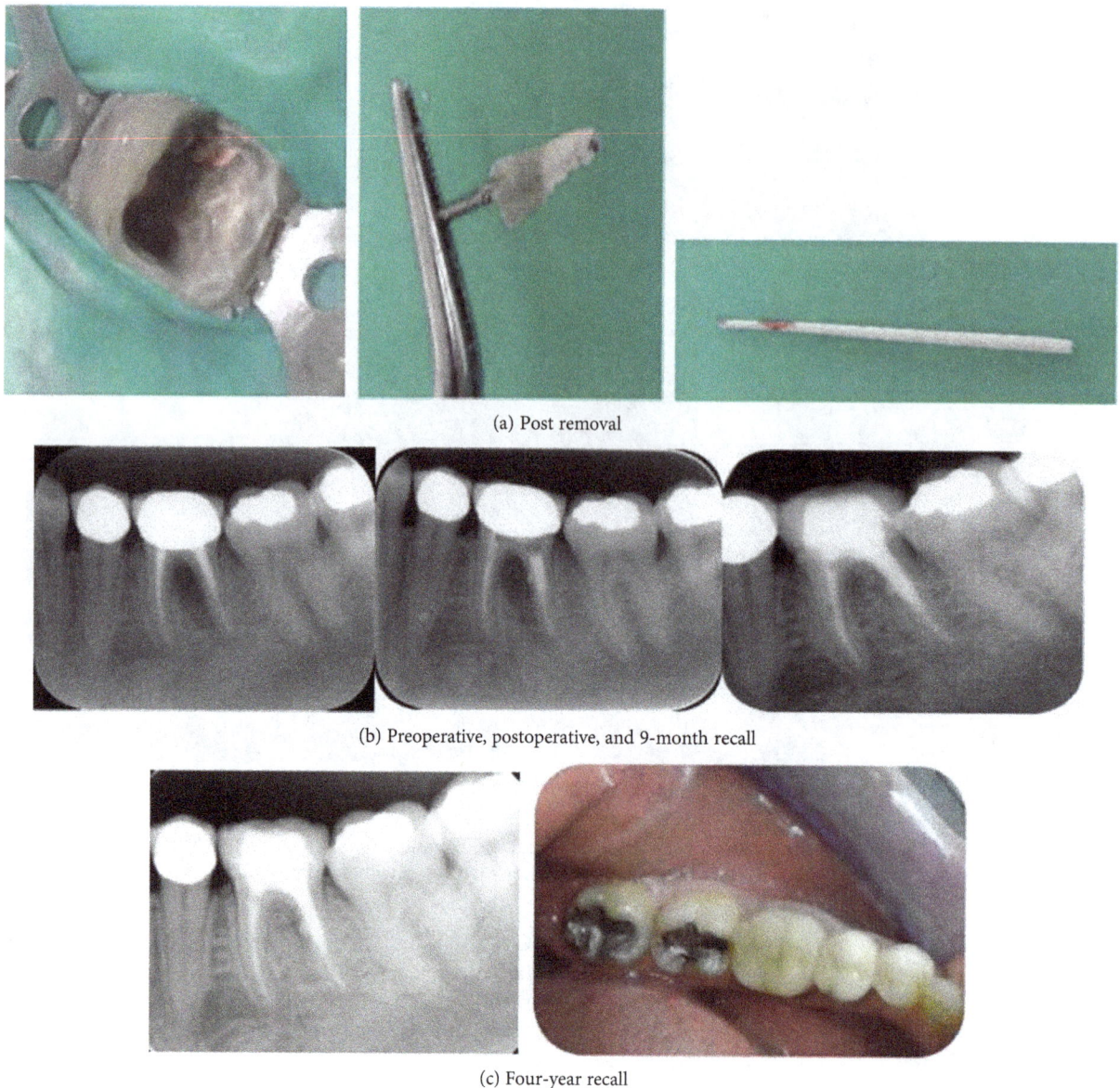

FIGURE 2: (a) Tooth #36 has a perforation in the distal root. The post is shown after removal, as is a paper point with a blood spot. (b) The mineral trioxide aggregate (MTA) repair. The recall examinations show osseous regeneration in the furcation. (c) The follow-up clinical photograph of tooth #36 shows the final crown and normal soft tissue.

The classification of the first case was a primary endodontic lesion with drainage through the periodontal ligament through a fistula. The pulp was necrotic and there was a deep and narrow pocket in one tooth aspect. All of these factors confirmed the diagnosis and led to the correct treatment modality, which was endodontic treatment alone. The other cases were diagnosed as iatrogenic periodontal lesions that resulted from the treatment modality: by tooth perforation (as shown in the second case) or by dental trauma caused by orthodontic treatment, which is not mentioned in the Al-Fouzan classification [4]. The authors of the current study suggest adding this category to Al-Fouzan's classification under "iatrogenic periodontal lesions" because trauma from orthodontic movement can cause pulp necrosis and thereby lead to periodontal disease and pocket formation.

Root perforation is an unnatural communication between the root canal system and the supporting tissues of the teeth or the oral cavity [9]. One study [10] reported that 53% of iatrogenic perforations occur during the insertion of posts. Factors that affect the perforation prognosis depend on the location of the perforation, its duration, size of the perforation and tooth, sterilization of the perforation site, and the material used to seal the perforation. Immediate sealing of small perforations away from the coronal attachment of the tooth under aseptic conditions with compatible materials are the most important factors for a good prognosis [11, 12].

Mineral trioxide aggregate is a bioceramic material, composed of tricalcium silicate, tricalcium aluminate, tricalcium oxide, and silicate oxide, that forms a colloidal

(a)

(b) (i) Preoperative image. (ii) Calcium hydroxide [Ca(OH)$_2$] placement.
(iii) Postoperative image. (iv) The 30-month recall image

(c)

(d)

(e)

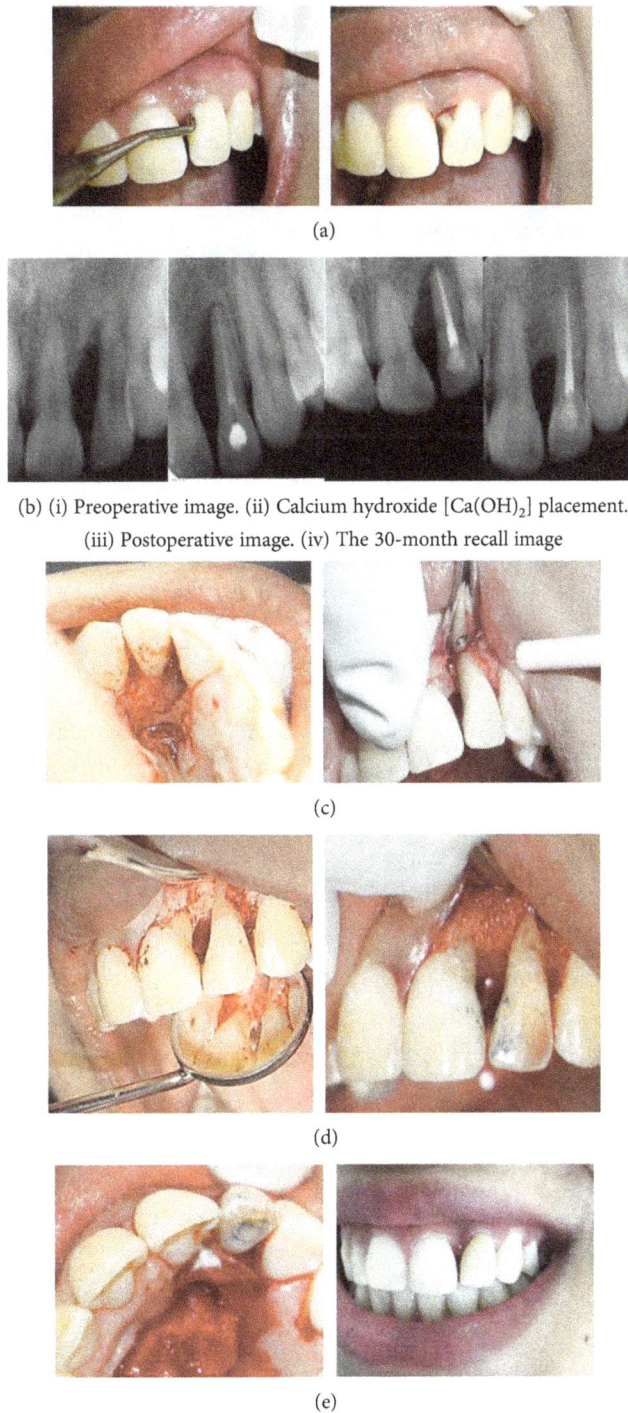

FIGURE 3: (a) A deep periodontal pocket and drainage of pus through the gingival sulcus are visible. (b) Radiographs of tooth #22 exhibit (i) a large lateral radiolucency on the mesial tooth surface extending from the bone crest to the root apex, (ii) calcium hydroxide [Ca(OH)2] placement, (iii) root canal obturation, and (iv) bone healing. (c) Surgical exposure of tooth #22 shows calculus accumulation and granulation tissue mesially with the absence of buccal bone. (d) Removal of calculus and granulation tissues and placement of the bone graft. (e) Placement of the barrier membrane; the 30-month recall photograph shows normal gingival tissue.

gel on hydration and solidifies in approximately 3 hours. The calcium oxide in MTA reacts with tissue fluids to form calcium hydroxide, which may then encourage hard tissue deposition because of its high pH. In addition, several studies [13–15] have demonstrated the sealing ability of MTA.

Dental pulp is a soft connective tissue encased in a rigid, noncompliant chamber; therefore, changes in pulpal blood flow or vascular tissue pressure can have serious effects on the health of the pulp. Many studies [16, 17] have explained the effects of orthodontic forces on teeth.

These forces influence blood flow and cellular metabolism and lead to degenerative and/or inflammatory responses in the dental pulp. Spector et al. [18] reported two cases in which teeth were devitalized during orthodontic therapy. Hamersky et al. [19] used a radiorespirometric method to demonstrate a significant depression in the pulpal respiratory rate when a tooth underwent orthodontic movement. In addition, as a person's age increased, the relative amount of pulpal respiratory rate depression increased. Moreover, orthodontic forces may induce more rapid aging processes within the pulp because of blood flow interruption, and thereby reduce the pulp's ability to withstand future forces [16]. Orthodontically treated teeth also show histologic findings similar to those of periodontally involved teeth.

In endodontic-periodontal lesions, the cause of the lesion is endodontic or periodontal in origin, and the patient may benefit from undergoing root canal therapy first [20, 21] because pulpal infection could promote marginal epithelial downgrowth along the root surfaces of the teeth [22]. Unhealed lesions with persistent infection were further managed through endodontic-periodontal surgery or through periodontal regenerative surgery alone. This sequence of treatment conveys a good chance for primary healing, a better assessment of the periodontal conditions of the involved teeth, and controls reinfection by bacteria or their by-products [20].

Regenerative techniques involve cell differentiation, cell proliferation and induction, and/or tissue formation conduction. All of these factors work together to complete the healing of damaged periapical tissues. This healing can be obtained by using bone grafts (e.g., autografts, allografts, alloplasts, and xenografts), periodontal membranes (e.g., nonabsorbable or absorbable of the natural or synthetic type), growth factors, or a combination of these [7, 23].

In the first two cases, soft and hard tissue healing commenced with administering root canal therapy alone or perforation repair. However, in the third case, follow-up for 3 months after completing the root canal revealed a persistent bone defect and periodontal pocket, which indicated the need for a further treatment modality to restore the health of the periodontal tissues.

Von Arx and Cochran [24], Dietrich et al. [25], and Kim and Kratchman [26] described various classifications of periradicular lesions to ensure the best treatment modalities for such lesions. The last classification was reported by Von Arx and AlSaeed in 2011 [27] and is based on the type of periradicular lesion. Their classification was as follows: (i) the lesion is limited to the periapical area; (ii) the lesion erodes the lingual/palatal cortex (with or without erosion of the buccal cortex) and has caused a through-and-through (i.e., tunnel) defect; and (iii) the apicomarginal lesion has complete denudation of the buccal root surface. Investigators in clinical and experimental studies have concluded that only tunnel and apicomarginal defects could benefit from a regenerative treatment protocol [28, 29]. In the third case, there was an absence of buccal bone at tooth #22 after surgical exposure. Thus, the labial root surface was exposed to the root apex. The root surface was covered with calculus and granulation tissues. The calculus and granulation tissues were removed with ultrasonic scaling, followed by placing a bone graft and barrier membrane, which led to complete healing. Some studies have reported considerable success rates in managing such apicomarginal defects [26, 30, 31].

Controversial findings challenge the current understanding of the ideal interval between endodontic treatment and periodontal surgery. It has been reported that root canal treatment performed 10 weeks, 3 months, or 6 months before periodontal surgery did not impair periodontal healing [32–34]. In the third case, root canal treatment was performed 3-4 months before the periodontal surgery and showed no disruptive effect on complete bone healing. In conclusion, all cases presented in this report were successfully treated and showed great promise in managing endodontic-periodontal lesions, which are a very challenging disease condition that requires all possible treatment modalities reported in the literature such as endodontic therapy, periodontal therapy, and regenerative procedures to ensure satisfactory and complete healing. In this paper, we have added a modification to the latest endodontic-periodontal classification and highlighted the importance of using a step-by-step systematic approach for managing such complex lesions.

Acknowledgments

The authors would like to thank Editage (http://www.editage.com/) for English language editing.

References

[1] M. Zehnder, S. I. Gold, and G. Hasselgren, "Pathologic interactions in pulpal and periodontal tissues," *Journal of Clinical Periodontology*, vol. 29, no. 8, pp. 663–671, 2002.

[2] M. Simring and M. Goldberg, "The pulpal pocket approach: retrograde periodontitis," *Journal of Periodontology*, vol. 35, no. 1, pp. 22–48, 1964.

[3] J. H. S. Simon, D. H. Glick, and A. L. Frank, "The relationship of endodontic–periodontic lesions," *Journal of Endodontics*, vol. 39, no. 5, pp. e41–e46, 2013.

[4] K. S. Al-Fouzan, "A new classification of endodontic-periodontal lesions," *International Journal of Dentistry*, vol. 2014, Article ID 919173, 5 pages, 2014.

[5] J. M. Hirsch, U. Ahlstrom, P. A. Henrikson, G. Heyden, and L. E. Peterson, "Periapical surgery," *International Journal of Oral Surgery*, vol. 8, no. 3, pp. 173–185, 1979.

[6] N. Imura, E. T. Pinheiro, B. P. F. A. Gomes, A. A. Zaia, C. C. R. Ferraz, and F. J. Souza-Filho, "The outcome of endodontic treatment: a retrospective study of 2000 cases performed by a specialist," *Journal of Endodontics*, vol. 33, no. 11, pp. 1278–1282, 2007.

[7] J. D. Bashutski and H. L. Wang, "Periodontal and endodontic regeneration," *Journal of Endodontics*, vol. 35, no. 3, pp. 321–328, 2009.

[8] D. E. Arens, M. Torabinejad, N. Chivian, and R. Rubinstein, *Practical Lessons in Endodontic Surgery*, vol. 1, Quintessence Publishing Co., Chicago, IL, USA, 1998.

[9] American Association of Endodontists, *Glossary of Endodontic Terms*, American Association of Endodontists, Chicago, IL, USA, 7th edition, 2003.

[10] I. Kvinnsland, R. J. Oswald, A. Halse, and A. G. Grønningsæter, "A clinical and roentgenological study of 55 cases of root perforation," *International Endodontic Journal*, vol. 22, no. 2, pp. 75–84, 1989.

[11] Z. Fuss and M. Trope, "Root perforations: classification and treatment choices based on prognostic factors," *Dental Traumatology*, vol. 12, no. 6, pp. 255–264, 1996.

[12] I. Tsesis and Z. Fuss, "Diagnosis and treatment of accidental root perforations," *Endodontic Topics*, vol. 13, no. 1, pp. 95–107, 2006.

[13] C. Main, N. Mirzayan, S. Shabahang, and M. Torabinejad, "Repair of root perforations using mineral trioxide aggregate: a long-term study," *Journal of Endodontics*, vol. 30, no. 2, pp. 80–83, 2004.

[14] S. J. Lee, M. Monsef, and M. Torabinejad, "Sealing ability of a mineral trioxide aggregate for repair of lateral root perforations," *Journal of Endodontics*, vol. 19, no. 11, pp. 541–544, 1993.

[15] J. Kennethweldonjr, D. Pashley, R. Loushine, R. Normanweller, and W. Frankkimbrough, "Sealing ability of mineral trioxide aggregate and super-EBA when used as furcation repair materials: a longitudinal study," *Journal of Endodontics*, vol. 28, no. 6, pp. 467–470, 2002.

[16] S. Seltzer and I. B. Bender, *The Dental Pulp*, J. B. Lippincott Company, Philadelphia, PA, USA, 3rd edition, 1984.

[17] R. E. Unsterseher, L. G. Nieberg, A. D. Weimer, and J. K. Dyer, "The response of human pulpal tissue after orthodontic force application," *American Journal of Orthodontics and Dentofacial Orthopedics*, vol. 92, no. 3, pp. 220–224, 1987.

[18] J. Spector, B. Rothenhaus, and R. Herman, "Pulpal necrosis following orthodontic therapy. Report of two cases," *New York State Dental Journal*, vol. 40, no. 1, pp. 30–32, 1974.

[19] P. A. Hamersky, A. D. Weimer, and J. F. Taintor, "The effect of orthodontic force application on the pulpal tissue respiration rate in the human premolar," *American Journal of Orthodontics*, vol. 77, no. 4, pp. 368–378, 1980.

[20] I. Rotstein and J. H. Simon, "The endo-perio lesion: a critical appraisal of the disease condition," *Endodontic Topics*, vol. 13, no. 1, pp. 34–56, 2006.

[21] E. Y. Kwon, Y. Cho, J. Y. Lee, S. J. Kim, and J. Choi, "Endodontic treatment enhances the regenerative potential of teeth with advanced periodontal disease with secondary endodontic involvement," *Journal of Periodontal & Implant Science*, vol. 43, no. 3, pp. 136–140, 2013.

[22] L. Blomlof, A. Lengheden, and S. Lindskog, "Endodontic infection and calcium hydroxide-treatment. Effects on periodontal healing in mature and immature replanted monkey teeth," *Journal of Clinical Periodontology*, vol. 19, no. 9, pp. 652–658, 1992.

[23] L. Lin, M. Y. H. Chen, D. Ricucci, and P. A. Rosenberg, "Guided tissue regeneration in periapical surgery," *Journal of Endodontics*, vol. 36, no. 4, pp. 618–625, 2010.

[24] T. von Arx and D. L. Cochran, "Rationale for the application of the GTR principle using a barrier membrane in endodontic surgery: a proposal of classification and literature review," *International Journal of Periodontics & Restorative Dentistry*, vol. 21, no. 2, pp. 127–139, 2001.

[25] T. Dietrich, P. Zunker, D. Dietrich, and J. P. Bernimoulin, "Apicomarginal defects in periradicular surgery: classification and diagnostic aspects," *Oral Surgery, Oral Medicine, Oral Pathology, Oral Radiology, and Endodontology*, vol. 94, no. 2, pp. 233–239, 2002.

[26] S. Kim and S. Kratchman, "Modern endodontic surgery concepts and practice: a review," *Journal of Endodontics*, vol. 32, no. 7, pp. 601–623, 2006.

[27] T. von Arx and M. AlSaeed, "The use of regenerative techniques in apical surgery: a literature review," *The Saudi Dental Journal*, vol. 23, no. 3, pp. 113–127, 2011.

[28] M. L. Marin-Botero, J. S. Dominguez-Mejia, J. A. Arismendi-Echavarria, A. L. Mesa-Jaramillo, G. A. Florez-Moreno, and S. I. Tobon-Arroyave, "Healing response of apicomarginal defects to two guided tissue regeneration techniques in periradicular surgery: a double-blind, randomized-clinical trial," *International Endodontic Journal*, vol. 39, no. 5, pp. 368–377, 2006.

[29] T. Dietrich, P. Zunker, D. Dietrich, and J. P. Bernimoulin, "Periapical and periodontal healing after osseous grafting and guided tissue regeneration treatment of apicomarginal defects in periradicular surgery: results after 12 months," *Oral Surgery, Oral Medicine, Oral Pathology, Oral Radiology, and Endodontics*, vol. 95, no. 4, pp. 474–482, 2003.

[30] E. Kim, J. S. Song, I. Y. Jung, S. J. Lee, and S. Kim, "Prospective clinical study evaluating endodontic microsurgery outcomes for cases with lesions of endodontic origin compared with cases with lesions of combined periodontal–endodontic origin," *Journal of Endodontics*, vol. 34, no. 5, pp. 546–551, 2008.

[31] J. Douthitt, J. Gutmann, and D. Witherspoon, "Histologic assessment of healing after the use of a bioresorbable membrane in the management of buccal bone loss concomitant with periradicular surgery," *Journal of Endodontics*, vol. 27, no. 6, pp. 404–410, 2001.

[32] S. Perlmutter, M. Tagger, E. Tagger, and M. Abram, "Effect of the endodontic status of the tooth on experimental periodontal reattachment in baboons: a preliminary investigation," *Oral Surgery, Oral Medicine, and Oral Pathology*, vol. 63, no. 2, pp. 232–236, 1987.

[33] J. L. C. de Miranda, C. M. M. Santana, and R. B. Santana, "Influence of endodontic treatment in the post-surgical healing of human class II furcation defects," *Journal of Periodontology*, vol. 84, no. 1, pp. 51–57, 2013.

[34] N. A. Alnemer, H. Alquthami, and L. Alotaibi, "The use of bone graft in the treatment of periapical lesion," *Saudi Endodontic Journal*, vol. 7, no. 2, pp. 115–118, 2017.

20

Application of Immediate Dentoalveolar Restoration in Alveolus Compromised with Loss of Immediate Implant in Esthetic Area

Rafael de Lima Franceschi [1,2,3] **Luciano Drechsel,** [1,3,4] **and Guenther Schuldt Filho** [5]

[1] *Brasilian Association of Dental Surgeons, Curitiba, PR, Brazil*
[2] *Dental Institute of the Americas, Balneário Camboriú, SC, Brazil*
[3] *São Leopoldo Mandic University, Curitiba, PR, Brazil*
[4] *Brazilian Dental Association (ABO), Ponta Grossa, PR, Brazil*
[5] *Federal University of Santa Catarina, Florianópolis, SC, Brazil*

Correspondence should be addressed to Rafael de Lima Franceschi; odontorafael@yahoo.com.br

Academic Editor: Konstantinos Michalakis

In the reported clinical case, the immediate dentoalveolar restoration (IDR) technique was applied to reconstruct the buccal bone wall, with autogenous graft of the maxillary tuberosity, which had been lost due to a root fracture, and to provide the necessary bone substrate for the installation of an implant and its provisioning. One of the greatest risks inherent in the survival of immediate implants is the maintenance of their stability during the healing period. In this case, due to a mechanical trauma in sports activity in the first postoperative month, there was a total failure in the osseointegration process, confirmed by tomographic examination of both the implant and the bone graft. The deleterious effects of this accident were compensated with a new approach and reapplication of IDR technique using a smaller-diameter implant and with conical macrogeometry in conjunction with the new bone reconstruction under the same compromised alveolus; associated, after the period of osseointegration, with the maneuvers of volume increase of the gingival tissue by subepithelial connective tissue graft. The tomographic result demonstrated the success of the surgical procedures, and the clinical/photographic analysis obtained showed the stability of the gingival margin without compromising the esthetic result of the prosthetic restoration.

1. Introduction

Esthetic dentistry has currently reached a level of excellence that no longer allows teeth subject to exodontia for reasons such as trauma and bacterial infections, resulting in prosthetic works that do not adequately mimic homologous teeth and the surrounding gingival tissues. The challenge of removing a dental element and facing the events that occur on the protective and sustaining tissues requires deep knowledge in the areas of periodontics, surgery, and dental prosthesis [1].

Partial or total loss of the vestibular bone wall potentiates the deleterious effects on the periodontal tissues that occur in a postextraction alveolus and indicate the need for preservation and simultaneous alveolar reconstruction to the exodontia, allowing the stability of these tissues and enhancing their

clinical predictability [2]. The possibility of installing an immediate implant and its adequate provisioning are is a factor that contributes to the maintenance of esthetics and peri-implant health, and when associated with the autogenous graft, the osteogenic, osteoinductive, and osteoconductive capacity of this material results in a more rapid vascularization and incorporation, with no immune response, being the gold standard of regenerative procedures [3].

Immediate loading, even in infraocclusion, to which immediate implants are installed postexodontia in esthetic areas, increases the risks of postoperative failures and complications [4]. If the loss of a dental element is already bad, an immediate implant is even worse because the bone bed has already been milled, and failure in the osseointegration process results in a rapid formation of granulation tissue; alteration of local irrigation; formation of areas of necrosis, in short, a severe collapse of the peri-implant tissues with increased bone remodeling; and alteration in the vestibular gingival margin, compromising the esthetic result of the procedure [5, 6].

The immediate dentoalveolar restoration (IDR) technique aims at regenerating, via the autogenous bone of the maxillary tuberosity, the postextracting alveolus that has one or more compromised bone walls, allowing the installation of an immediate implant and its provisioning. In the situation of loss of one immediate implant with total loss of the vestibular bone wall, IDR would be a viable tool to repair the alveolus, creating a clinical situation that allows the installation of a new implant and its prosthesis, immediately recovering the esthetics of the patient who can subsequently receive regenerative procedures aimed at maintaining or improving the level and contours of the peri-implant soft tissues, which are critical for esthetics and long-term success [7].

2. Case Report

A male patient, thirty-five years of age, attended the clinic for care after reporting intense pain during chewing in which he reported hearing a fractured tooth 11 and its subsequent mobility. He received a ceramic crown (metal-free) rehabilitation on the upper teeth two years ago. The clinical examination revealed that the gingival biotype was thick, there was a small active fistula on the vestibular surface, and the depth of probing in this area was 7 mm, with mobility of the crown in the vestibular-palatine direction (Figure 1).

After a CBCT scan, the diagnosis of vertical root fracture and invasion of the biological space with a compromised vestibular bone wall was confirmed (Figure 2(a)). The treatment proposed to the patient was an immediate dentoalveolar restoration with grafting material from the right maxillary tuberosity, implant, and immediate provision.

According to the protocol of the technique, the antibiotic therapy with amoxicillin 500 mg every 8 hrs was initiated five days before surgery and afterwards for another 7 days in order to reduce and modulate the inflammatory process aided by dexamethasone 4 mg 2 tablets 1 hour before surgery and 1 tablet every 8 hours for 3 days and paracetamol 750 mg every 8 hours for 3 days.

After an infiltrative anesthesia in the vestibule and the palatine region of tooth 11 with 2% mepivacaine and epinephrine 1 : 100,000 (DFL), an intrasulcular incision was made with a 15C (Swann-Morton) blade with the aid of a peritoneum, apical levers, and delicate forceps, minimally invasive exodontia was performed (Figure 2(b)) without compromising the integrity of the papillae. Thorough curettage and irrigation were performed until all granulation tissue was removed.

A mapping of the vestibular wall defect was performed using a millimeter probe inside the fresh alveolus and the milling sequence started at 5 mm from the cervical margin of the palatal bone wall and a cylindrical Cone Morse (Intraoss, Brazil) implant with a diameter of 4.0 mm × 13.0 mm to 3 mm infrabony, in a more palatinate position. Primary stability was achieved with a torque record of 35 Ncm. Altering

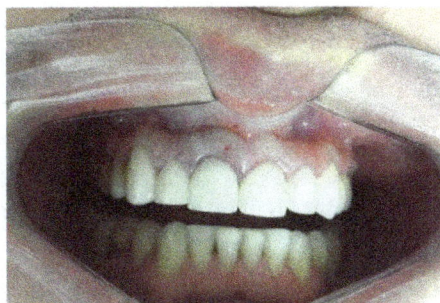

FIGURE 1: Presence of ceramic restorations in the upper anterior teeth with swollen gingival area on the vestibular face of element 11.

the original technique advocated the preparation of the provisional crown at this time, using a titanium UCLA directly in the internal connection of the implant, and due to the objective of using an intermediate prosthetic abutment between the implant and the provisional crown, this phase was postponed until after bone reconstruction.

Anesthesia was performed in the region of the right tuft (2% mepivacaine, epinephrine 1 : 100,000) in the vestibular and ischemic anterior region at the crest and palatine area. A supracrestal incision was performed until the periosteum and subsequent total displacement of the flap until the relaxing incisions in the region corresponding to the position where the third molar is generally located. With the aid of a surgical hammer and a goose chisel number 08, the cortical-medullary bone sheet was removed and taken to a glass plate where it was carved in the shape of the defect to be reconstructed (Figure 3(a)). The blade was then fitted into the defect, and the gap between the implant and the blade was filled with the remainder of the bone material collected from the tuberosity which was particulate with a delicate and properly condensed alveoli.

The implant cover was removed and an intermediate pillar of 1.5 mm height was installed (Figure 3(b)). A stock tooth facet was captured under a titanium UCLA duly prepared with flow resin (Opallis, FGM) and Z-350 A1B composite resin (3M Espe). Adequate adjustments were made in the emergency profile and in the disocclusion guides with incisal height reduction. The reconstruction allowed the complete closure of the spaces and there was no need for sutures in tooth region 11 (Figures 4(a) and 4(b)). Only the tuft was adequately sutured with 4.0 silk thread (Ethicon).

Postoperative guidelines were followed in relation to a soft diet without using the tooth in question. The patient was monitored every 7 days, with total remission of the vestibular fistula.

Twenty-two days after the initial surgical procedure, the patient scheduled emergency care. He also reported that when doing a jiu-jitsu class, he received an elbow in the operated tooth with bleeding and pain after the trauma (Figures 5(a) and 5(b)).

After the clinical examination, a change was observed in the three-dimensional position of the implant/crown with vestibularization and gyroversion of the same. The crown was removed, and small fragments of bone abduction were

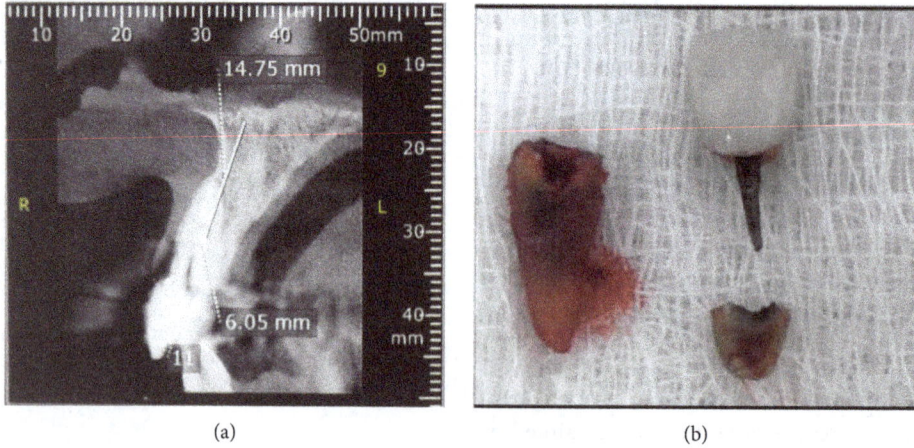

(a)

(b)

FIGURE 2: Root fracture and its subsequent bacterial contamination caused the vestibular wall to become impaired. (a) Tomography demonstrating the loss of vestibular bone wall in element 11. (b) The root fracture and invasion of the biological space generated inflammation on the vestibular face.

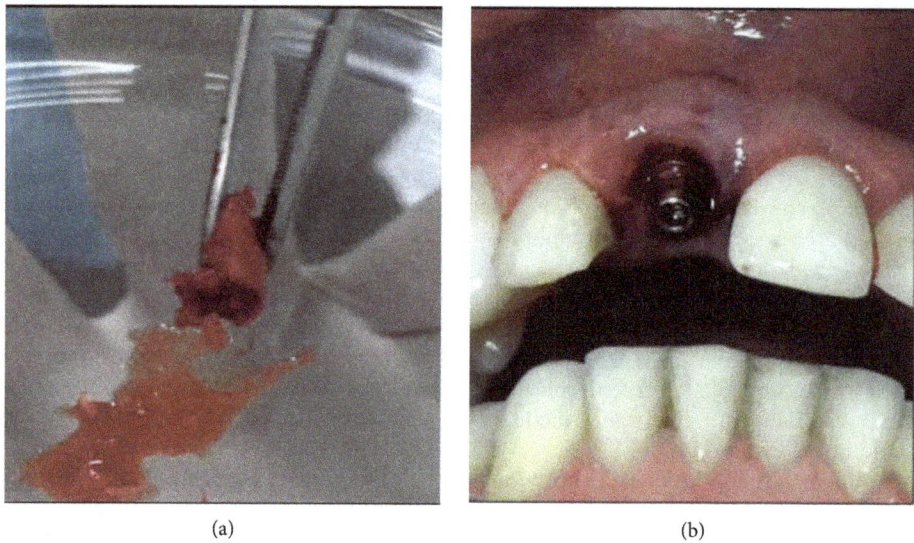

(a)

(b)

FIGURE 3: IDR surgical phase. (a) Cortical-medullary blade removed from the right maxillary tuberosity. (b) Cone Morse implant installation and pillar height test.

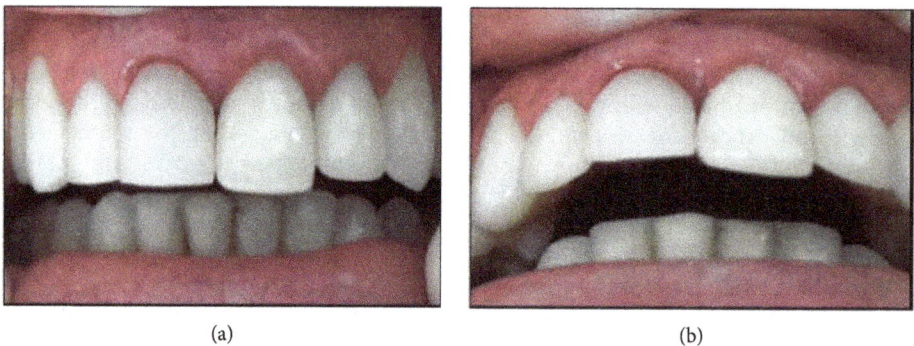

(a)

(b)

FIGURE 4: Immediate postoperative preserving the protective tissues with maintenance of vestibular volume and gingival margin. (a) Front view of the IDR. (b) Occlusal view with incisal relief.

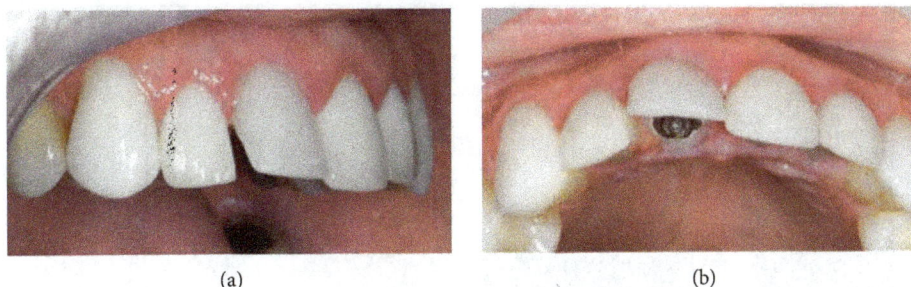

(a)   (b)

FIGURE 5: Trauma during sports procedure in the immediate implant region. (a) Due to the trauma, there was vestibularization. (b) Implant-crown turning compromising the entire osseointegration process.

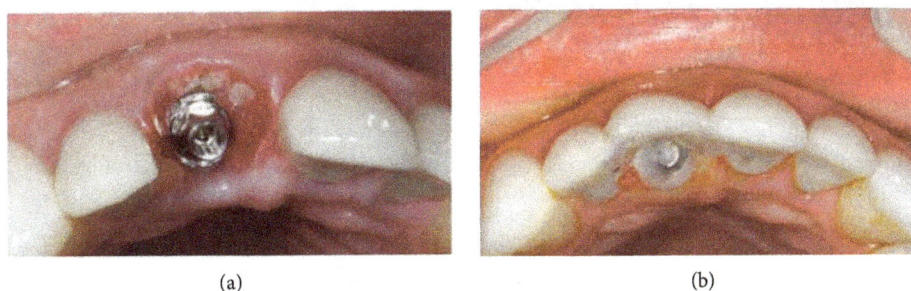

(a)   (b)

FIGURE 6: The provisional crown was removed and then reinstalled and attached to the neighboring teeth. (a) Presence of bone sequestration arising from the reconstruction of the vestibular wall. (b) Repositioning of the crown and union to the neighboring teeth with resinous cement.

found in the abutment region (Figure 6(a)). It was reinstalled and through the crown fixing screw, the entire structure was manipulated towards the palatal in an attempt to reposition it as close as possible to the original position. Temporary union with U-200 resin cement (3M Espe) of the acrylic crown was performed on the neighboring teeth 12 and 21 (Figure 6(b)). An implant tomography was ordered to assess the extent of the problem.

After ten days of trauma, the tomographic image analysis recorded that the three-dimensional positioning of the implant was out of the proper position, compromising the entire reconstruction of the vestibular wall. The loss of implant stability is directly related to the absence of supporting bone tissue in the vestibular area (Figures 7(a) and 7(b)).

Several treatment alternatives were then presented to the patient to remove the implant and to perform alveolar preservation through grafting of biomaterials and membranes for guided bone regeneration. However, it was a consensus among the surgeons that any of the cases presented could lead to a change and instability of the vestibular gingival margin, further compromising the esthetic outcome of the case. Alternatively, the possibility of retreatment through a new IDR was suggested. Although there were no reports of this, the idea behind the treatment was to consider the implant lost as if it were a root compromised with total loss of the vestibular bone wall, aided at this time by the absence of the infectious process.

With the endorsement of the patient, all the steps of the protocol of the technique were initiated through previous antibiotic therapy, and the surgical sequence was the same

as previously described with only the following modifications: total curettage of the alveolus with removal of all the bone fragments and granulation tissue gift was performed; the new implant had a smaller diameter, 3.5 × 13 mm (Intraoss, Brazil), and its macrogeometry was conical; its insertion was searching the center of the alveolus, even if it was not possible to make a screwed prosthesis; and the maxillary tuberosity that provided the material for grafting was the left tuft.

After implanting the implant with 45 Ncm torque, reconstruction of the buccal bone wall was performed with the insertion of medullary bone compacted at the apex of the implant up to half its length, only after the cortical-medullary lamina was positioned throughout the vestibular region leaving a 3 mm gap of the lamina to the implant that was filled by a new insertion of compacted medullary bone. A new 2.5 mm height abutment was installed with a torque of 32 Ncm, and immediate provisioning was still possible with a screwed crown even though the prosthetic connection of the abutment was in a more vestibularized position (Figures 8(a) and 8(b)).

The tubal suture was identical to the previous report, and the postoperative care was reinforced and amplified even with the use of an acrylic total plate in the upper arch to protect against any new trauma. The patient was monitored weekly until the ninety days of the surgical intervention and then every two weeks for a further two months. In this period, two CBCT scans were performed: the first ten days after the new IDR (Figures 9(a) and 9(b)) and the second after five months, confirming the osseointegration of the

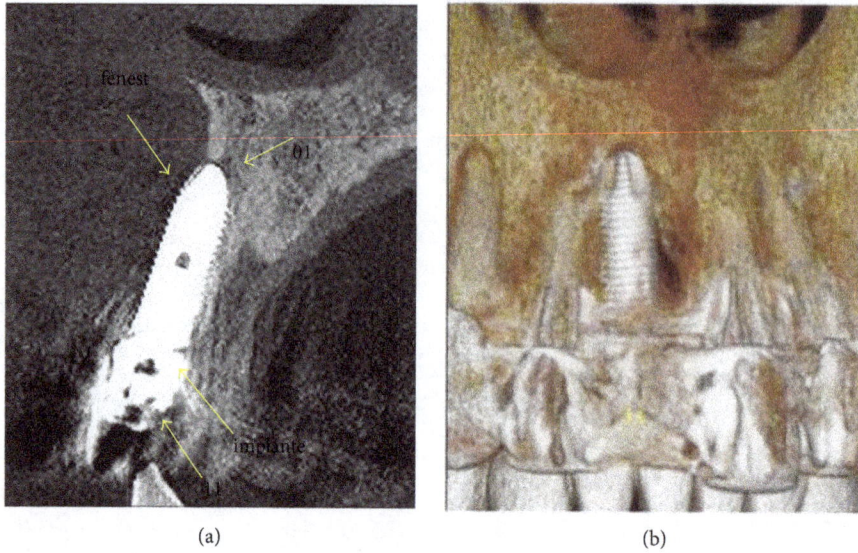

(a)

(b)

FIGURE 7: Radiographic analysis ten days after the trauma. (a) The tomographic image registers the implant in an inadequate three-dimensional position. (b) Loss of vestibular wall that had been rebuilt.

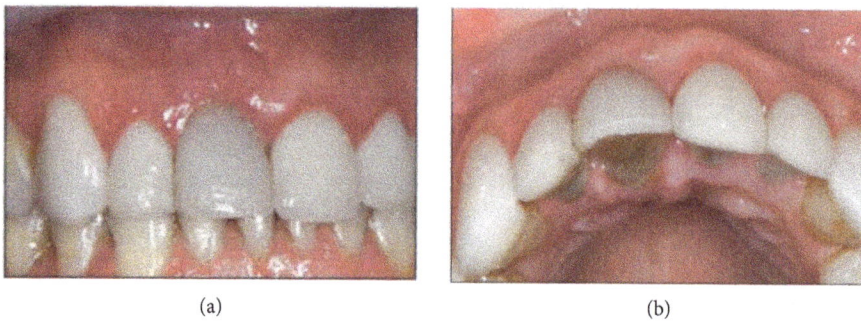

(a)

(b)

FIGURE 8: Immediate postoperative of the second IDR applied to element 11 with peri-implant tissue normality. (a) Immediate frontal view and (b) occlusal view demonstrating the maintenance of vestibular volume.

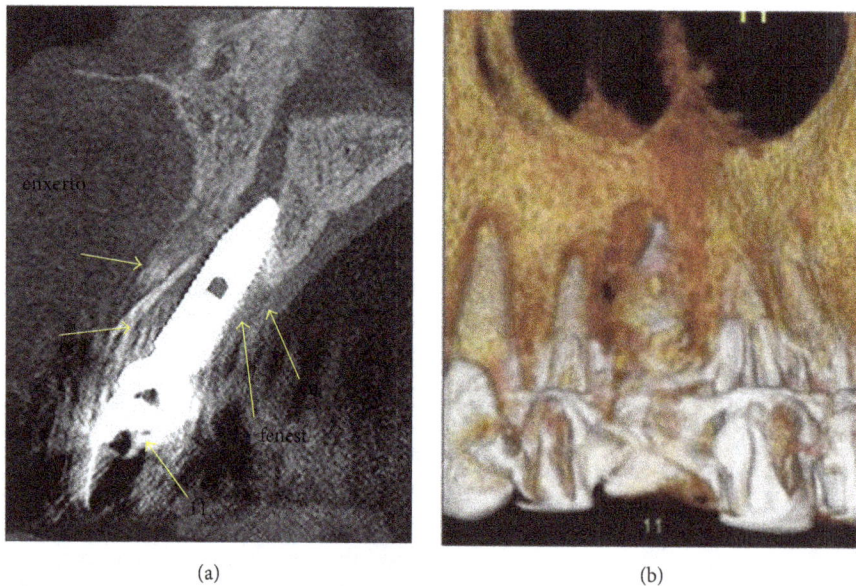

(a)

(b)

FIGURE 9: Tomography 10 days after surgery to visualize the 3D position of the implant and the presence of the cortical-medullar lamina. (a) Tomographic section where it is possible to visualize the grafted bone tissue. (b) Image recording bone reconstruction.

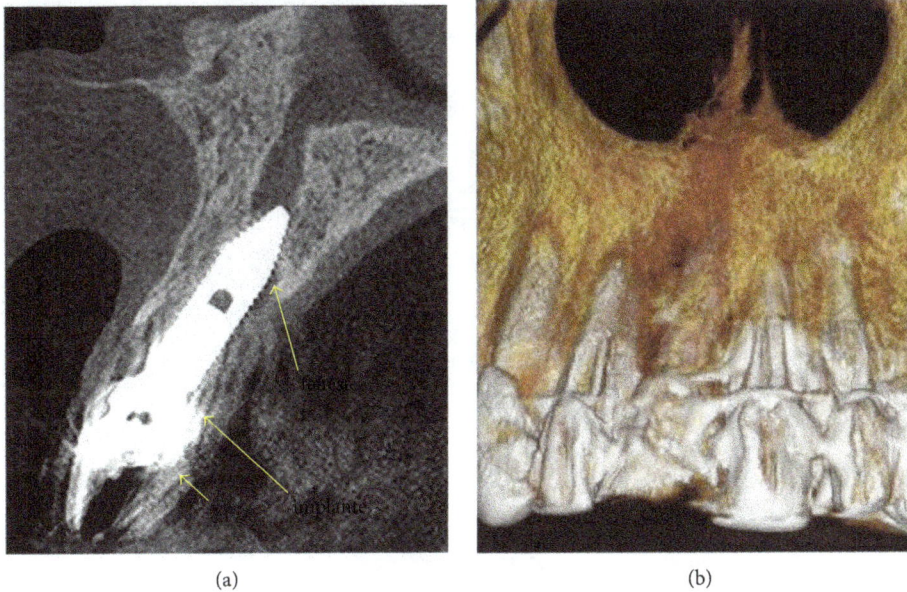

(a)

(b)

FIGURE 10: Tomography after five months of the second IDR. (a) Tomography performed with oral retractor to reveal soft tissues. (b) Recording of total graft incorporation and presence of a new vestibular bone wall.

implant and maintenance of the new vestibular bone wall (Figures 10(a) and 10(b)).

In the sixth month after the new intervention, the screw crown was removed to evaluate the peri-implant soft tissue emergence and visualization profile. The pillar torque that continued with 32 Ncm was also verified. At this time, an esthetic evaluation of the gingival margin was made, and it was found that in the operated region, there was a smaller volume, and the gingival margin was more apical than the other incisors (Figure 11).

Even though he was satisfied with the result, the patient reported that he would like to improve his case as much as possible and that he would go through further interventions if necessary. Then, the possibility of a subepithelial connective tissue graft that would improve the height of the gingival margin and give more volume to the peri-implant tissues was presented to him, being of great value in the maintenance and stability of these tissues in the long term.

After his endorsement, a new surgical procedure was scheduled. Anesthesia of the vestibular and ischemic fundus was performed in the vestibular region of tooth 11 and in the palatine region of teeth 14 to 16 with 3% articaine and epinephrine 1 : 100,000 (DLF). An intrasulcular incision with 15 C lamina (Swann-Morton) was performed around the implant, and the tissue division was done with the aid of tunneling. After mapping the amount to be grafted, the palate was accessed, and through an "L" incision, the connective tissue was removed (Figure 12(a)) and sutured in the vestibular region (Figure 12(b)) with 5.0 absorbable suture thread Technew. After the positioning of the graft with the flap moved to the incisor, the gingival margin was repositioned (Figures 13(a) and 13(b)), the crown was removed, the critical and subcritical area of the emergency profile was resized (Figures 14(a) and 14(b)), and the suspensory suture was made in the papillae

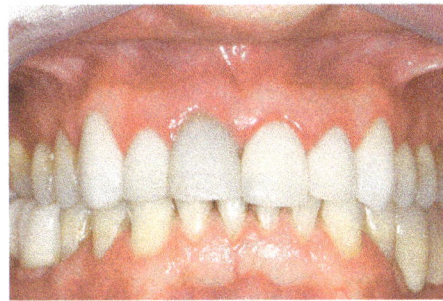

FIGURE 11: Result obtained after five months of healing. Despite clinical success, there was a slight discrepancy in the gingival margin of element 11.

and in the center of the margin and fixed directly to the acrylic crown with flow resin (Opallis, FGM) for better tissue stability. In the weeks following the removal of the points, the area of the emergency profile was checked and polished until complete visual healing of the peri-implant tissues.

Concluding this phase after ninety days, the provisional crown was removed, the final healing of the peri-implant tissues was evaluated, the pillar torque was checked, and the final crown was made (Figure 15).

The prosthetic phase begins with an additional silicone molding (Variotime, Heraeus/Kulzer) in an open tray with customization of the transfer abutment with acrylic resin (Pattern Resin LS, GC America Inc.) which copied the shape of the peri-implant tissues, achieved during the phase of the provisional crown.

After scanning of the model, an STL file was generated, and the analysis of the positioning of the implant/abutment complex was analyzed by the CAD of the Zirkonzahn

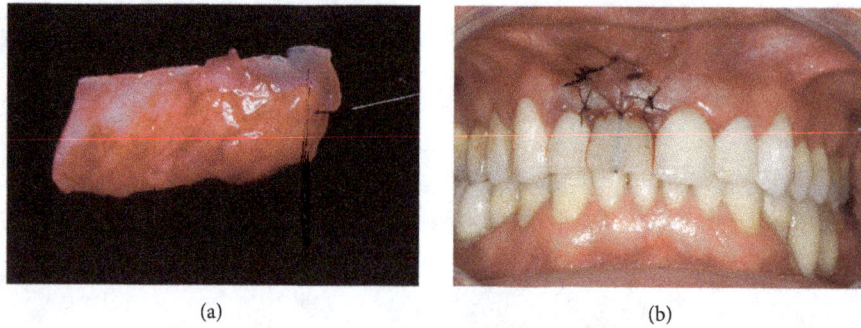

(a)

(b)

FIGURE 12: Connective tissue graft. (a) Subepithelial connective tissue removed from the palate. (b) Suture of the graft divided into the vestibular flap using the provisional crown as a foundation for better position and support of the gingival margin.

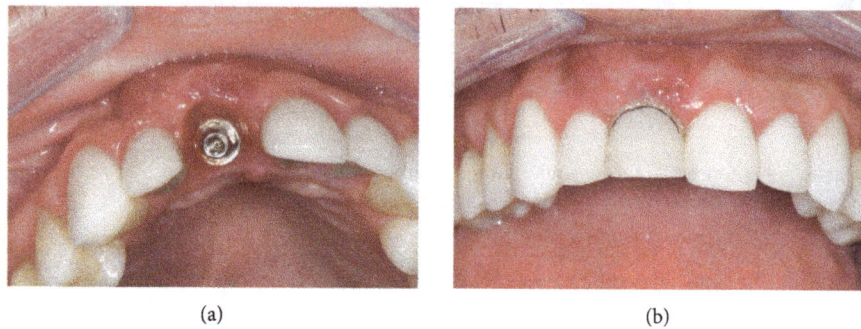

(a)

(b)

FIGURE 13: Grafted tissue in maturation process. (a) Occlusal view of the scar area after 30 days with increased volume. (b) Positioning of the new vestibular gingival margin.

(a)

(b)

FIGURE 14: Correct delineation of the emergency profile is crucial to the long-term success of the technique. (a) Concave emergency profile in the cervicovestibular region. (b) The critical line corresponds to the position of the gingival margin, and below it is the subcritical area that should accommodate and maintain healthy peri-implant soft tissues.

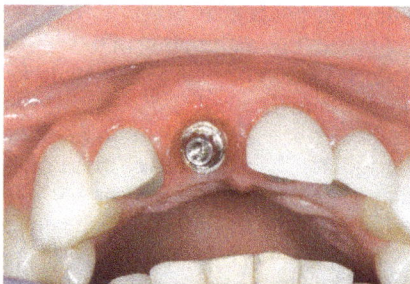

FIGURE 15: Occlusal view where the volume and quality of the peri-implant tissues obtained after the completion of the IDR with connective graft can be visualized.

system. It was decided by a cemented crown so that the technician had enough space to apply ceramic layers that reproduced the contralateral tooth in relation to shape and color.

A custom screwed pillar and a coping, both using zirconia (Figures 16(a) and 16(b)), were milled (CAM, Zirkonzan). After the necessary tests and adjustments of the infra-structures, there was the application of stratified ceramics (Figure 17). The zirconia abutment was radiographed to confirm its adaptation and screwed with 32 Ncm torque, the screw hole was closed with Teflon tape (PTFE), the crown was cemented with U-200 resin cement (3M, Espe), and extreme attention was given to the cementation line

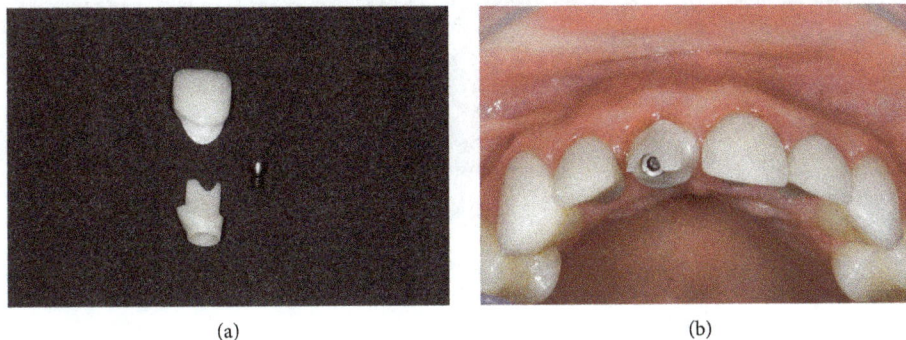

<table>
<tr><td>(a)</td><td>(b)</td></tr>
</table>

FIGURE 16: Prosthetic phase using custom zirconia abutment. (a) Screwed zirconia abutment and pure ceramic crown. (b) Occlusal view of the abutment screwed with the screw in the incisal line of the other incisors proving the more vestibular positioning of the prosthetic connection.

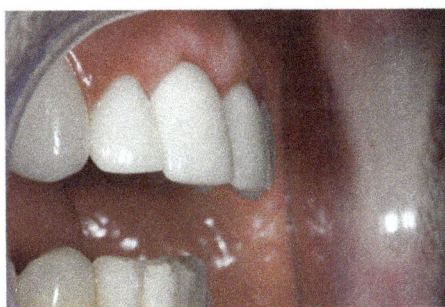

FIGURE 17: Lateral view of the abutment test and the stratified ceramic crown demonstrating adaptation to the peri-implant tissues, appropriate color, and shape.

so that there was no infiltration into the peri-implant tissues (Figure 18(a)). All occlusal adjustments were reviewed, and the disocclusion guides were checked (Figure 18(b)). A new tomography was performed with a buccal retractor in order to record the measurements of the hard and soft tissues in the vestibular region after twelve months of the IDR reapplication to determine the zero (follow-up zero) momentum, serving as a basis for follow-up and future comparisons (Figures 19(a) and 19(b)). Measurements at two points on the vestibular wall (cervical 4.6 mm and apical 6.3 mm at the implant) recorded the formation of the new vestibular wall with a considerable increase of the bone tissue, mainly in relation to the homologous tooth (21), whose measurements at similar points recorded a typical buccal bone board as described in the literature with values lower than 1 mm in the cervical and median and only in the apical region of the root with a measurement of 2.3 mm. In relation to the soft tissues, the subepithelial connective tissue graft practically doubled the values found in the contralateral tooth (8.2 mm versus 4.6 mm cervical, 11.2 mm versus 6.9 mm apical), being of paramount importance for maintaining a stable gingival margin and avoiding possible recessions that can affect the vestibular face of the immediate implants.

The end result in relation to the reconstruction of support and protection tissues projects clinical success in the long term (Figure 20).

3. Discussion

The literature describes that the buccal bone plate has on average less than 1 mm thickness and that the bone remodeling that occurs after the exodontia will alter the vestibular gingival margin independent of the installation of an immediate implant [8, 9].

Among the various methods to prevent spontaneous remodeling of tissues and to preserve the alveolar ridge, the most used is through biomaterials of low rate of reabsorption and protection with membranes, called guided bone regeneration (GBR) [10].

The major challenge for performing immediate implants is when one or more bone walls are lost. Clinically, the most common is the total or partial loss of the buccal bone wall, and IDR is presented as an alternative for the use of GBR. The idea of the technique is similar, and in the case of IDR, the cortical-medullary bone graft installed in the shape of the defect to be reconstructed will be a barrier to stabilize the particulate bone graft that will exist in the gap between the implant and the new bone wall. The use of the autogenous bone material of the maxillary tuberosity provides factors different from traditional biomaterials [11]. As the vascular pattern is vital for the success of bone grafts, the medullary nature of the grafts harvested at this site indicates that there is indeed a possibility of transferring bone material with viable and high-capacity osteoprogenitor cells into the receptor bed which provides faster and more effective healing with minimal alteration to the involved tissues. In addition to early and low-intensity stimulation that does not compromise mechanical stability, increased blood flow and contact osteogenesis will accelerate the full incorporation of the bone graft, ensuring the substrate necessary for the success of the implant and peri-implant tissues [12, 13].

The risks inherent in immediate loading techniques such as a minimally traumatic and flapless surgery, a 3D implant position, a gap filling, and its provisioning may not prevent postexodontic alveolar changes, and recessions may compromise the gingival margin and longevity of supporting and protective tissues [14].

The alveolus-dental topography in the anterior maxilla region, due to the inclination of the teeth, results in a very thin vestibular bone board and a thicker and more robust

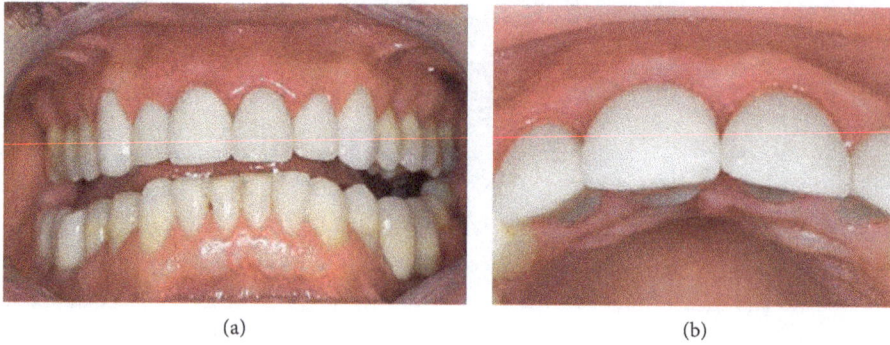

(a)   (b)

FIGURE 18: Final result after cementation with resin cement. (a) Front view of the cemented crown. (b) Occlusal view showing the correct 3D positioning of the prosthetic crown.

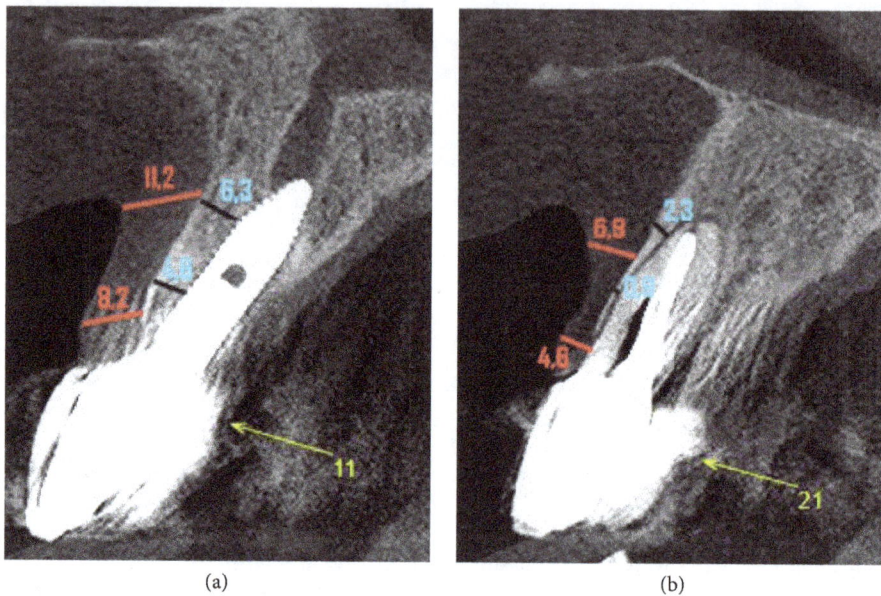

(a)   (b)

FIGURE 19: CBCT scan of the follow-up of the IDR reapplication. (a) Tomography with measures of bone and gingival tissue in the vestibule of implant 11 which was reconstructed by the surgical procedures. (b) Tomography where it is possible to compare the volumes of bone and gingival tissue in the vestibular area of a healthy tooth 21.

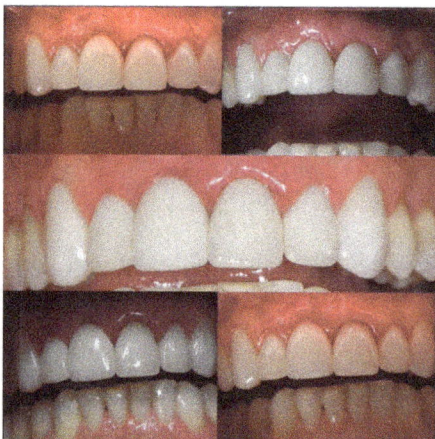

FIGURE 20: Case completed. Photo of the case with different light intensities, after one year of IDR reapplication, demonstrating the normality of the peri-implant tissues and the maintenance of the final gingival margin compatible with esthetic rehabilitation.

palatine bone wall [15]. The bone perforation for implant installation should always be in a palatal approach where greater primary stability is obtained. The preparation of the bone bed in this position allows the formation of a gap between the implant and the buccal wall that should be filled by grafting material. Its filling confers a substrate site for the osteoblasts to secrete a new bone matrix [16]. The materials most used for this purpose are autogenous bone and xenogenic hydroxyapatite. Both are important sources in reconstructive procedures and can often even be associated according to the need of the recipient site [17].

Proper positioning of the implant in the mesiodistal direction allows the preservation of the papilla, in the vestibular-palatine sense, determines the dimensions of the prosthetic crown, and is a preponderant factor in the choice of definitive restorations, whether cemented or screwed [18].

A vestibular wall approximately 2 mm thick is ideal for long-term esthetic success, as it allows peri-implant soft tissue stability. In cases of impairment of the buccal bone plate, the use of smaller-diameter implants concomitant with the regeneration of hard tissues will favor the maintenance of theses tissues [19, 20].

When mucosal deficiencies compromise planning and outcome, regenerative techniques should be associated to restore proper contour and volume. One of the measures is to optimize the presence of keratinized mucosa around the implants [21]. In these cases, it is recommended to perform a subepithelial connective tissue graft to prevent the vertical and horizontal volumetric loss of the peri-implant tissues. The presence of keratinized mucosa will provide texture and tone similar to natural teeth, hiding the tooth/crown interface and facilitating biofilm control [22–24].

The provisioning phase is one of the key factors for the immediate implants since it maintains the normal gingival architecture after the removal of a dental element [25]. The prosthetic crown loaded under the implant defines the shape of the gingival tissue relative to the bone crest and the mesial/distal contact points, the emergence profile of the provisional crown favors the maturation of the peri-implant tissues during the period of osseointegration of the implant, and the sculpture of the subcritical area determines the stability of the vestibular gingival margin [26, 27].

The analysis of the final tomography of this case shows that the IDR technique provided a significant increase of the vestibular bone wall when compared to the homologous tooth, whereas the healthy buccal bone of tooth 21 is less than 1 mm and the new vestibular bone wall of implant 11 is more than 2 mm. In addition to the fact that the subepithelial connective tissue graft created a new gingival biotype due to the increase in the volume and thickness of the peri-implant tissues, it can be affirmed that the necessary factors were created for the stabilization of the gingival margin in a position that did not compromise the esthetic results in the short and long term, according to the most recent studies described in the literature.

4. Conclusion

In spite of the intercurrences in the first phase of the IDR technique application, failure in osseointegration of the implant/bone graft complex allowed the clinical opportunity to measure the challenges of reapplying the IDR in an alveolus involved with the variables of the inflammatory events that occur with loss of an immediate implant. The result of success obtained significantly increases the possibilities of application of the technique and is of great assistance to the surgeon who, at the moment, is increasingly involved with the immediate implants in an esthetic area.

Funding

This study was self-financed by the authors.

References

[1] R. A. Levine, J. Ganeles, L. Gonzaga et al., "10 keys for successful esthetic-zone single immediate implants," *The Compendium of Continuing Education in Dentistry*, vol. 38, no. 4, pp. 248–260, 2017.

[2] S. Chen and D. Buser, "Esthetic outcomes following immediate and early implant placement in the anterior maxilla—a systematic review," *The International Journal of Oral & Maxillofacial Implants*, vol. 29, pp. 186–215, 2014.

[3] J. C. M. Rosa, A. C. P. O. Rosa, C. M. Zardo et al., *Immediate Dentoalveolar Restoration – Immediately Loaded Implants in Compromised Sockets*, Quintessence, São Paulo, 2014.

[4] M. Esposito, G. Zucchelli, G. Canizzaro et al., "Immediate, immediate-delayed (6 weeks) and delayed (4 months) post-extractive single implants: 1-year post-loading data from a ramdomised controlled trial," *European Journal of Oral Implantology*, vol. 10, no. 1, pp. 11–26, 2017.

[5] T. Jemt, M. Karouni, J. Abitbol, O. Zouiten, and H. Antoun, "A retrospective study on 1592 consecutively performed operations in one private referral clinic: part II: peri-implantitis and implant failures," *Clinical Implant Dentistry and Related Research*, vol. 19, no. 3, pp. 413–422, 2017.

[6] F. Zuffetti, M. Capelli, F. Galli, M. del Fabbro, and T. Testori, "Post-extraction implant placement into infected versus non-infected sites: a multicenter retrospective clinical study," *Clinical Implant Dentistry and Related Research*, vol. 19, no. 5, pp. 833–840, 2017.

[7] J. C. M. Rosa, A. C. P. O. Rosa, D. Rosa, and C. M. Zardo, "Immediate dentoalveolar restoration of compromised sockets: a novel technique," *International Journal of Esthetic Dentistry*, vol. 8, no. 3, pp. 432–443, 2013.

[8] P. Weigl and A. Strangio, "The impact of immediately placed and restored single-tooth implants on hard and soft tissues in the anterior maxilla," *European Journal of Oral Implantology*, vol. 9, Supplement 1, pp. 89–106, 2016.

[9] G. Huynh-Ba, B. E. Pjetursson, M. Sanz et al., "Analysis of the socket bone wall dimensions in the upper maxilla in relation to immediate implant placement," *Clinical Oral Implants Research*, vol. 21, no. 1, pp. 37–42, 2010.

[10] M. G. Araújo, E. Linder, and J. Lindhe, "Bio-Oss Collagen in the buccal gap at immediate implants: a 6-month study in the dog," *Clinical Oral Implants Research*, vol. 22, no. 1, pp. 1–8, 2011.

[11] R. S. de Molon, E. D. de Avila, L. A. B. de Barros-Filho et al., "Reconstruction of the alveolar buccal bone plate in compromised fresh socket after immediate implant placement followed by immediate provisionalization," *Journal of Esthetic and Restorative Dentistry*, vol. 27, no. 3, pp. 122–135, 2015.

[12] L. Cannullo, J. C. M. Rosa, V. S. Pinto, C. E. Francischone, and W. Gotz, "Inwards-inclined implant platform for the amplified platform-switching concept: 18-month follow-up report of a prospective randomized matched-pair controlled trial," *International Journal of Oral and Maxillofacial Implants*, vol. 27, no. 4, pp. 927–934, 2012.

[13] A. C. P. de Oliveira Rosa, J. C. M. da Rosa, L. A. V. D. Pereira, C. E. Francischone, and B. S. Sotto-Maior, "Guidelines for selecting the implant diameter during immediate implant placement of a fresh extraction socket: a case series," *The International Journal of Periodontics & Restorative Dentistry*, vol. 36, no. 3, pp. 401–407, 2016.

[14] D. P. Tarnow, S. J. Chu, and M. A. Salama, "Flapless postextraction socket implant placement in the esthetic zone: part 1. The effect of bone grafting and/or provisional restoration on facial-palatal ridge dimensional change—a retrospective cohort study," *The International Journal of Periodontics & Restorative Dentistry*, vol. 34, no. 3, pp. 323–331, 2014.

[15] D. E. Azar, "Minimally invasive single-implant treatment in the esthetic zone," *The Compendium of Continuing Education in Dentistry*, vol. 38, no. 4, article 28368132, pp. 241–247, 2017.

[16] S. T. Chen, I. B. Darby, E. C. Reynolds, and J. G. Clement, "Immediate implant placement postextraction without flap elevation," *Journal of Periodontology*, vol. 8, no. 91, pp. 163–172, 2009.

[17] L. W. Vasconcelos, D. A. Hiramatsu, L. G. P. Paleckis, C. E. Francischone, R. C. B. Vasconcelos, and T. G. Chaves, "Implante imediato e preservação de alvéolo com Bio-Oss Collagen® em área estética," *The International Journal of Oral & Maxillofacial Implants*, vol. 1, no. 3, pp. 472–480, 2016.

[18] U. Grunder, "Crestal ridge width changes when placing implants at the time of tooth extraction with and without soft tissue augmentation after a healing period of 6 months: report of 24 consecutive cases," *The International Journal of Periodontics & Restorative Dentistry*, vol. 31, no. 1, pp. 9–17, 2011.

[19] G. O. Sarnachiaro, S. J. Chu, E. Sarnachiaro, S. L. Gotta, and D. P. Tarnow, "Immediate implant placement into extraction sockets with labial plate dehiscence defects: a clinical case series," *Clinical Implant Dentistry and Related Research*, vol. 18, no. 4, pp. 821–829, 2016.

[20] B. Gjelvold, J. Kisch, B. R. Chrcanovic, T. Albrektsson, and A. Wennerberg, "Clinical and radiographic outcome following immediate loading and delayed loading of single-tooth implants: randomized clinical trial," *Clinical Implant Dentistry and Related Research*, vol. 19, no. 3, pp. 549–558, 2017.

[21] S. Yoshino, J. Y. K. Kan, K. Rungcharassaeng, P. Roe, and J. L. Lozada, "Effects of connective tissue grafting on the facial gingival level following single immediate implant placement and provisionalization in the esthetic zone: a 1-year randomized controlled prospective study," *The International Journal of Oral & Maxillofacial Implants*, vol. 29, no. 2, pp. 432–440, 2014.

[22] J. Cosyn, H. De Bruyn, and R. Cleymaet, "Soft tissue preservation and pink aesthetics around single immediate implant restorations: a 1-year prospective study," *Clinical Implant Dentistry and Related Research*, vol. 15, no. 6, pp. 847–857, 2013.

[23] G. Paniz and F. Mazzocco, "Tratamento cirúrgico-protético de defeitos de tecidos moles vestibulares em próteses sobre implantes unitários anteriores," *The International Journal of Esthetic Dentistry*, vol. 1, no. 1, pp. 142–155, 2016.

[24] K. M. Chochlidakis, A. Geminiani, P. Papaspyridakos, N. Singh, C. Ercoli, and C. J. Chen, "Buccal bone thickness around single dental implants in the maxillary esthetic zone," *Quintessence International*, vol. 48, no. 4, pp. 295–308, 2017.

[25] I. Gamborema and M. B. Blatz, *Evolution: Protocols for Anterior Single-Tooth Implants*, Quintessence, Chicago, 2015.

[26] H. Su, O. González-Martin, A. Weisgold, and E. Lee, "Considerations of implant abutment and crown contour: critical contour and subcritical contour," *The International Journal of Periodontics & Restorative Dentistry*, vol. 30, no. 4, pp. 335–343, 2010.

[27] T. Waki and J. Y. K. Kan, "Instalação e provisionalização imediatas de implante unitário anterossuperior com procedimentos de regeneração óssea guiada, enxerto de tecido conjuntivo e retalho posicionado coronalmente," *The International Journal of Esthetic Dentistry*, vol. 1, no. 3, pp. 442–453, 2016.

21

Localized Bone Loss Resulted from an Unlikely Cause in an 11-Year-Old Child

Bianca Tozi Portaluppe Bergantin,[1] Daniela Rios ⓘ,[1] Daniela Silva Barroso Oliveira,[2] Edmêr Silvestre Pereira Júnior,[3] João Adolfo Costa Hanemann ⓘ,[3] and Heitor Marques Honório ⓘ[1]

[1]Department of Pediatric Dentistry, Orthodontics and Public Health, Bauru School of Dentistry, University of São Paulo, Bauru, SP, Brazil
[2]Department of Clinic and Surgery, Federal University of Alfenas, Rua Gabriel Monteiro da Silva, 700, 37130000 Alfenas, MG, Brazil
[3]Department of Clinic and Surgery, Pediatric Dentistry, Federal University of Alfenas, Rua Gabriel Monteiro da Silva, 700, 37130000 Alfenas, MG, Brazil

Correspondence should be addressed to Heitor Marques Honório; heitorhonorio@usp.br

Academic Editor: Gavriel Chaushu

Periodontal diseases have several causes, amongst them, by foreign bodies. In this case report, an 11-year-old child who lived in a rural area and has never been treated by a dentist presented an extensive horizontal bone loss and edema on the region of tooth 44. The diagnosis of foreign body was obtained after biopsy, since an elastic band around the middle of the root tooth was found. The elastic band was not radiopaque, and the patient did not inform that she found the elastic band on the floor of the school and introduced the tooth by herself. Based on the case reported, it is concluded that anamnesis and clinical and radiographic examination are fundamental strategies to obtain the diagnosis, but sometimes, especially in children, there may be inconsistencies that can be elucidated by a biopsy.

1. Introduction

The term "periodontal disease" includes every pathological condition that causes damages to support and/or protection periodontium [1, 2]. Basically, these damages start with an inflammation of these tooth-supporting tissues [3], followed by the differentiation of osteoclasts induced by inflammatory cells that degrade the mineralized matrix, generating bone resorption [4], causing exposure of the roots, mobility, and tooth loss [5].

Periodontal diseases are not limited to adults [5, 6], and the occurrence of radiographic bone loss in children (2–11 years) has a significant prevalence (8.88%) [7]. The inflammation that generates bone resorption may be the consequence of several factors, among them the foreign body reaction that is a local gingival inflammatory condition due

to the introduction of foreign materials into the gingival connective tissue, causing ruptures in the epithelium. The most common examples of foreign bodies in the literature are amalgam restorations or penetration of materials during clinical procedures [8], such as elastic bands for tooth separations for orthodontic treatment [9].

The literature describes bone loss and mobility resulted from orthodontic elastic bands along the roots [10–17]. The early diagnosis improves the chance for a successful treatment [18]; however, when the patient reports no previous orthodontic treatment and the elastic band is radiolucent, it is very difficult to diagnose. This case report is of interest in that an 11-year-old child, who lived in a rural area, has never been treated by a dentist, presented an extensive horizontal bone loss and vestibular and lingual edema on the region of tooth 44, caused by an elastic band.

2. Case Report

An 11-year-old girl with no pain complaint and adequate oral hygiene reported mobility on the 44 teeth (Figure 1). Clinically, a reddish edema around the teeth, sessile, with an irregular surface, and no local irritant was found (Figure 2). In the anamnesis, the parents reported that the child had never been to a dentist. In addition, the child said that she did not put any object in the affected region. The radiography showed an extensive horizontal bone loss on the mesial and distal areas of tooth 44 (Figure 3). After clinical examination and anamnesis, the probable diagnosis of *pyogenic granuloma* was discarded because no trauma or local irritant [19] was found or reported. In the first visit, the professional irrigated the site with sodium iodide 2% and hydrogen peroxide, and beyond that, subgingival scaling was made. After these procedures, no foreign body was removed or identified. Therefore, a biopsy and the granuloma removal were planned in the next visit. The surgery started with anesthesia of the alveolar, lingual, and buccal nerve block, incision with scalpel blade, and tissue removal by excisional biopsy (Figure 4). During the surgery, the foreign body, an orthodontic elastic band, was found around the root's tooth (Figure 5). The elastic band was removed (Figure 6), the root scaling was performed, and the soft tissues were sutured (Figure 7). After 7 days, the patient returned for the suture removal, showing adequate healing (Figure 8). The patient never attended to the subsequent control schedules.

3. Discussion

Bone loss can be caused by accumulation of bacteria that release lipopolysaccharides that are recognized by toll-like receptors, initiating a signaling cascade and inducing secretion of proinflammatory proteins. However, this causal factor is rarer in children, being the more common bone loss caused by foreign body reaction, in which the presence of foreign materials lead to rupture of the epithelium and contact with the connective tissue generating local inflammatory reactions. In any of these cases, bone loss is a consequence of a degradation of tissue matrix proteins and immunoglobulins due to the differentiation of osteoclasts precursors in osteoclasts, causing a bone resorption and apical migration of the tissue (consequently of the foreign body) [2, 4]. According to the American Academy of Pediatric Dentistry, bone loss can also occur in the absence of local factors such as aggressive periodontitis, which is considered a disease of adolescents and young adults, and it can begin at any age and usually affects the entire dentition, with a generally genetic cause. In the case presented, the patient presented gingival edema witch discarded the diagnosis of pyogenic granuloma [20] by the presence of a periodontal pocket, with horizontal bone loss observed radiographically. However, clinically, it was not possible to observe the presence of supra and subgingival biofilm, which excluded the hypothesis of aggression by the presence of bacteria; on the other hand, as the bone loss was located in a single dental element, the hypothesis of the presence of periodontal

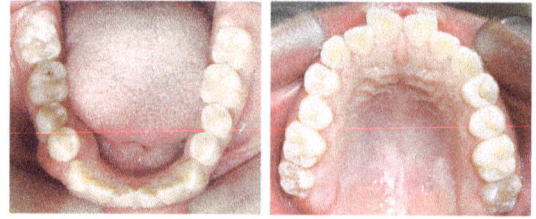

FIGURE 1: Adequate oral hygiene aspect.

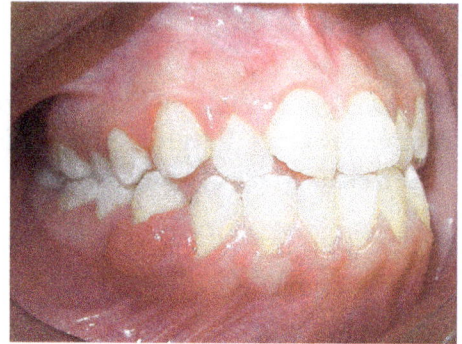

FIGURE 2: Edema around the 44 region.

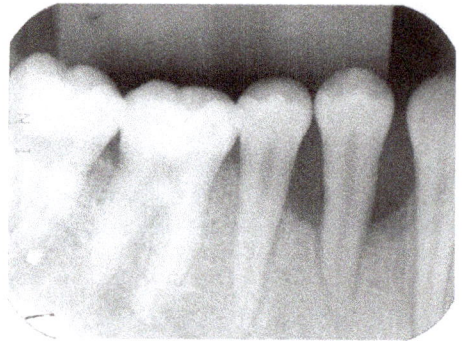

FIGURE 3: The radiographic image, where we can observe the extensive horizontal bone loss.

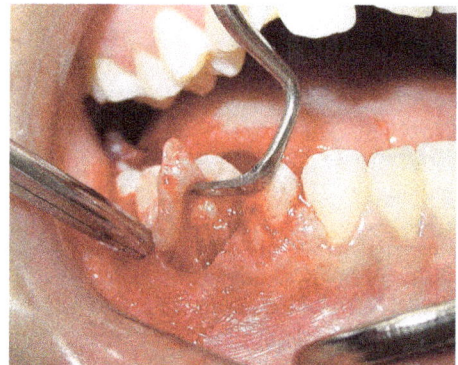

FIGURE 4: Excisional biopsy.

disease was also eliminated. Therefore, the remaining possible causal factor was foreign body or other type of oral lesion.

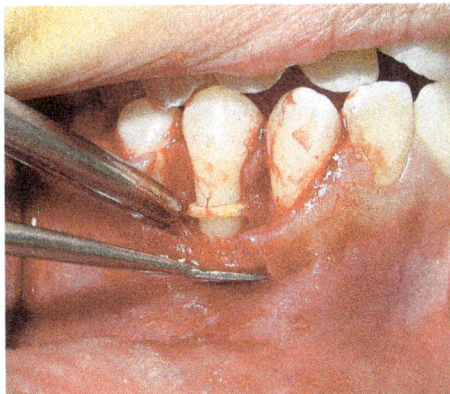

FIGURE 5: The orthodontic elastic band found.

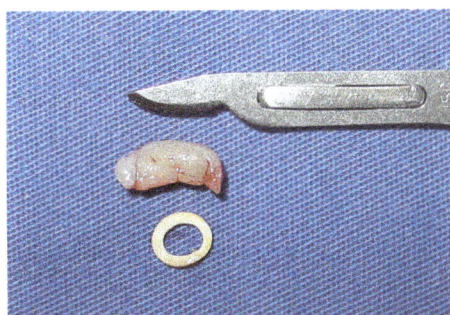

FIGURE 6: The elastic band and the tissue removed.

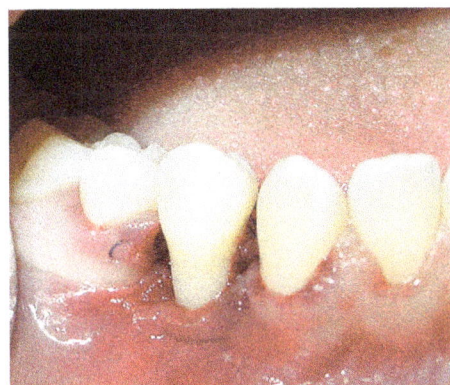

FIGURE 7: Immediate postoperative aspect.

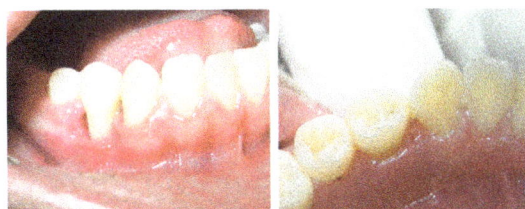

FIGURE 8: Aspect after seven days postoperative.

Orthodontic elastics are widely used for diastema correction, separation of teeth for band placement, and crossbite correction [21, 22]. These are left in place for a maximum of 1 week [19]. In cases where the elastic band is left over for a longer period, iatrogenic situations may occur [9], in which there is a great loss of bone and, in more severe cases, leads to loss of the dental element [19]. In the clinical case presented, the patient was from a rural area and reported having no previous experience with dental care, which made the hypothesis on the iatrogenic placement of the elastic discarded, since in the cases reported in the literature this was due to failure of the surgeon dentist [9–14]. Given the difficulty of diagnosis through clinical and radiographic examination, it was decided to perform the biopsy for histological analysis of the specimen. However, during the surgery, the presence of an orthodontic elastic band was detected around the tooth. After the dentist questioned the child of whom would have put the elastic band, she reported that she had forgotten to say it in the anamnesis, but she herself had put the elastic band found on the school floor.

In view of the above, we can observe that even if a good anamnesis is performed, children are often not able to adequately report the facts, due to oblivion or omission. Another point to be discussed is the quality of the orthodontic elastic band, which ideally must be radiopaque, allowing its detection in the radiographic exam. In addition, it might be also nontoxic, reducing the tissue adverse reaction [23]. However, this type of material is often illegally marketed, not following quality standards. In addition, the elastics are being used widely, due to the higher prevalence of malocclusions and, consequently, higher necessity of orthodontic treatment [24], causing unlikely use, as in the present case in which the child placed the elastic band, found on the school floor, which is equal to children who used appliance.

Although the biopsy, especially in children, seems to be a very invasive treatment, there are situations in which it is indicated and fundamental for the diagnosis. However, oftentimes, professionals opt for less invasive treatments, delaying the procedure, which can lead to worsening of the condition, making it difficult to treat [22]. Based on the case reported, it is concluded that anamnesis and clinical and radiographic examination are fundamental strategies to obtain the diagnosis, but sometimes, especially in children, there may be inconsistencies that can be elucidated by a biopsy.

References

[1] B. L. Pihlstrom, B. S. Michalowicz, and N. W. Johnson, "Periodontal diseases," *Lancet*, vol. 366, no. 9499, pp. 1809–1820, 2005.

[2] M. J. Novak, "Classification of disease and conditions affecting the periodontium," in *Carranza's Clinical Periodontology*, M. G. Newman and H. H. Takei, Eds., pp. 64–73, W. B. Saunders Company, San Diego CA, USA, 9th edition, 2002.

[3] H. Al-Ghutaimel, H. Riba, S. Al-Kahtani, and S. Al-Duhaimi, "Common periodontal diseases of children and adolescents," *International Journal of Dentistry*, vol. 2014, Article ID 850674, 7 pages, 2014.

[4] S. C. Holt, L. Kesavalu, S. Walker, and C. A. Genco, "Virulence factors of porphyromonas gingivalis," *Periodontology 2000*, vol. 20, no. 1, pp. 168–238, 1999.

[5] The American Academy of Periodontology, "Periodontal diseases of children and adolescences," *Journal of Periodontology*, vol. 67, pp. 57–62, 1996.

[6] M. R. Moreira, "Lesões bucais em pacientes pediátricos: estudo retrospectivo de 620 biópsias registradas no Laboratório de Patologia Bucal da Universidade Federal de Uberlândia-MG-Brasil," in *2006. 64 f. Dissertação (Mestrado em Ciências da Saúde)*, Universidade Federal de Uberlândia, Uberlândia, 2006.

[7] M. do Carmo Machado Guimarães, V. M. de Araújo, M. R. Avena, D. R. da Silva Duarte, and F. V. Freitas, "Prevalence of alveolar bone loss in healthy children treated at private pediatric dentistry clinics," *Journal of Applied Oral Science*, vol. 18, no. 3, pp. 285–290, 2010.

[8] J. E. Hirichs and M. J. NovakCarranza, Periodontia Clínica, "Classificação e epidemiologia das doenças periodontais," Elsevier, Rio de Janeiro, 2011.

[9] S. Tandon, A. Ahad, A. Kaur, F. Faraz, and Z. Chaudhary, "Orthodontic elastic embedded in gingiva for 7 years," *Case Reports in Dentistry*, vol. 2013, Article ID 212106, 4 pages, 2013.

[10] N. I. Zager and M. L. Barnett, "Severe bone loss in a child initiated by multiple orthodontic rubber bands: case report," *Journal of Periodontology*, vol. 45, no. 9, pp. 701–704, 1974.

[11] A. R. Goldstein and M. Schpero, "Retained ligature wire and periodontal health: report of a case," *American Journal of Orthodontics*, vol. 86, no. 4, pp. 315–318, 1984.

[12] Y. Zilberman, A. Shteyer, and B. Azaz, "Iatrogenic exfoliation of teeth by the incorrect use of orthodontic elastic bands," *Journal of the American Dental Association*, vol. 93, no. 1, pp. 89–93, 1976.

[13] I. Rubel, "Avulsion of central incisors by elastic bands with subsequent orthodontic treatment," *Journal of the American Dental Association*, vol. 100, no. 2, pp. 211-212, 1980.

[14] C. R. Caldwell, F. W. Worms, and D. J. Gatto, "Orthodontic and surgical intervention to arrest tooth loss secondary to subgingival elastic," *American Journal of Orthodontics*, vol. 78, no. 3, pp. 273–278, 1980.

[15] V. A. Marino, H. R. Fry, and R. G. Behrents, "Severe localized destruction of the periodontium secondary to subgingival displacement of an elastic band," *Journal of Periodontology*, vol. 59, no. 7, pp. 472–477, 1988.

[16] R. L. Finkbeiner, L. S. Nelson, and J. Killebrew, "Accidental orthodontic elastic band-induced periodontitis: orthodontic and laser treatment," *Journal of the American Dental Association*, vol. 128, no. 11, pp. 1565–1569, 1997.

[17] T. Becker and A. Neronov, "Orthodontic elastic separator-induced periodontal abscess: a case report," *Case Reports in Dentistry*, vol. 2012, Article ID 463903, 3 pages, 2012.

[18] A. R. Goldstein and M. Schpero, "Retained ligature wire and periodontal health," *American Journal of Orthodontics*, vol. 86, no. 4, pp. 315–318, 1984.

[19] A. da Costa Monini, M. de Sousa Guimarães, L. G. G. Júnior, L. Santos-Pinto, and J. Hebling, "Tooth separation: a risk-free procedure?," *American Journal of Orthodontics and Dentofacial Orthopedics*, vol. 142, no. 3, pp. 402–405, 2012.

[20] R. Kamal, P. Dahiya, and A. Puri, "Oral pyogenic granuloma: various concepts of etiopathogenesis," *Journal of Oral and Maxillofacial Pathology*, vol. 16, no. 1, pp. 79–82, 2012.

[21] W. F. Waggoner and K. D. Ray, "Bone loss in the permanent dentition as a result of improper orthodontic elastic band use: a case report," *Quintessence International*, vol. 20, no. 9, pp. 653–656, 1989.

[22] M. N. Al-Qutub, "Orthodontic elastic band-induced periodontitis – a case report," *The Saudi Dental Journal*, vol. 24, no. 1, pp. 49–53, 2012.

[23] M. M. Pithon, R. L. Santos, M. V. I. Oliveira, G. S. Mendes, and M. T. V. Romanos, "Avaliação da citotoxicidade de elásticos ortodônticos intermaxilares," *Matéria*, vol. 14, no. 1, pp. 689–693, 2009.

[24] P. Kumar, S. M. Londhe, A. Kotwal, and R. Mitra, "Prevalence of malocclusion and orthodontic treatment need in schoolchildren - an epidemiological study," *Medical Journal Armed Forces India*, vol. 69, no. 4, pp. 369–374, 2013.

22

Diode Laser-Assisted Surgical Therapy for Early Treatment of Oral Mucocele in a Newborn Patient: Case Report and Procedures Checklist

Marina Consuelo Vitale,[1] **Maria Francesca Sfondrini** ⓘ,[1] **Giorgio Alberto Croci,**[2] **Marco Paulli,**[2] **Lorenzo Carbone,**[1] **Paola Gandini,**[1] **and Andrea Scribante** ⓘ[1]

[1]Unit of Orthodontics and Paediatric Dentistry, Section of Dentistry, Department of Clinical, Surgical, Diagnostic and Paediatric Sciences, University of Pavia, Pavia, Italy
[2]Unit of Anatomic Pathology, Department of Molecular Medicine, University of Pavia and Fondazione IRCCS Policlinico San Matteo, Pavia, Italy

Correspondence should be addressed to Andrea Scribante; andrea.scribante@unipv.it

Academic Editor: Pia L. Jornet

Mucocele (also known as ranula or salivary gland mucous cyst) of the newborn is a lesion present on the intraoral cavity, with the potential to interfere with respiration and feeding. In the present report, a case of mucocele in a 4-month female patient has been described. As conventional surgery can be followed by several complications such as intraoperative bleeding, difficulties in wound healing, and maintenance of sterility during surgery, in the present case, the use of diode laser has been planned. A topic anesthesia with lidocaine gel was performed. A diode laser (810 nm wavelength, continuous wave mode, power output of 3 watt, and 0.4 mm diameter fiber optic) was set for excising the lesion. The tip was directed at an angle of 10 to 15°, moving around the base of the lesion with a circular motion. The procedure was completed in 3 minutes. The patient was visited with a follow-up of 2 weeks and 4 months after excision. The intraoral wound healed without complications, and no signs of infection or mass recurrence were noted. The histopathological examination confirmed the diagnosis of mucocele. On the basis of the results of the present case report, the use of diode laser can be easily performed also in a noncompliant newborn patient for successful excision of mucocele lesions, and checklist of clinical procedures has been described.

1. Introduction

Mucocele (also known as ranula or salivary gland mucous cyst) of the newborn has been extensively reported in Literature [1–3]. This benign lesion of the oral cavity could potentially interfere with respiration and feeding [4]. This condition in neonates represents a situation often creating anxiety and apprehension among parents. Early examination and prompt diagnosis can aid in prudent management and serve as baseline against the future course of the disease [5]. It is difficult for the clinician to establish an accurate diagnosis based only on clinical symptoms, so a biopsy with histological examination is necessary to exclude other lesions [6].

Conventional treatment of mucocele involves a surgical approach for excision with general or local anesthesia. This procedure can be followed by several complications such as intraoperative bleeding, difficulties in wound healing, and maintenance of sterility during surgery [7].

Some authors described the efficacy of lasers in the treatment of oral tissues problems for photodynamic therapy [8, 9] and surgical procedures [1, 10, 11]. Diode laser (with wavelengths varying between 800 and 980 nm) is poorly absorbed by hard dental tissue, is safe, and well indicated for soft oral tissue surgeries for cutting, vaporization, curettage, blood coagulation, and hemostasis in the oral region [12].

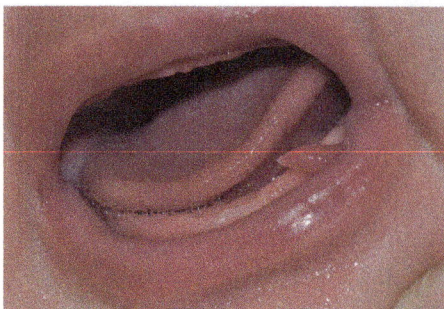

FIGURE 1: Initial intraoral photograph (age: 4 months).

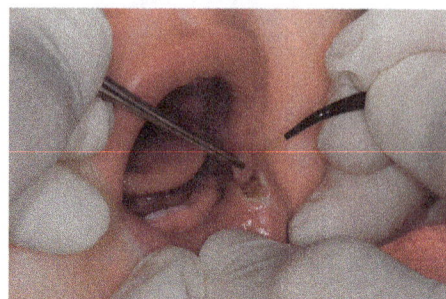

FIGURE 3: Laser-assisted lesion excision (age: 6 months).

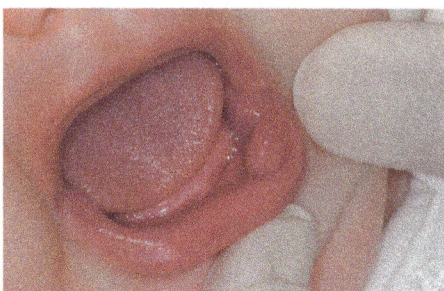

FIGURE 2: Intraoral photograph (age: 6 months).

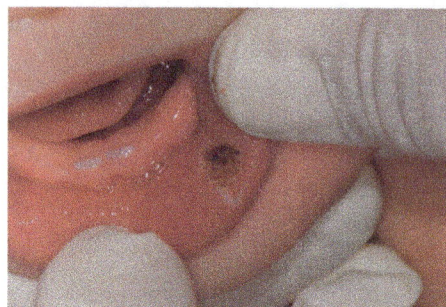

FIGURE 4: Intraoral photograph immediately after intervention.

To our knowledge, case reports presented in Literature concerning chairside laser treatments of mucocele are related to child, adolescent, and adult patients [1], but no case reports have been presented with newborn patients yet. The approach in newborn patients, due to their lack of compliance, has been reported in general anesthesia, with the relative problems and risks [4].

Therefore, the aim of the present manuscript was to present a case report about the use of a diode laser for chairside treatment of a mucocele in a newborn patient as a conservative and nonstressful method. The case has been described, and a checklist of clinical operative procedures has been proposed.

2. Case Report

2.1. Diagnosis and Etiology. A baby female, aged 4 months, was referred to our Orthodontics and Paediatric Dentistry Unit. The patient was receiving breast-feeding since birth. Her parents reported, during the first months of life, the spontaneous formation of a pink oblong vesicle in the left internal part of the lower lip (Figure 1). The color [13], the localization [14], and the shape [15] have been considered coherent with a mucocele lesion; however, a conclusive diagnosis requires histopathological examination. As spontaneous regression of these oral lesions has been reported [16], the parents planned only a further control.

After a month, the patient returned, and the lesion had a significant growth with a shape modification and appeared as a more regular bulla (Figure 2). Therefore, the excision intervention was planned. The size of lesion in the moment of surgery was about 10 mm × 6 mm.

2.2. Treatment Objectives. The objective of the treatment was mucocele treatment with topic anesthesia and laser-assisted excision.

2.3. Treatment Alternatives. The first possible alternative to the treatment was the delay of the intervention, thus planning only further controls, with the risk of lesion growth and feeding problems. Another alternative consisted in a conventional lancet surgical approach, with the consequent risks of intra- and postoperative bleeding and potential difficulties in wound healing. The last option was marsupialization that would allow lesion drainage without excision, but this technique is more fitted for larger lesions.

2.4. Treatment Progress. Written informed consent was obtained from the patient's parents to proceed with lesion excision with laser surgery. The patient and the whole staff wore protective glasses to prevent eye damage [17]. Local topic anesthesia was performed with lidocaine gel local application for one minute. Diode laser (Diode Laser, DMT Lissone, Italy) at 810 nm wavelength, continuous wave mode with a power output of 3 watt, and a 0.4 mm diameter fiber optic were set for excising the lesion. The tip was directed at an angle of 10 to 15°, moving around the base of the lesion with a circular motion [18] (Figure 3). It took 3 minutes to complete the procedure. The diode laser provided a combination of clean cutting of the tissue and hemostasis (Figure 4). The patient was discharged with necessary postoperative instructions for maintenance of good oral hygiene and keeping the area clean. No additional analgesic or antibiotic was recommended.

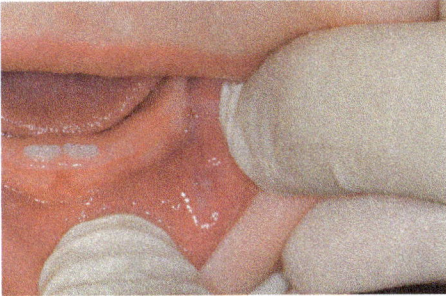

FIGURE 5: Healing (age: 6.5 months).

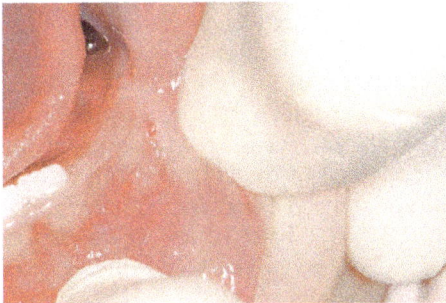

FIGURE 6: Follow-up (age: 10 months).

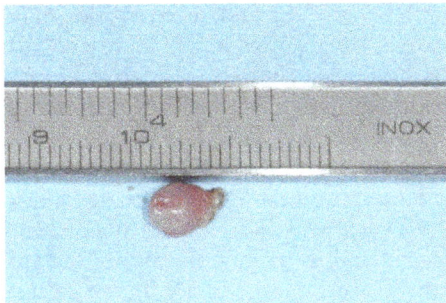

FIGURE 7: The lesion measured about 1 cm maximal length, displayed a polypoid fashion, and was covered by a smooth mucosal layer.

After excision, the lesion was immersed in formalin and then was sent to histopathologic service for evaluation.

2.5. Treatment Results. After excision, the patient had no signs of respiratory distress and no feeding difficulty was reported from the parents. The patient was visited with a follow-up of 2 weeks and 3 months. After 2 weeks follow-up (Figure 5), the intraoral wound healed without complications and no signs of infection or mass recurrence were noted. After 4 months (Figure 6) follow-up, the lesion healed completely and the patient had a functionally and developmentally normal mucosa without lesion recurrence. The patient demonstrated age-appropriate weight gain.

The histopathological examination confirmed the initial clinical diagnosis of mucocele. Grossly, the lesion displayed a polypoid fashion and was covered by a smooth mucosal layer (Figure 7). Histologic examination revealed a process

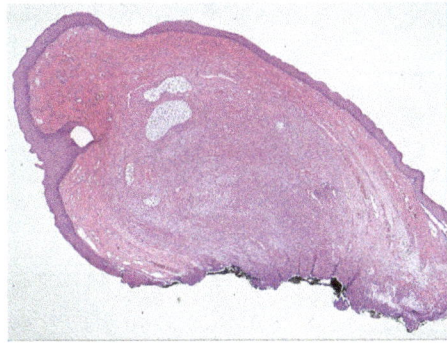

FIGURE 8: Histologic examination revealed a process deep seated within the submucosal connective tissue (HE, ×2 magnification).

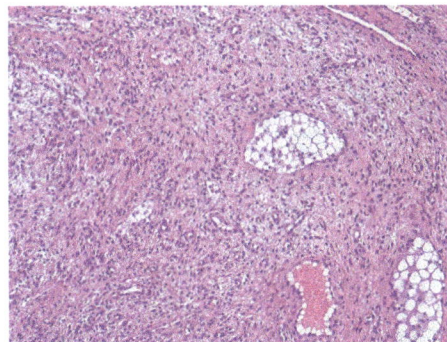

FIGURE 9: The lesion consisted of newly formed capillary vessels intermingled with a chronic, lymphohistiocytic inflammatory infiltrate and associated with deposition of extracellular mucin (HE, ×10 magnification).

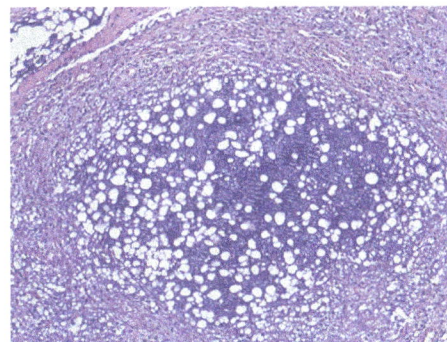

FIGURE 10: Extracellular mucin resulted Alcian blue positive (Alcian-PAS, ×20 magnification).

deep seated within the submucosal connective tissue (Figure 8), consisting of newly formed capillary vessels intermingled with a chronic, lymphohistiocytic inflammatory infiltrate and associated with deposition of extracellular mucin (Figure 9), the latter which resulted Alcian blue positive (Figure 10). Thus, the histopathologic picture was consistent with stromal reaction to extravasated mucin, possibly related to an injured, salivary gland mucous cyst (mucocele).

TABLE 1: Brief review of the dosimetry and techniques used in previous clinical reports.

Authors	Laser	Mode	Power setting	Wavelength
Kato and Wijeyeweera [10]	CO_2	Continuous	3 W or 4 W	$10.6\,\mu m$
Pedron et al. [24]	Diode	Continuous	2 W	810 nm
Wu et al. [1]	CO_2	Continuous	5 W	NA
Agarwal et al. [25]	Diode	Pulsed (10 ms)	1.3 W	940 nm
Chinta et al. [26]	Diode	Pulsed (50 ms)	2 W	810 nm
Ramkumar et al. [11]	Diode	Continuous	1.5 W	940 nm
Ahad et al. [27]	Diode	Pulsed (30 ms)	2 W	810 nm

3. Discussion

In the present report, a mucocele lesion in a baby female, aged 6 months, was treated with laser excision. Clinically, this lesion usually appears as an asymptomatic vesicle or bulla with a pink or bluish color [15]. The size can extend from 1 mm to some centimeters [19] and are most frequently located on the lower lip [14]. Mucocele lesions can be of two types: extravasation and retention mucoceles, the former affecting the lower lip most frequently [3].

In the present case, the lesion was pink, bulla-shaped with a size of 10 mm approximately, and was situated on the lower lip. These characteristics are coherent with typical aspects of these lesions, and for this reason, the diagnosis before the histologic report was of "suspected mucocele." This lesion is commonly due to alterations in the minor salivary glands and is occurring with a prevalence of 0.2 cases per 1,000 persons. Approximately 2.7% of patients are under the age of one [20]. However, the real frequency of oral mucocele is difficult to calculate, as many of these lesions recede spontaneously [16].

As occasional spontaneous regression has been reported for these lesions [21], the frequent monitoring for regression may be used as a management option. However, if the lesion continues growing or if it interferes with respiration or deglutition, conservative excision under anesthesia is recommended as the traditional treatment [13]. For these reasons, in the present report, parents, after the first visit, decided to plan only a control after a couple of months. During the second control, the lesion showed a significant increase in dimensions and volume so the parents accepted to plan an intervention.

We decided to avoid both marsupialization that is often planned for larger lesions [15] and conventional lancet surgical approach, with the consequent risk of bleeding and potential difficulty in wound healing [1]. Therefore, a laser-assisted excision was planned. The advantages of this technique over conventional surgical approach are multiple.

The first advantage is related to anesthesia. From a clinical point of view, a topic on anesthesia has been reported to be sufficient for pain control during laser application on soft tissue as lidocaine-containing products play an integral role in mucous anesthesia by providing patient comfort with minimal side effects [22]. This possibility allows the clinicians to avoid more invasive techniques, such as the injection, the sedation, and the general anesthesia.

The second advantage is related to procedure speed. The laser-assisted procedure is reported to require significant less time than the conventional approach during surgical excision of oral lesions, thus reducing patient discomfort [10]. Indeed, pain and time reduction are crucial aspects during therapy, especially for paediatric patients.

The third advantage is the lack of bleeding. Lasers provide cut and coagulation in one time so no bleeding is present during intervention. Moreover, no sutures are required at the end of the surgical procedure [23]. Previous authors showed laser-assisted mucocele excision [1, 10, 11, 24–27]. A brief review of the dosimetry and techniques used in previous clinical studies is reported in Table 1.

In the present study, after excision, the parents reported no problems in feeding, the intraoral alveolar wound healed without complications, and no signs of infection or mass recurrence were noted. Laser-assisted excision of oral lesions has been extensively reported in Literature, and no particular side effects have been showed [3]. A risk of recurrence is reported with mucoceles [1]. In the present report, at a follow-up of 4 months, the lesion showed no recurrence. Moreover, in the present report, the minor salivary gland that caused the mucocele has been presumably removed. However, the cauterization produced by laser either in the tissue removed and in the oral mucosa of the patient does not allow the total excision certainty. Therefore, a recurrence risk is always present, with a 5% to 7% risk [1, 15] for the anatomic region that has been treated.

On the basis of the present case report and Literature review, in clinical cases with a mucocele suspect, a procedure checklist could be considered as follows:

(i) Check the lesion coherence with mucocele characteristics (asymptomatic, bulla shape, pink or bluish color, 1 mm to several cm diameter, and location on the lower lip predominantly) [15].

(ii) If the lesion does not heal spontaneously after two weeks, the excision could be planned [21].

(iii) Intervention consist in topic anesthesia [22], protective glasses wearing [17], and lesion excision [18] with either diode (continuous or pulsed mode, 810 nm to 940 nm wavelength, and 1.3 to 3 W power output), or CO_2 (continuous mode, $10.6\,\mu m$ wavelength, and 3 W to 5 W power output) laser with a 0.4 mm fiber diameter and tip angulation of $10°$–$15°$approximately.

(iv) Surgical piece can be stored in formalin, if anatomopathological exam is needed.

(v) Check for recurrence after 1 to 6 months.

Certainly, before excision planning, the evaluation of lesion dimension and location is crucial. In fact, bigger manifestations (with a diameter of some centimeters) and lesions localized in hard-to-reach areas (such as the sublingual mucosa) are deserved for a conventional general surgery approach.

4. Conclusions

After topical anesthesia, diode laser excision of mucocele lesions could be applied also in newborn patients with a few-minute surgical approach. This procedure is particularly safe and effective.

Ethical Approval

The study was approved by the Unit Internal Review Board Committee (2016/0318).

Consent

The patient was treated after parental approval and in agreement with international guidelines.

References

[1] C. W. Wu, Y. H. Kao, C. M. Chen, H. J. Hsu, C. M. Chen, and I. Y. Huang, "Mucoceles of the oral cavity in pediatric patients," *Kaohsiung Journal of Medical Sciences*, vol. 27, no. 7, pp. 276–279, 2011.

[2] P. R. Martins-Filho, T. de Santana Santos, M. R. Piva et al., "A multicenter retrospective cohort study on pediatric oral lesions," *Journal of Dentistry for Children*, vol. 82, no. 2, pp. 84–90, 2015.

[3] S. Patil, R. S. Rao, B. Majumdar, M. Jafer, M. Maralingannavar, and A. Sukumaran, "Oral lesions in neonates," *International Journal of Clinical Pediatric Dentistry*, vol. 9, pp. 131–138, 2016.

[4] M. M. George, O. Mirza, K. Solanki, J. Goswamy, and M. P. Rothera, "Serious neonatal airway obstruction with massive congenital sublingual ranula and contralateral occurrence," *Annals of Medicine and Surgery*, vol. 4, no. 2, pp. 136–139, 2015.

[5] H. Rodríguez, R. De Hoyos Parra, G. Cuestas, J. Cambi, and D. Passali, "Congenital mucocele of the tongue: a case report and review of the literature," *Turkish Journal of Pediatrics*, vol. 56, no. 2, pp. 199–202, 2014.

[6] O. K. Adegun, P. H. Tomlins, E. Hagi-Pavli, D. L. Bader, and F. Fortune, "Quantitative optical coherence tomography of fluid-filled oral mucosal lesions," *Lasers in Medical Science*, vol. 28, no. 5, pp. 1249–1255, 2013.

[7] G. R. Fritz, P. J. Stern, and M. Dickey, "Complications following mucous cyst excision," *Journal of Hand Surgery*, vol. 22, no. 2, pp. 222–225, 1997.

[8] J. C. Tsai, C. P. Chiang, H. M. Chen et al., "Photodynamic therapy of oral dysplasia with topical 5-aminolevulinic acid and light-emitting diode array," *Lasers in Surgery and Medicine*, vol. 34, no. 1, pp. 18–24, 2004.

[9] A. R. Barcessat, I. Huang, F. P. Rosin, D. dos Santos Pinto Jr., D. Maria Zezell, and L. Corrêa, "Effect of topical 5-ALA mediated photodynamic therapy on proliferation index of keratinocytes in 4-NQO-induced potentially malignant oral lesions," *Journal of Photochemistry and Photobiology B: Biology*, vol. 126, pp. 33–41, 2013.

[10] J. Kato and R. L. Wijeyeweera, "The effect of CO_2 laser irradiation on oral soft tissue problems in children in Sri Lanka," *Photomedicine and Laser Surgery*, vol. 25, no. 4, pp. 264–268, 2007.

[11] S. Ramkumar, L. Ramkumar, N. Malathi, and R. Suganya, "Excision of mucocele using diode laser in lower lip," *Case Reports in Dentistry*, vol. 2016, Article ID 1746316, 4 pages, 2016.

[12] M. B. Amaral, I. Z. Freitas, H. Pretel, M. H. Abreu, and R. A. Mesquita, "Low level laser effect after micro-marsupialization technique in treating ranulas and mucoceles: a case series report," *Lasers in Medical Science*, vol. 27, no. 6, pp. 1251–1255, 2012.

[13] R. Conrad and M. C. Perez, "Congenital granular cell epulis," *Archives of Pathology & Laboratory Medicine*, vol. 138, no. 1, pp. 128–131, 2014.

[14] M. Shapira and S. Akrish, "Mucoceles of the oral cavity in neonates and infants–report of a case and literature review," *Pediatric Dermatology*, vol. 31, no. 2, pp. e55–e58, 2014.

[15] C. M. Piazzetta, C. Torres-Pereira, and J. M. Amenábar, "Micro-marsupialization as an alternative treatment for mucocele in pediatric dentistry," *International Journal of Paediatric Dentistry*, vol. 22, no. 5, pp. 318–323, 2012.

[16] D. T. Oliveira, A. Consolaro, and F. J. Freitas, "Histopathological spectrum of 112 cases of mucocele," *Brazilian Dental Journal*, vol. 4, no. 1, pp. 29–36, 1993.

[17] C. Sweeney, "Laser safety in dentistry," *General Dentistry*, vol. 56, no. 7, pp. 653–659, 2008.

[18] M. Asnaashari, S. Azari-Marhabi, S. Alirezaei, and N. Asnaashari, "Clinical application of 810 nm diode laser to remove gingival hyperplasic lesion," *Journal of Lasers in Medical Sciences*, vol. 4, no. 2, pp. 96–98, 2013.

[19] I. Mínguez-Martinez, C. Bonet-Coloma, J. Ata-Ali-Mahmud, C. Carrillo-García, M. Peñarrocha-Diago, and M. Peñarrocha-Diago, "Clinical characteristics, treatment, and evolution of 89 mucoceles in children," *Journal of Oral and Maxillofacial Surgery*, vol. 68, no. 10, pp. 2468–2471, 2010.

[20] A. F. Gatti, M. M. Moreti, S. V. Cardoso, and L. V. Loyola, "Mucus extravasation phenomenon in newborn babies: report of two cases," *International Journal of Paediatric Dentistry*, vol. 11, no. 1, pp. 74–77, 2001.

[21] P. Ritwik, R. B. Brannon, and R. J. Musselman, "Spontaneous regression of congenital epulis: a case report and review of the literature," *Journal of Medical Case Reports*, vol. 4, no. 1, pp. 331–334, 2010.

[22] K. Greveling, E. P. Prens, L. Liu, and M. B. van Doorn, "Non-invasive anaesthetic methods for dermatological laser procedures: a systematic review," *Journal of the European Academy of Dermatology and Venereology*, vol. 31, no. 7, pp. 1096–1110, 2017.

[23] A. Karimi, F. Sobouti, S. Torabi et al., "Comparison of carbon dioxide laser with surgical blade for removal of epulis fissuratum. A randomized clinical trial," *Journal of Lasers in Medical Sciences*, vol. 7, no. 3, pp. 201–204, 2016.

[24] I. G. Pedron, V. C. Galletta, L. H. Azevedo, and L. Corrêa, "Treatment of mucocele of the lower lip with diode laser in pediatric patients: presentation of 2 clinical cases," *Pediatric Dentistry*, vol. 32, no. 7, pp. 539–541, 2010.

[25] G. Agarwal, A. Mehra, and A. Agarwal, "Laser vaporization of extravasation type of mucocele of the lower lip with 940-nm diode laser," *Indian Journal of Dental Research*, vol. 24, no. 2, p. 278, 2013.

[26] M. Chinta, A. J. Saisankar, C. Birra, and P. K. Kanumuri, "Successful management of recurrent mucocele by diode laser and thermoplasticised splint as an adjunctive therapy," *BMJ Case reports*, pii: bcr2016216354, 2016.

[27] A. Ahad, S. Tandon, A. K. Lamba, F. Faraz, P. Anand, and A. Aleem, "Diode laser assisted excision and low level laser therapy in the management of mucus extravasation cysts: a case series," *Journal of Lasers in Medical Sciences*, vol. 8, no. 3, pp. 155–159, 2017.

23

Gingival Reactive Lesions in Orally Rehabilitated Patients by Free Revascularized Flap

Gianluca Tenore (ID), **Ahmed Mohsen** (ID), **Giorgio Pompa**, **Edoardo Brauner** (ID), **Andrea Cassoni**, **Valentino Valentini**, **Antonella Polimeni** (ID), **and Umberto Romeo** (ID)

Department of Oral and Maxillofacial Sciences, "Sapienza" University of Rome, Rome, Italy

Correspondence should be addressed to Ahmed Mohsen; ahmed.mohsen@uniroma1.it

Academic Editor: Jose López-López

The aim is to discuss four cases of gingival reactive hyperplastic lesions in patients with a history of excision of oral neoplastic lesions and rehabilitation by a free revascularized flap of the iliac crest. One female and 3 male patients were referred due to the presence of exophytic lesions at the rehabilitated sites. The clinical examination revealed that the poor oral hygiene was the common trigger factor in all the cases, in addition to trauma from the upper left second molar in the first case, pericoronitis related to a partially erupted lower right third molar in the third case, and poor stability of an upper removable partial denture in the fourth case. All the cases were subjected to elimination of these suspected triggering factors, exclusion of dysplasia, excisional biopsy by CO2 laser, and five follow-up visits. The histological examination of all the cases confirmed the diagnosis of pyogenic granuloma. These presented cases suggest that the limitations in oral functions and maintaining the oral hygiene measures following the free revascularized flap reconstruction surgery probably played a role in the development of gingival reactive hyperplastic lesions with presence of trigger factors such as local trauma, chronic infection, or inadequate prosthesis.

1. Introduction

Reactive hyperplastic lesion is defined as an excessive proliferation of connective tissue in response to chronic irritation. In the oral cavity, the gingival reactive hyperplastic lesions are pyogenic granuloma (PG), peripheral fibroma, fibroepithelial hyperplasia, peripheral ossifying fibroma, and peripheral giant-cell granuloma. The gingival reactive hyperplastic lesions are commonly described as "epulides," which is a Greek word, means "on the gingiva." However, this commonly used term is only describing lesions clinically present on the gingiva without specifying the nature of the lesion [1, 2].

PG was firstly described in 1897 by Poncet and Dor [3]. It is defined to be an inflammatory hyperplasia that usually exists in response to local low-grade irritants, traumatic injury, hormonal change, or certain medications. Focal epithelial hyperplasia is preferred instead of its classic term "PG" because the lesion is not precisely a granuloma or an infection [1, 4].

PG has a more female incidence than male with a ratio of 3 : 2. The most common site is the keratinized gingiva in about 75% of cases, followed, respectively, by tongue, lips, and buccal mucosa. It occurs more commonly in the maxilla than in the mandible and in the anterior region than the posterior [4]. Presence of periodontal disease and dental calculus are frequently suspected as initiating causative factors. In the last few years, PG and peripheral giant-cell granuloma have been considered the most common reactive lesions that appeared in association with implants. Elimination of triggering factors and surgical removal are recommended in the management protocol [1, 2].

The reconstruction of bone continuity defects and solving some complications such as facial contour disfigurement by a free revascularized flap (FRF) have become a valuable part in the management of head and neck cancers. The idea of FRF is the transplantation of bone segment with muscle and skin allowing a simultaneous reconstruction of hard and soft tissues [5].

The high success rate of FRF reconstruction is about 95–97% due to the refinement of microvascular and magnification instruments; however, rare complications still occur. The complications are divided into recipient site and donor site complications. The most common complications of recipient site are related to vascular thrombosis [6].

Many cases of hyperplastic/inflammatory response and formation of granulation tissues around implant abutments in the orally rehabilitated sites by FRF are reported. Some authors speculate that the unsuitability of skin tissues around implants and the negative reaction of the skin in the oral cavity may be the reason of this complication [5].

Presented here are four cases of gingival reactive lesions (mainly PG) in patients with a history of excision of oral neoplastic lesions and rehabilitation by a FRF of the iliac crest.

2. Materials and Methods

The cases are 1 female and 3 males. The management was started with full clinical examination consisting of medical, dental history, and radiographic investigation.

Suspected triggering factors were diagnosed and eliminated for each patient. Conventional blade incisional biopsy was performed after two weeks of the first visit. All the collected biopsy samples were fixed in a 10% neutral buffered formalin solution. The histopathological evaluation confirmed the absence of dysplasia in all the samples.

All the patients were informed about the advantages and disadvantages of laser surgery, signed an informed consent, and managed by the same surgeon.

Excisional biopsies were performed with local anesthesia (mepivacaine) by carbon dioxide (CO_2) laser (wavelength of 10,600 nm; model SMART US-20D, DEKA®, Florence, Italy), with these parameters: power of 1.5–1.7 watts on pulsed wave (PW), frequency of 100 Hz, (power density 1432.12 W/cm^2, energy density 14.32 J/cm^2), and spot diameter of 400 μm [7].

A 0.2% chlorhexidine spray (Corsodyl spray, GlaxoSmithKline Consumer Healthcare S.p.A., Baranzate, Milan, Italy) and a 0.5 ml of amino acids and sodium hyaluronate gel (Aminogam gel, Errekappa Euroterapici Spa, Milan, Italy) were prescribed three times daily for one week. The patients were informed to eat cold and soft food and to avoid hot and spicy food on the day of the intervention.

Five follow-up visits were performed according to this schedule: one week, three weeks, three months, six months, and one year after the surgery, in order to evaluate the healing process and the possibility of recurrence.

3. Case Series

3.1. Case I. A 28-year-old female complained of an intraoral swelling in the lower left region. This swelling appeared few months ago. There was a complaint of bleeding on brushing without pain. Regarding her medical and dental history, she was suffering from ossifying fibroma at the left premolar-molar region of the mandible (Figure 1). It was excised and

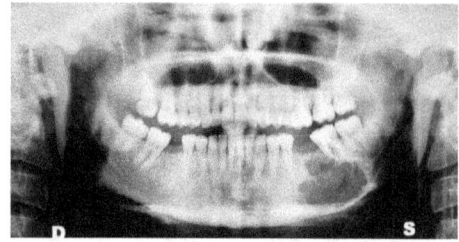

FIGURE 1: Panoramic X-ray before the excision of ossifying fibroma.

simultaneously rehabilitated by a FRF of iliac crest in 2013 (Figure 2).

The oral examination revealed that an erythematous exophytic sessile lesion with granulomatous appearance and soft-elastic consistency on the lower left retromolar region. This lesion developed after approximately 2 years of the reconstruction by FRF (Figure 3).

A presence of mechanical irritation at the lesion area related to the upper second left molar was observed. Radiographic investigation did not show any bone resorption in relation to the lesion.

The provisional diagnosis was probably a reactive lesion like PG or peripheral giant-cell granuloma. Routine blood tests, exclusion of dysplasia by cold-blade incisional biopsy, and elimination of contributing triggering factors were done. Smoothing of the cusp tips of the upper left second molar was done in addition to improvement of the oral hygiene.

Complete excision of the lesion by CO_2 laser was performed under local anesthesia with the help of Allis forceps. The histological examination of the excised lesion confirmed the diagnosis of PG (Figure 4).

3.2. Case II. A 58-year-old male had a history of ameloblastoma at the right side of the body of the mandible. Excision and hemimandibulectomy were performed in 2011 with simultaneous reconstruction by a FRF of the iliac crest. It was rehabilitated with five prosthetic implants eight months later. He came for consultation of an intraoral swelling in the lower right area that appeared a few months ago after about 3 years of the reconstruction by FRF.

The oral examination showed an exophytic lesion, mostly sessile with granulomatous appearance and soft-elastic consistency related to the implants in the right incisors bicuspids region, from the lower right central incisor region to the first molar region on the same side. The radiographic investigation did not show any bone resorption in relation to the lesion around the implants.

Routine blood tests, exclusion of dysplasia by cold-blade incisional biopsy, and elimination of contributing triggering factors were performed. It was suggested that the triggering factor was the poor oral hygiene, thus the prosthetic crowns and bridge were removed for three weeks to facilitate the control of bacterial infection and to promote better tissue regeneration. Complete excision of the lesion by CO_2 laser was performed under local anesthesia with the help of suture 3-0.

Another surgical intervention was performed with CO_2 laser for recontouring the gingiva around the implants and to facilitate the cementing of implant prosthesis.

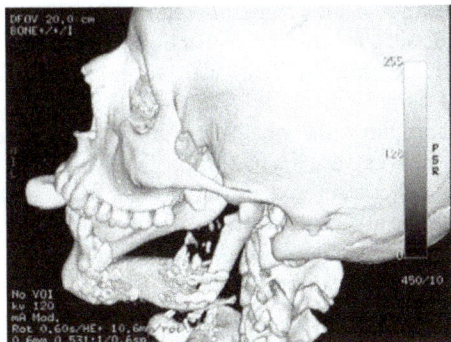

FIGURE 2: Radiographic image after reconstruction by FRF.

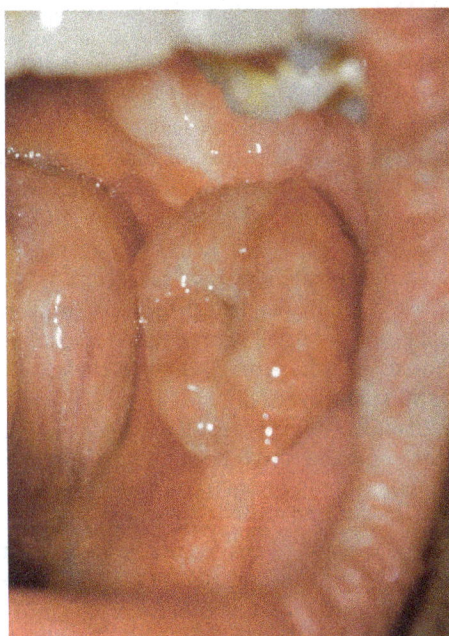

FIGURE 3: Clinical preoperative.

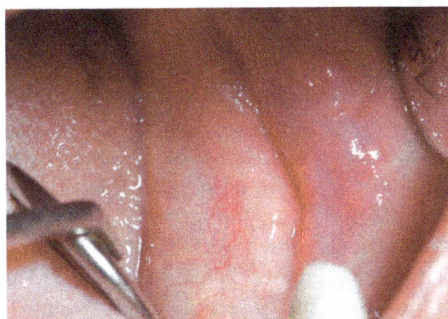

FIGURE 4: One-year follow-up.

In the three-month follow-up visit, a recurrence was observed. A further intervention was performed by CO_2 laser, with motivating the patient on the importance of maintaining the oral hygiene measures in order to ascertain the complete elimination of triggering factors. The histological examination confirmed the diagnosis of PG.

3.3. Case III. A 19-year-old male was referred for consultation of a painless mass in the right retromolar area that developed few weeks ago. The medical and dental history revealed that in 2015 an excision of moderately differentiated mucoepidermoid carcinoma at the upper right posterior molar region and hemimaxillectomy were carried out with simultaneous reconstruction by a FRF of the iliac crest (Figures 5 and 6).

The oral examination revealed an exophytic, mostly pedunculated lesion, with irregular granulomatous appearance and elastic consistency on the lower right retromolar area related to a partially erupted lower right third molar (Figure 7). The radiographic investigation did not show any bone resorption at the site of the lesion.

Routine blood tests, exclusion of dysplasia by cold-blade incisional biopsy, and elimination of contributing triggering factors were performed. It was decided to excise the lesion by CO_2 laser under local anesthesia and to extract the lower right third molar which might be the cause of chronic irritation.

The histological examination revealed a benign lesion with vascular structures and diffuse inflammatory infiltrate of granulocytes and neutrophils (Figure 8).

3.4. Case IV. A 21-year-old male was examined in our outpatient clinic complaining of a painless swelling in the upper left posterior region. Regarding his medical and dental history, left hemimaxillectomy, adenoidectomy, and partial removal of zygoma were carried out in 2001 due to a rhabdomyosarcoma in the left maxillary sinus. It was simultaneously reconstructed by a FRF of iliac crest, followed by radiotherapy and chemotherapy before and after the surgical intervention.

The oral examination showed exophytic, mostly pedunculated lesion with irregular granulomatous appearance and elastic consistency on the upper left posterior region related to the buccal flange and the fitting surface of the upper removable partial denture (RPD). The radiographic investigation did not show any bone resorption at the site of the lesion.

Contributing triggering factor was the poor stability of RPD. It was decided not to wear the RPD for two weeks. Routine blood tests, exclusion of dysplasia by cold-blade incisional biopsy, and the excision of the lesion by CO_2 laser under local anesthesia were performed. The histological examination revealed a benign lesion with vascular structures and diffuse inflammatory infiltrate of granulocytes and neutrophils, in addition to focal aspects of abscess formation.

Deepening of the buccal vestibule by CO_2 laser after the three-week follow-up has been done responding to a request from the prosthodontic department, to remake the RPD with better stability.

4. Discussion

The management of head and neck cancer has been improved by the introduction of microvascular surgery and FRF reconstruction. The ability of tissue transfer from a distant site enables the surgeons to reconstruct the bone and the

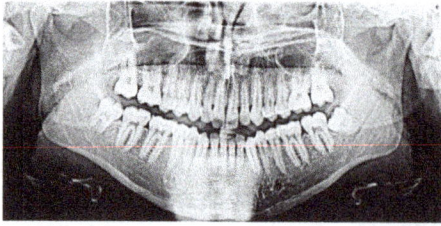

FIGURE 5: Panoramic X-ray before the excision of mucoepidermoid carcinoma.

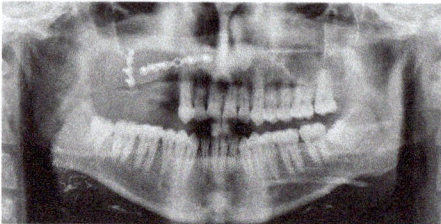

FIGURE 6: Panoramic X-ray after reconstruction by FRF.

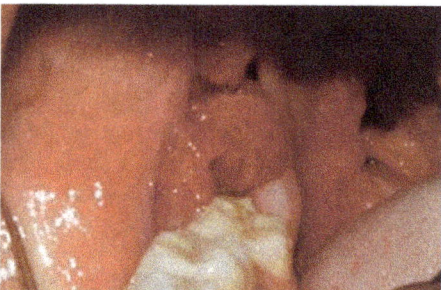

FIGURE 7: Clinical preoperative.

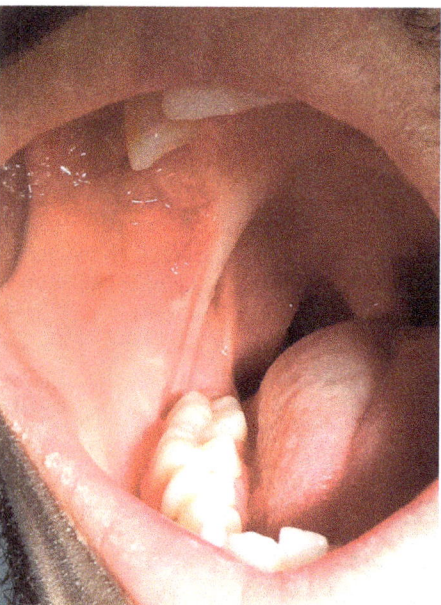

FIGURE 8: One-year follow-up.

soft tissues in a single-staged procedure [8]. The most common donor sites for the reconstruction of maxilla and mandible with FRF are the iliac crest, scapula, radial forearm, and fibula flap [5].

Few complications of FRF in the recipient sites are reported such as vascular thrombosis and second primary squamous cell carcinoma (SCC). Many factors have been proposed to be associated with the development of complications after FRF reconstruction such as patients' age, tobacco use, and prolonged surgical time [8–10].

There are four suggested hypotheses for the development of SCC as a complication of FRF; which are the presence of cancer cells into the flap during the implementation of tumor ablation, lymphatic dissemination of the original tumor, the existence of another tumor in the donor site before raising the flap, and the exposure of the skin of the flap to a stimulus in the oral environment that is not normally experienced [8].

The etiology of PG is still unclear. About 30–50% of the patients with PG have a history of local trauma. Infection and poor oral hygiene are frequently reported as triggering factors. Also, the hormonal cause may be added to these factors [4].

In a retrospective study by Jané-salas et al., it is suggested adding incorrect or inadequate prosthesis (implant cap or healing cap, poorly adjusted suprastructures, etc.) as possible causative factors [1]. In general, the association of PG with implants is still controversial.

In the literature, it is reported a presence of hyperplastic/inflammatory response and formation of granulation tissues around implant abutments that are implemented in orally rehabilitated sites by FRF [5]. Anitua and Pinas stated that the implant-related PG seems to be a response to the same stimulus that triggers tooth-related PG. They confirmed the absence of significant correlation between PG and the marginal bone loss around dental implants [6].

In the presented cases, there is only one case of PG around implants in the rehabilitated sites. The poor oral hygiene was the common trigger factor in all the cases, in addition to trauma from the upper left second molar in the first case, pericoronitis related to a partially erupted lower right third molar in the third case, and the poor stability of an upper RPD in the fourth case.

The incidence of recurrence of PG is estimated to be between 2.9 and 8.2%, with a slight increase in cases associated with implants [1]. In the second case, the recurrence was observed probably due to the incomplete elimination of suspected triggering factors. While in the other three cases, the recurrence was not observed. These suggest that the reconstruction by a FRF may be an aggravating condition rather than being a triggering factor of PG.

It seems that the triggering factors are aggravated due to the limitation in oral functions, the difficulty of maintaining the oral hygiene measures following the reconstruction surgery, and the difference in nature between the skin of flap and the normal oral tissues when they are subjected to stimuli, resulting in the development of PG in relation to the site of reconstruction rather than in the common sites that are reported in the literature.

PG is histologically characterized by a prominent capillary growth in hyperplastic granulation tissue. The presence of little vascular fibrotic septa separating a clustered or medullary pattern of the blood vessels leads sometimes to considering PG as a polypoid form of capillary hemangioma [6].

The histological reports of the third and the fourth cases were not with a definitive diagnosis; therefore, these cases were confirmed to be PG through the consultation of an oral pathologist and the clinical picture.

The differential diagnosis of PG includes peripheral giant-cell granuloma, peripheral ossifying fibroma, hemangioma, conventional granulation tissue, and hyperplastic gingival inflammation. In some cases, malignant lesions, such as metastatic carcinoma, melanotic melanoma, or non-Hodgkin's lymphoma, can be a differential diagnosis [3].

5. Conclusion

These presented cases suggest that the limitations in oral functions and the difficulty of maintaining the oral hygiene measures due to the FRF reconstruction surgery with the presence of trigger factors such as local trauma, chronic infection, or inadequate prosthesis probably played a role in the development of gingival reactive hyperplastic lesions.

Consent

Written informed consent was obtained from all the patients.

Authors' Contributions

All the authors contributed to the work-up of this case series and the manuscript has been reviewed and approved by all the authors.

References

[1] E. Jané-salas, R. Albuquerque, A. Font-muñoz, B. González-navarro, A. Estrugo Devesa, and J. López-López, "Pyogenic granuloma/peripheral giant-cell granuloma associated with implants," *International Journal of Dentistry*, vol. 2015, Article ID 839032, 9 pages, 2015.

[2] P. K. Verma, R. Srivastava, H. C. Baranwal, T. P. Chaturvedi, A. Gautam, and A. Singh, "Pyogenic granuloma - hyperplastic lesion of the gingiva: case reports," *The Open Dentistry Journal*, vol. 6, pp. 153–156, 2012.

[3] R. Fekrazad, H. Nokhbatolfoghahaei, F. Khoei, and K. A. Kalhori, "Pyogenic granuloma: surgical treatment with Er:YAG laser," *Journal of Lasers in Medical Sciences*, vol. 5, no. 4, pp. 199–205, 2014.

[4] I. Dojcinovic, M. Richter, and T. Lombardi, "Occurrence of a pyogenic granuloma in relation to a dental implant," *Journal of Oral and Maxillofacial Surgery*, vol. 68, no. 8, pp. 1874–1876, 2010.

[5] M. Chiapasco, F. Biglioli, L. Autelitano, E. Romeo, and R. Brusati, "Clinical outcome of dental implants placed in fibula-free flaps used for the reconstruction of maxillo-mandibular defects following ablation for tumors or osteoradionecrosis," *Clinical Oral Implants Research*, vol. 17, no. 2, pp. 220–228, 2006.

[6] E. Anitua and L. Pinas, "Pyogenic granuloma in relation to dental implants: clinical and histopathological findings," *Journal of Clinical and Experimental Dentistry*, vol. 7, no. 4, pp. e447–e450, 2015.

[7] G. Palaia, A. Del Vecchio, A. Impellizzeri et al., "Histological ex vivo evaluation of peri-incisional thermal effect created by a new-generation CO_2 superpulsed laser," *The Scientific World Journal*, vol. 2014, Article ID 345685, 6 pages, 2014.

[8] E. M. Genden, A. Rinaldo, C. Suárez, W. I. Wei, P. J. Bradley, and A. Ferlito, "Complications of free flap transfers for head and neck reconstruction following cancer resection," *Oral Oncology*, vol. 40, no. 10, pp. 979–984, 2004.

[9] Y. S. Lim, J. S. Kim, N. G. Kim, K. S. Lee, J. H. Choi, and S. W. Park, "Free flap reconstruction of head and neck defects after oncologic ablation: one surgeon's outcomes in 42 cases," *Archives of Plastic Surgery*, vol. 41, no. 2, pp. 148–152, 2014.

[10] K. Bozikov and Z. M. Arnez, "Factors predicting free flap complications in head and neck reconstruction," *Journal of Plastic, Reconstructive & Aesthetic Surgery*, vol. 59, no. 7, pp. 737–742, 2006.

24

Garre's Osteomyelitis of the Mandible Caused by Infected Tooth

Hayati Murat Akgül,[1] Fatma Çağlayan,[1] Sevcihan Günen Yılmaz,[2] and Gözde Derindağ [ID][1]

[1]Department of Oral and Maxillofacial Radiology, Faculty of Dentistry, Ataturk University, Erzurum, Turkey
[2]Department of Oral and Maxillofacial Radiology, Faculty of Dentistry, Akdeniz University, Antalya, Turkey

Correspondence should be addressed to Gözde Derindağ; gozde.derindag@atauni.edu.tr

Academic Editor: Tommaso Lombardi

Aim. Garre's osteomyelitis is a local thickening of the periosteum caused by a slight irritation or infection. We aimed to present the extraoral, intraoral, and radiographic findings and postoperative pursuits of two patients diagnosed with Garre's osteomyelitis. In this case report, although clinical findings indicate infection source, these clinical findings are strongly supported by cone-beam computed tomography images. In addition, it can be seen that when we have followed the case I, we have chosen the right path in treatment. *Case Reports*. Two patients presented to our clinic due to severe swelling and facial asymmetry in the right and left mandibular region. As a result of the clinical and radiological examinations, the patients were diagnosed with Garre's osteomyelitis. Infected teeth that were responsible for the formation of Garre's osteomyelitis were extracted under antibiotic treatment in both cases. A complete improvement in postoperative control was observed in case I. On the other hand, the other case could not be followed up postoperatively. *Conclusion*. In Garre's osteomyelitis, new bone formation can occur in many pathological conditions. Therefore, it should be distinguished from other pathologies that cause new bone formation, such as Ewing's sarcoma, Caffey disease, and fibrous dysplasia.

1. Introduction

Garre's osteomyelitis, which was first described by Carl Garre in 1893, is a chronic nonsuppurative sclerotic bone inflammation characterized by a rigid bony swelling at the periphery of the jaw [1–4]. It is most commonly seen in men aged below 30 years [1, 2, 5, 6]. The mandible is more often affected than the maxilla, and it is most generally seen at the lower margin of the mandible in the mandibular first molar region [1, 3, 4, 6, 7]. There is typically a nontender swelling on the medial and lateral sides of the jaw [1, 5, 8, 9]. The size of the swelling may vary from 1-2 cm to the involvement of the entire length of the jaw on the affected side; the thickness of the cortex can reach 2-3 cm [1].

Clinically, Garre's osteomyelitis results in facial asymmetry, since the lesion unilaterally expands to the outer surface of the bone [3–5, 8, 9]. Pain is not a characteristic finding, although severe pain can occur if the lesion is secondarily infected [1, 6]. While it is referred to as nonsuppurative, Garre's osteomyelitis has sometimes been seen to result in a fistula on the skin [3, 6]. The other symptoms are fever, lymphadenopathy, and leukocytosis [1, 3].

There is no macroscopically suppurative lithic area in cases of Garre's osteomyelitis, although histopathological examinations have detected microabscesses and microsequesters [7, 10].

The radiographic appearance varies with the duration of the lesion and the degree of calcification. During the early period, a thin crust-like convex layer appears over the cortex. As the event continues, the cortex is thickened as a result of successive new bone deposits. This lamellar structure is referred to as "onion skin" on radiographs [1, 2, 6, 7]. The adjacent spongiosa bone may exhibit a mixed structure, with some osteolytic areas within the sclerotic field, normal, or sclerotic area [1].

We aimed to present the extraoral, intraoral, and radiographic findings and postoperative pursuits of two patients diagnosed with Garre's osteomyelitis.

2. Case Reports

2.1. Case I. Our patient, an eight-year-old girl, presented to our clinic, with severe swelling and facial asymmetry on the right mandibular molar region. We were informed that the patient developed the swelling as a result of an infection three months previously. The patient had been treated with antibiotics, but as that treatment had not proved successful, she was referred to our clinic. In addition, a passed or congenital disease was not specified in the patient's medical history. Clinical examination revealed severe swelling without fluctuation upon palpation and submandibular lymphadenopathy in the right mandibular region. The patient's skin was of normal color and appearance. In the oral examination, the right mandibular first molar tooth was found to have a deep caries cavity and to not be mobile. The other parts of the oral mucosa were normal. The radiographic examination revealed a deep caries cavity and a radiolucent area in the apical region of the right mandibular first molar tooth. There was also a lamellar appearance on the external cortical surface of the mandible as well as at the lower edge of the mandibular corpus, showing focal new bone formation (Figure 1(a)). When the axial and cross sections were evaluated during the examination with cone-beam computed tomography (CBCT), a tunnel-like defect was identified in the cortical bone in the vestibule surface of the inflamed bone, starting from the apical region of the right mandibular first molar tooth. Bone deposition at the radiolucent area in the center was observed at the lower edge of the mandible as well as the vestibule surface in this region (Figure 2(a)). When all these findings were evaluated, it was concluded that the pathologic lesion was Garre's osteomyelitis due to the periapical infection of the right mandibular first molar tooth. In this case, endodontic treatment was considered primarily to retain the infected tooth in the mouth. However, as the patient had come from a remote rural area and could not accept such a treatment due to the prohibitive cost, she was transferred to the surgical clinic, where the most appropriate treatment method was considered to be dental extraction.

The postoperative examination four months later revealed that the bone contours had returned to normal, the asymmetry of the face had disappeared, and the cortical bone thickness had decreased and been remodeled to the previous normal appearance (Figures 1(b) and 2(b)).

2.2. Case II. A 16-year-old girl similarly presented to our clinic with severe swelling and facial asymmetry in the left mandibular premolar region. No pathology could be determined from her clinical and medical history. Clinical examination revealed severe swelling without fluctuation upon palpation, submandibular lymphadenopathy, and a deep caries cavity in the left mandibular second premolar tooth. Additionally, in the radiologic examination, a deep caries cavity was found in the left mandibular second premolar tooth, while a radiolucent area was found in its apical region. However, no change could be detected at the lower edge of the mandibular corpus on these conventional radiographs (Figure 3). For this reason, a sectional examination using CBCT was required. When the axial and coronal sections were evaluated, in addition to the inflammation in the apical region of this tooth, bone deposition was observed horizontally on the vestibule surface of the mandible (Figure 4). When all these findings were evaluated, it was concluded that the pathologic lesion was Garre's osteomyelitis due to the

periapical infection of the left mandibular second premolar tooth. Considering the age of the patient, endodontic treatment was considered to retain the infected tooth in the mouth. However, since the patient refused that treatment for similar reasons as in the previous case, the patient was sent to the surgical clinic. Although we wanted her to return to our clinic for a postoperative check-up a few months after the tooth extraction, we were unable to contact her again.

3. Discussion

Garre's osteomyelitis is a localized periosteal thickening caused by mild irritation or infection [1, 4, 9, 11]. Although it is sometimes idiopathic, it is known that a moderate infection (such as dental decay, periodontal disease, or soft tissue disease), starting from the spongiosa layer of the jaw and extending into the periosteum, is the result of stimulating bone formation. However, in order for this pathological condition to occur, the balance between the virulent bacteria and oral flora must be impaired, while the periosteal osteoblastic activity must also be high [1, 12].

There is no need for a biopsy during the diagnosis of Garre's osteomyelitis, except the cause is unknown [4, 6]. Conventional radiographic methods or CT images are sufficient for diagnosis [3, 4, 9, 10]. As our two cases exhibited obvious clinical and radiographic features, a biopsy was not required.

In addition to Garre's osteomyelitis, new bone formation can occur in many pathological conditions. Therefore, it should be distinguished from other pathologies that cause new bone formation, including Ewing's sarcoma, Caffey disease, fibrous dysplasia, Paget's disease, osteosarcoma, and hard, nodular, or pedunculated masses seen in the mandible (peripheral osteomas, torus and exostoses, ossifying subperiosteal hematoma, etc.) [3, 4, 6, 10].

Caffey disease presents in a similar view to Garre's osteomyelitis due to the "onion skin" appearance in the bone. However, Caffey disease is distinguished from Garre's osteomyelitis due to the early age of onset (prior to two years of age), it is being more common in the ramus and angulus region of the mandible with bilateral involvement and occurrence in multiple bones [1].

Ewing's sarcoma is similar to Garre's osteomyelitis in terms of the subperiosteal bone formation and appearance in young people. However, Ewing's sarcoma can also be distinguished from Garre's osteomyelitis due to producing osteophytes with a "sun ray" appearance, causing bone enlargement too rapidly and causing more osteolytic reactions in the bone, as well as the occurrence of frequent complications such as facial neuralgia and lip paresthesia [1, 10].

Osteosarcoma can also produce a hard bone mass on the bone surface. However, it is distinguished from Garre's osteomyelitis due to showing the characteristic features of malign tumors, such as new bone formation with a "sun ray" appearance and periosteal reactions in the form of a Codman triangle in radiography [1, 12].

Another pathologic condition requiring a differential diagnosis is fibrous dysplasia. Fibrous dysplasia is seen at younger ages, which is similar to Garre's osteomyelitis, and

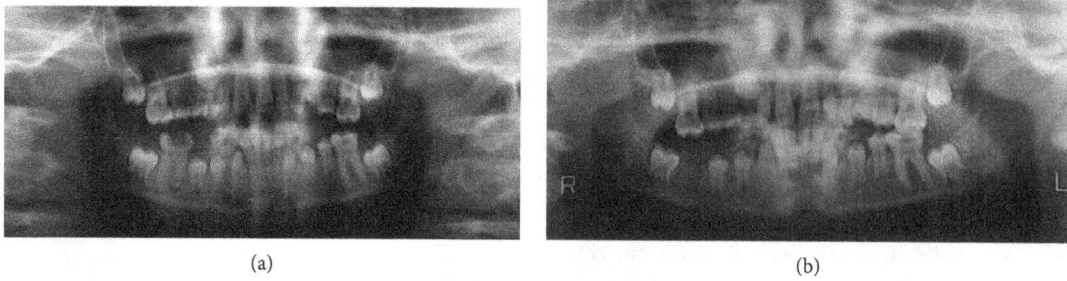

(a)   (b)

FIGURE 1: Orthopantomographic image showing a deep caries cavity in the right mandibular first molar tooth, a radiolucent area in its mesial root, and subperiosteal new bone formation below the lower border of the mandible (a). Orthopantomographic image taken four months after tooth extraction showing the return of normal bone contours (b).

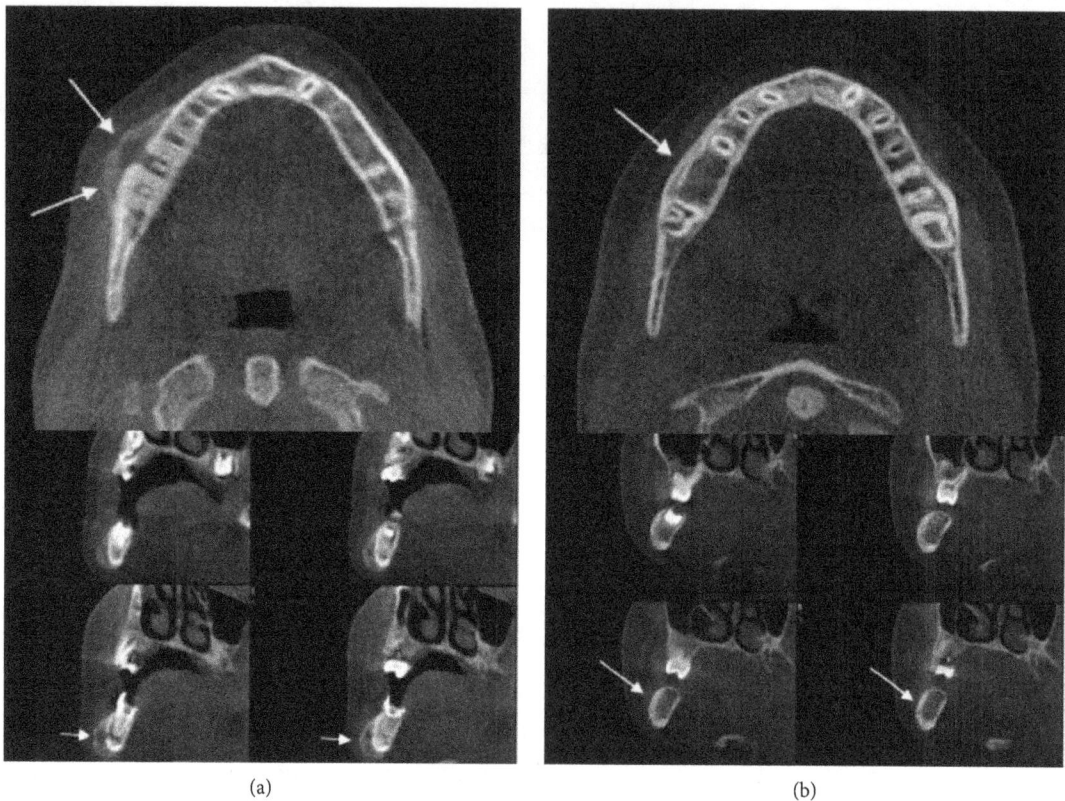

(a)   (b)

FIGURE 2: Axial and cross sections in CBCT showing new bone formation and a tunnel-like defect in the vestibule cortical surface of the inflamed bone starting from the apical region of tooth number 46 (a). CBCT image showing decreased cortical bone thickness and the presence of the original cortex within the enlarged portion of the jaw in the postoperative control (b).

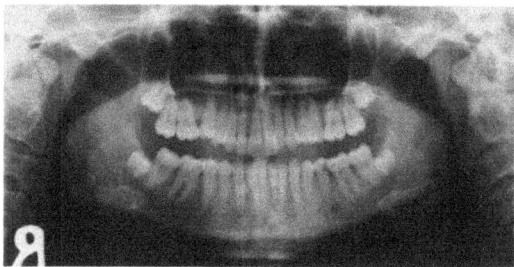

FIGURE 3: Orthopantomographic image showing a deep caries cavity in the left mandibular second premolar tooth and a radiolucent area in its apical region.

the resulting bone mass is similar in both shape and volume. Yet, fibrous dysplasia is distinguished from Garre's osteomyelitis due to the "ground glass appearance" as well as the thinning seen in the cortex. Further, unlike Garre's osteomyelitis, it is not associated with any dental infection. In addition, the enlargement is seen in the internal structure of the bone in fibrous dysplasia, whereas the enlargement of the bone in Garre's osteomyelitis is seen on the outer surface of the cortex, while the presence of the original cortex can be detected within the enlarged portion of the jaw in a careful examination [1, 4, 6, 10].

Hard, nodular, or pedunculated masses, such as peripheral osteomas, torus, and exostosis, are radiographically seen

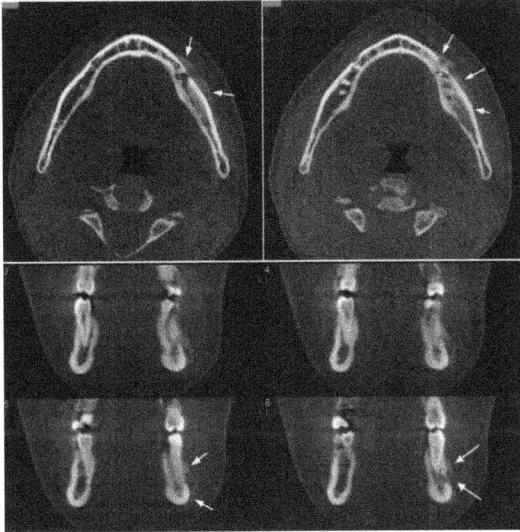

FIGURE 4: Axial and cross sections showing horizontal bone deposition on the vestibule surface of the mandible.

as a dense, uniform radiopaque mass extending outward from the cortex. However, Garre's osteomyelitis has regular contours. The clinical appearance of ossifying subperiosteal hematoma may also be similar to that of Garre's osteomyelitis. However, it does not exhibit uniform radiopacity, but can instead be distinguished by the mottled appearance or trabecular structure and trauma story [1].

Different opinions exist regarding the most appropriate treatment for Garre's osteomyelitis. Although hyperbaric oxygen therapy and endodontic treatment have proved successful, the most commonly accepted treatment is the administration of antibiotics and the extraction of the infected tooth [8, 9]. Considering the difficulties associated with applying endodontic treatments in both our cases, antibiotic therapy and tooth extraction were performed. In the first case, the improvement in the bone contours was confirmed in the control films taken four months after the tooth extraction.

Ethical Approval

All procedures followed were in accordance with the ethical standards of the responsible committee on human experimentation (institutional and national) and with the Helsinki Declaration of 1975, as revised in 2008.

Consent

Informed consent was obtained from all patients for being included in the study.

Authors' Contributions

All of the authors contributed to the formation of the article.

References

[1] F. R. Karjodkar, *Textbook of Dental and Maxillofacial Radiology*, Jaypee, Panama City, Panama, 2nd edition, 2009.

[2] P. Çelenk and H. M. Akgül, "Garre's osteomyelitis (a case report)," *Journal of Ondokuz Mayıs University Dental Faculty*, vol. 3, pp. 29–31, 2000.

[3] H. Nakano, T. Miki, K. Aota, T. Sumi, K. Matsumoto, and Y. Yura, "Garré's osteomyelitis of the mandible caused by an infected wisdom tooth," *Oral Science International*, vol. 5, no. 2, pp. 150–154, 2008.

[4] R. Suma, C. Vinay, M. C. Shashikanth, and V. V. Subba Reddy, "Garre's sclerosing osteomyelitis," *Journal of the Indian Society of Pedodontics and Preventive Dentistry*, vol. 25, pp. 30–33, 2007.

[5] M. Erişen, Ö. F. Bayar, and G. Ak, "Garre osteomyelitis: a case report," *The Journal of Dental Faculty of Atatürk University*, vol. 9, pp. 49–53, 2014.

[6] M. Gonçalves, D. P. Oliveira, E. O. Oya, and A. Gonçalves, "Garre's osteomyelitis associated with a fistula: a case report," *The Journal of Clinical Pediatric Dentistry*, vol. 26, no. 3, pp. 311–313, 2002.

[7] S. K. Kannan, G. Sandhya, and R. Selvarani, "Periostitis ossificans (Garrè's osteomyelitis) radiographic study of two cases," *International Journal of Paediatric Dentistry*, vol. 16, no. 1, pp. 59–64, 2006.

[8] A. Jayasenthil, P. Aparna, and S. Balagopal, "Non-surgical endodontic management of Garre's osteomyelitis: a case report," *British Journal of Medicine and Medical Research*, vol. 9, no. 3, pp. 1–4, 2015.

[9] M. T. Brazao-Silva and T. N. Pinheiro, "The so-called Garrè's osteomyelitis of jaws and the pivotal utility of computed tomography scan," *Contemporary Clinical Dentistry*, vol. 8, no. 4, pp. 645–646, 2017.

[10] S. C. White and M. J. Pharoah, *Oral Radiology: Principles and Interpretation*, Mosby, St. Louis, MO, USA, 6th edition, 2009.

[11] D. Singh, P. Subramaniam, and P. D. Bhayya, "Periostitis ossificans (Garrè's osteomyelitis): an unusual case," *Journal of the Indian Society of Pedodontics and Preventive Dentistry*, vol. 33, no. 4, pp. 344–346, 2015.

[12] Y. Suei, A. Taguchi, and K. Tanimoto, "Diagnosis and classification of mandibular osteomyelitis," *Oral Surgery, Oral Medicine, Oral Pathology, Oral Radiology, and Endodontology*, vol. 100, no. 2, pp. 207–214, 2005.

25

Management of Crown-Root Fracture in Primary Canine by Surgical Extrusion: A Case Report with 1-Year Follow-Up

I. Kanimozhi,[1] **Mahesh Ramakrishnan,**[2] **Dhanalakshmi Ravikumar** (iD),[2] **and Ningthoujam Sharna**[3]

[1]*Government Medical College, Tuticorin, Tamil Nadu, India*
[2]*Department of Pedodontics and Preventive Dentistry, Saveetha Dental College, Chennai, Tamil Nadu, India*
[3]*Private Pratice, Imphal, Manipur, India*

Correspondence should be addressed to Dhanalakshmi Ravikumar; dhana9677@gmail.com

Academic Editor: H. Cem Güngör

Complicated crown-root fractures of primary teeth often present with a greater challenge to the pediatric dentist. Extraction of the involved tooth is the routine treatment indicated. But, early loss of this primary tooth may lead to esthetic and psychological problems and also causes a detrimental effect on the development of occlusion and the alveolar bone. The present case report described the management of crown-root fracture in a primary canine by surgical extrusion and showed a satisfactory prognosis at one-year follow-up.

1. Introduction

Trauma to the teeth and orofacial region is most commonly encountered in children compared to adults. The child age and behaviour management play an important role in deciding the treatment protocol. The fracture line originates in the crown portion of the tooth, extends apically into the root in an oblique direction, and frequently exposes the pulp which is termed as a complicated crown fracture. The management protocol should consider both the function and the esthetics of the fractured tooth [1]. Various treatment approaches are indicated depending on the tooth fracture, the age of the child, and the location of the degree of level of fracture. When the fracture line extends below the gingival margin, there is a high chance of microleakage from the gingival crevicular fluid and difficulty in isolation for postendodontic restorations. In such cases, extraction of the fractured tooth is often indicated [1]. When the fracture involves the anterior teeth, it can lead to esthetic and psychological problems, but also bring detrimental effect on the development of occlusion and the alveolar bone [2]. Therefore, prevention of injury and conservation of severely traumatised teeth are eminently significant whenever possible [3].

Surgical tooth extrusion is considered to be one of the most favourable treatment options when the fracture line extends subgingivally. The procedure involves severing the bone root periodontal attachment utilising a surgical instrument to place the root in a more coronal position [1–4]. The extruded tooth is then stabilised using a semirigid splint for a maximum of 3 weeks for ideal periodontal healing. Surgical extrusion is a one-step procedure which is biologically acceptable and less time to consume than orthodontic extrusion in the management of horizontal and oblique root fracture [1–3]. Literature review identified case reports of successful management involving surgical extrusion in permanent teeth. But in cases involving primary teeth, the only treatment opinion available is extraction followed by space management.

The present article describes a case of management of crown-root fracture in a primary canine by surgical extrusion, when followed up for 12-month duration that showed a satisfactory prognosis.

2. Case Report

A 6-year-old girl presented to the Department of Pediatric and Preventive Dentistry with the history of trauma in her right upper front region of the jaw. She had a fall on the school ground while playing 1 hr before the presentation, had no symptoms of nausea, and did not have any discharge or bleeding from her nose. The medical history was unremarkable and did not have any history of daily medication. No gross facial asymmetry was evident. She had no abrasions on the lower or upper lip. Her temporomandibular joints were functioning within limits and with no clicking, pain, or any abnormal mandibular deviation. On intraoral examination, the patient had a complete set of primary dentition and had moderate oral hygiene, with mild plaque deposits at the gingival margins. There was a fracture in the right maxillary canine (tooth number 53) with the oblique fracture line extending subgingivally (Figure 1). Radiograph (IOPA) taken in the right anterior region of the jaw (tooth number 53) revealed evidence of fracture line running 2 mm below the cementoenamel junction and involving the pulp (Figure 2).

The treatment options and prognosis for tooth 53 were discussed with the patient's mother. Preoperative photographs were taken, and local anaesthesia was administered (2% xylocaine with 1 : 80,000 adrenaline) on the buccal and palatal aspects of tooth 53. The mobile tooth fragment was extracted, and the remaining tooth structure was surgically extruded using a maxillary anterior forceps (Figure 3). Occlusion was checked to ensure that there are no occlusal interferences. Acid etching of tooth numbers 51, 52, 53, and 54 was done. The bonding agent was applied, and a semirigid splint was placed and stabilised using a flowable composite (Figure 4). The patient was advised to consume a soft diet and to be meticulous with her oral hygiene. A 0.2% chlorhexidine gluconate mouthwash was also prescribed twice daily for the next two weeks. The patient was reviewed a day following her initial presentation, and pulpectomy was carried out on the next day and obturated using Metapex. Composite splinting was removed at the end of the third week, and polishing was done. Mobility was checked, and radiographs were taken. On eight weeks following trauma, a periapical radiograph and photograph were updated. The patient was followed up periodically at the 3rd month, 6th month, and 12th month (Figures 5 and 6).

3. Discussion

Crown-root fracture typically presents as a fracture line that originates in the crown portion of the tooth which extends apically in an oblique direction frequently with pulp exposure. The treatment protocol for primary teeth with crown-root fracture as recommended by IADT guidelines is to leave the tooth untreated if the coronal fragment is not displaced or extracting the coronal segment with repositioning and splinting might be considered [5]. In severe cases, when there is crown-root fracture which is extending into the subgingiva involving the primary teeth, it is indicated for extraction. As a result of this protocol, many root-fractured primary teeth were extracted in very young children. Loss of anterior teeth in these children will have negative effect on the social well-being affecting the quality of life. Surgical extraction has the potency to induce a certain amount of dental fear and anxiety

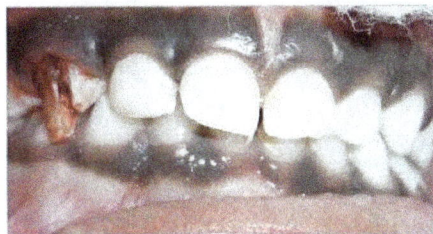

FIGURE 1: Preoperative photograph depicts fractured 53.

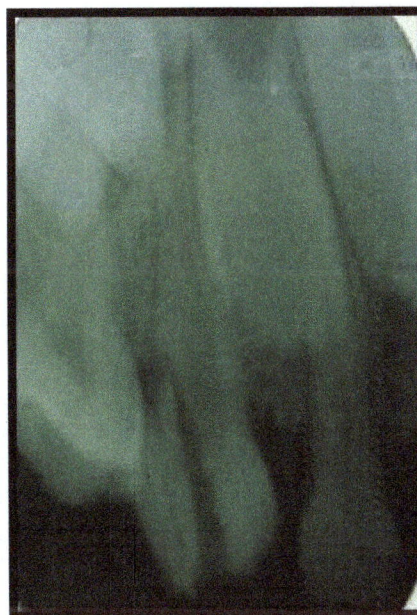

FIGURE 2: Preoperative radiograph depicts oblique crown-root fracture extending beyond cementoenamel junction.

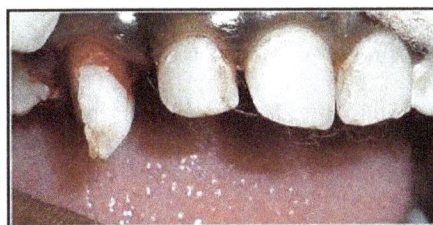

FIGURE 3: Surgically extruded 53.

in young children. Thus, a conservative approach, although it is controversial, could be adopted and attempts are made to save root-fractured primary teeth, with extraction as the last choice [6, 7].

The surgical extrusion is considered a viable alternative for the management of crown-root fracture, when the fractures extend subgingivally and periodontal surgery is not recommended owing to esthetic reason. When compared with orthodontic extrusion, which involves placing either post or brackets in the exposed tooth surface, this treatment option allows the detection of additional fractures at the root.

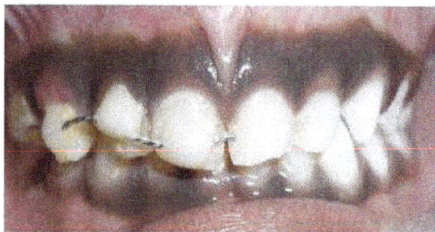

FIGURE 4: Surgically extruded 53 stabilised using composite splint.

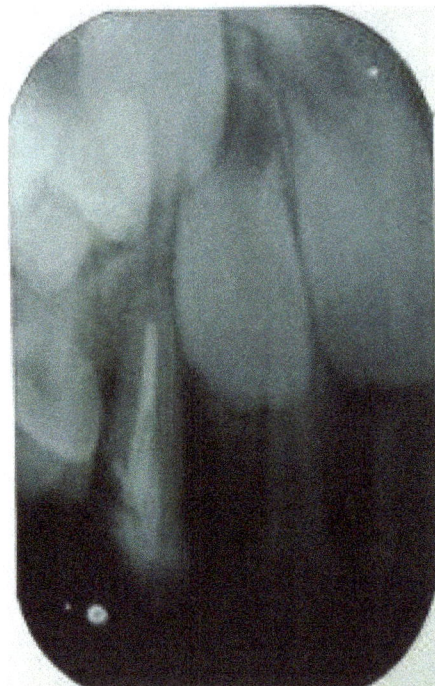

FIGURE 5: Radiograph taken at 6th-month follow-up.

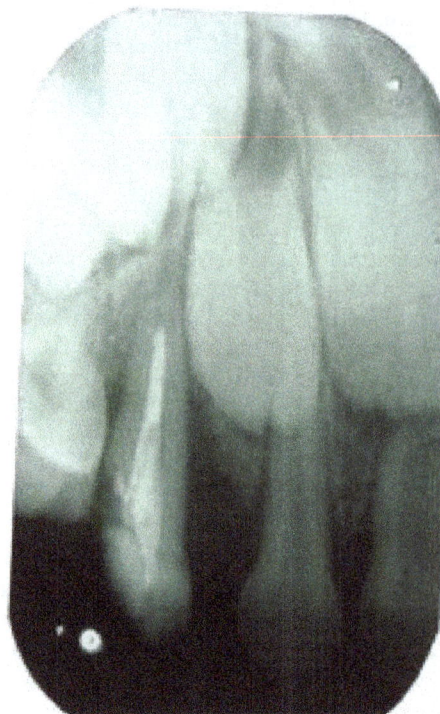

FIGURE 6: Radiograph taken at 12th-month follow-up.

Moreover, studies show that surgical extrusion has an acceptable prognosis; approximately 80% of teeth treated are still in working condition after five years [3, 4]. It is comparatively easier to get the patients' cooperation since it is a shorter-duration procedure, less expensive, and the tooth can be in function for a longer duration [1–4].

In the present case report, the traumatised teeth were surgically extruded followed by the extraction of mobile tooth fragment in the coronal portion, splinted and stabilised. In the next appointment, the teeth were treated with pulpectomy and coronal restoration. On eight-week follow-up, the tooth exhibited no clinical signs of failure, such as mobility, tenderness, or pain. The outcome was successful in this case at one year, as there was no underlying pathology in the follow-up period suggesting no risk for the underlying permanent tooth germ. The long-term success of surgical extrusion depends on the cooperation of the child, the condition of the periodontal ligament, the vitality of the teeth, and the time lapsed following trauma. Thus, the conservative approach in the management of crown-root fracture in primary dentition should be emphasised. Further more studies

of similar case reports are desirable in the management of crown-root fractures in primary dentition, before any recommendations to be made in the guidelines of the management of trauma.

In conclusion, this case report confirms that a multidisciplinary approach surgical extrusion is one of the alternative methods to manage the complicated crown-root fracture in a primary dentition.

References

[1] C.-S. Kim, S.-H. Choi, J.-K. Chai, C.-K. Kim, and K.-S. Cho, "Surgical extrusion technique for clinical crown lengthening: report of three cases," *The International Journal of Periodontics & Restorative Dentistry*, vol. 24, no. 5, pp. 412–421, 2004.

[2] W. Marcenes and U. Ryda, "Socio-psychological aspects of traumatic dental injuries," in *Textbook and Color Atlas of Traumatic Injuries to the Teeth*, J. O. Andreasen, F. M. Andreasen, and L. Andersson, Eds., pp. 197–206, Blackwell Munksgaard, Oxford, 4th edition, 2007.

[3] A. Sigurdsson, "Evidence-based review of prevention of dental injuries," *Journal of Endodontics*, vol. 35, no. 2, pp. 184–190, 2013.

[4] M. K. Calisskan, M. Turkun, and M. Gomel, "Surgical extrusion of crown-root-fractured teeth: a clinical review," *International Endodontic Journal*, vol. 32, no. 2, pp. 146–151, 1999.

[5] B. Malmgren, J. O. Andreasen, M. T. Flores et al., "International Association of Dental Traumatology guidelines for the management of traumatic dental injuries: 3. Injuries in primary dentition," *Dental Traumatology*, vol. 28, no. 3, pp. 174–182, 2012.

[6] A. Elkhadem, S. Mickan, and D. Richards, "Adverse events of surgical extrusion in treatment for crown–root and cervical root fractures: a systematic review of case series/reports," *Dental Traumatology*, vol. 30, no. 1, pp. 1–14, 2014.

[7] J. Roeters and J. P. Bressers, "The combination of a surgical and adhesive restorative approach to treat a deep crown-root fracture: a case report," *Quintessence International*, vol. 33, no. 3, pp. 174–179, 2002.

26

Aesthetic Rehabilitation of a Severe Dental Fluorosis Case with Ceramic Veneers: A Step-by-Step Guide

Aminah M. El Mourad

Department of Restorative Dental Sciences, King Saud University, Riyadh, Saudi Arabia

Correspondence should be addressed to Aminah M. El Mourad; amourad@ksu.edu.sa

Academic Editor: Mine Dündar

The selection of an appropriate treatment plan for cases of dental fluorosis depends on the severity of the condition. Ceramic veneers are considered the treatment of choice for moderate to severe cases of fluorosis given the optimum aesthetics, wear resistance, biocompatibility, and long-term results of these veneers. This case report describes a step-by-step rehabilitation of fluorosed teeth, using ceramic veneers in a 26-year-old Yemeni male. The patient presented at the restorative dentistry clinics at King Saud University complaining of an unpleasant smile and generalized tooth discoloration.

1. Introduction

Dental fluorosis is a tooth malformation characterized by outer hypermineralization and subsurface hypomineralization, and it is caused by the chronic ingestion of fluoride during tooth development [1].

Numerous studies have reported that water fluoridation is a safe and effective public health measure for reducing the occurrence of dental caries [2, 3]. However, excessive fluoride in drinking water, exceeding a concentration of 0.5–1.5 mg/l, can lead to metabolic alteration in ameloblasts; this results in a defective matrix and improper calcification of teeth, known as dental fluorosis [4].

Dental fluorosis becomes a cosmetic concern particularly if it affects the anterior teeth. Although the causes and characteristics of dental fluorosis have been widely reported, fewer studies have discussed the proper treatment of fluorosed teeth. The selection of an appropriate treatment plan depends on the severity of fluorosis [5]. Bleaching and microabrasion have been recommended for treating mild cases of fluorosis; however, in moderate to severe cases, bleaching and microabrasion are either ineffective or may lead to only transient improvement [6], while composite restorations are prone to discoloration, chipping, and debonding. Ceramic veneers are the restoration of choice for moderate to severe cases of fluorosis given their color maintainability, wear resistance, and biocompatibility [7].

This case report presents a step-by-step aesthetic rehabilitation of a patient with severe fluorosis by using ceramic veneers.

2. Case Report

A 26-year-old Yemeni male patient from Taiz Province was referred to the restorative dental clinics at King Saud University, Saudi Arabia. His chief complaint was an unpleasant smile caused by generalized tooth discoloration. His medical history was irrelevant. The fluoride level in the water around Taiz Province is >3.6 mg/l [8].

2.1. Clinical Examination. Clinical examination revealed generalized fluorosis with loss of the outermost enamel in irregular areas involving less than half of the entire surface, as well as changes in the morphology caused by merging pits and marked attrition (Figure 1). In this case, based on the Thylstrup and Fejerskov index (TFI) for dental fluorosis classification, the dental fluorosis was classified as TFI = 7 [9].

2.2. Treatment Plan. After the clinical examination, radiographs, preoperative photographs, and upper and lower

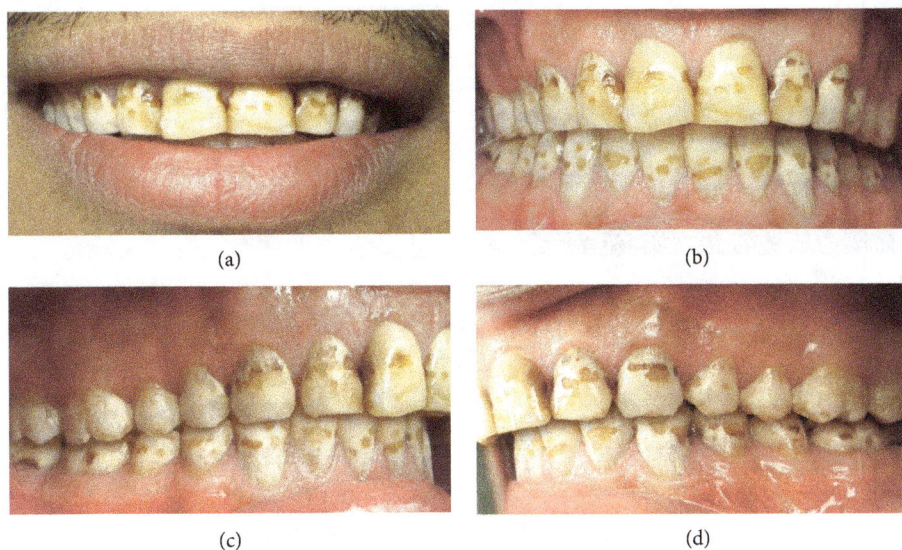

FIGURE 1: Preoperative clinical photographs: (a) smile, (b) frontal view, (c) lateral view: right side, and (d) lateral view: left side.

alginate impressions for diagnostic models were taken. The patient was presented with treatment options, which included ceramic or composite veneers, along with the advantages and disadvantages of each option. The patient agreed to smile enhancement using ceramic veneers for his upper teeth given that he desired an optimum aesthetic and a long-term result. The veneers would be placed on the patient's upper teeth, from his upper right 2nd premolar to upper left 2nd premolar. The patient decided to postpone veneering his lower teeth, given his limited financial capacity. Diagnostic models were analyzed to evaluate the occlusion, and a diagnostic wax-up was made of white-colored wax. The use of the wax-up allows the patient to preview the desired appearance of his teeth, and this wax-up is also essential for the fabrication of a clear matrix for temporary restorations.

2.3. Tooth Preparation.
The desired shade was selected using the VITAPAN classical shade guide (VITA Zahnfabrik, Germany). The enamel of the eight maxillary teeth was prepared using a flat-end tapered diamond bur to a depth of 0.5–0.75 mm facial reduction with 1.5 mm incisal reduction (Figure 2). A chamfer finish line was maintained at the level of the gingival margin. The proximal margin was extended into the facial and gingival embrasures.

2.4. Final Impression and Temporization.
Following tooth preparation, gingival retraction was achieved using retraction cords (Ultrapak Cord #00, Ultradent Products Inc., South Jordan, UT, USA) soaked in a hemostatic agent. Impressions were taken with a polyvinylsiloxane material (*Virtual*, Ivoclar Vivadent, Amherst, NY). The impression material was manipulated according to the manufacturer's instructions. Temporization was performed by spot etching on the facial surface of each prepared tooth with 37% phosphoric acid (Total Etch, Ivoclar Vivadent, Schaan, Liechtenstein). Bonding agent (OptiBond Solo Plus, Kerr, Orange, CA, USA) was

applied on the enamel-etched spots and light cured for 20 seconds using a high-intensity light-emitting diode (LED) curing light (Elipar S10, 3M ESPE, MN, USA). The clear matrix that was previously fabricated was loaded with a temporization material (Protemp Plus, 3M ESPE, MN, USA) and placed over the prepared teeth. Light curing was done for 10 seconds per tooth. Then, the matrix was gently teased away from the prepared teeth. A number 12 scalpel blade was used to remove the partially cured temporization material. Facial and lingual embrasures were refined with a thin diamond disk, the occlusion was adjusted, and the temporary restorations were polished using polishing discs and points (Figure 3).

2.5. Veneer Try-In and Cementation.
Ceramic veneers were fabricated with a lithium disilicate-reinforced glass ceramic material (IPS e.max Press, Ivoclar Vivadent, Schaan, Liechtenstein). Temporary veneers were removed, and the teeth were cleaned using pumice. Ceramic veneers were tried-in using a transparent shade try-in paste (Variolink Veneer try-in paste, Ivoclar Vivadent, Schaan, Liechtenstein) to assess marginal adaptation and shade.

Afterwards, veneers were prepared for bonding. Fitting surfaces of the veneers were etched with hydrofluoric acid (Porcelain Etchant 9.5%, Bisco Inc., Schaumburg, IL, USA) for 60 seconds, washed under running water for another 60 seconds, and dried with an air syringe. A layer of silane coupling agent (Monobond Plus, Ivoclar Vivadent, Schaan, Liechtenstein) was applied on the veneers' fitting surfaces and gently air-dried after one minute. Then, the prepared teeth were etched using 37% phosphoric acid for 30 seconds, rinsed, and dried. A clear mylar strip was placed interproximally to prevent inadvertent bonding to the adjacent tooth and to facilitate the subsequent removal of excess resin cement in the embrasures. A layer of bonding agent (Adhese Universal, Ivoclar Vivadent, Schaan, Liechtenstein) was applied on the prepared tooth surfaces and air-thinned.

(a)

(b)

(c)

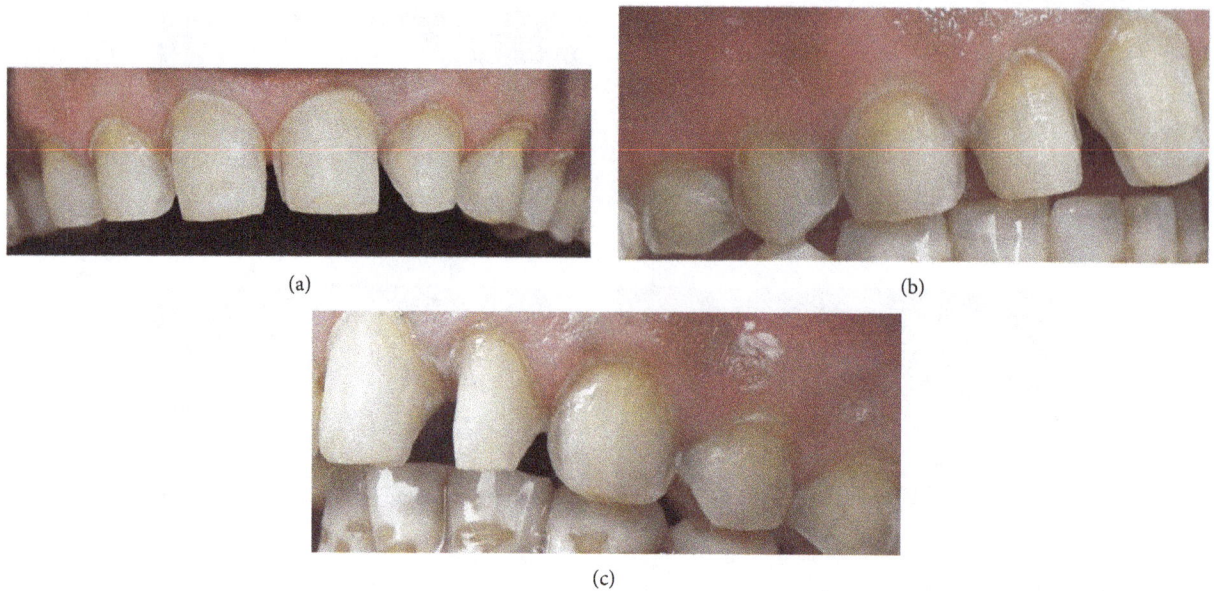

Figure 2: Maxillary tooth preparation: (a) frontal view, (b) lateral view: right side, and (c) lateral view: left side.

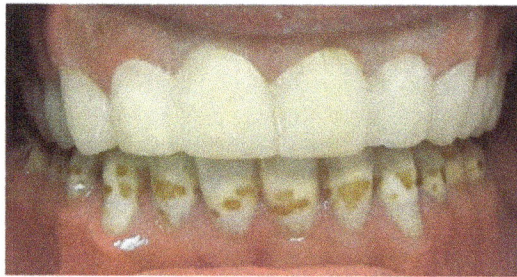

Figure 3: Temporary veneers.

Then, Heliobond (Ivoclar Vivadent, Schaan, Liechtenstein) was placed on the prepared tooth surfaces. The inner surface of the veneers was covered with light-cured resin cement (Variolink Veneer, transparent shade, Ivoclar Vivadent, Schaan, Liechtenstein). Veneers were positioned appropriately on the teeth by applying gentle pressure, following which excess resin cement was carefully removed with an explorer before light curing. Light curing was first performed for 2 seconds, and the excess resin cement was removed with a microbrush. After that, each veneer was light-cured from the facial aspect for 40 seconds and from the lingual aspect for 40 seconds. The two veneers of the central incisors were first simultaneously cemented. This was followed by cementation of the veneers of the two lateral incisors. Then, the veneers of the two canines were cemented. Finally, veneers for the first and second premolars were cemented simultaneously on each side.

Minimal gingival flash of the resin luting cement was removed with a number 12 scalpel blade. A flame-shaped fine diamond bur was used to finish the ceramic margins and to contour the embrasure surfaces. Occlusion was assessed and adjusted. Flossing was performed to ensure interproximal contact patency. Ceramic polishing was performed using a series of polishing cups and points (OptraFine polishing system, Ivoclar Vivadent, Schaan, Liechtenstein). Interproximal contacts were finished with finishing and polishing strips. Final surface lustre was achieved by using a diamond polishing paste with a rubber prophylaxis cup. The postoperative clinical photographs are shown in Figure 4. The patient was satisfied with the final result (Figure 5).

3. Discussion

The aim of the treatment in this case was to improve the patient's smile and aesthetic rehabilitation of teeth. This goal was achieved using ceramic veneers, which are the treatment of choice to mask tooth discoloration in cases of moderate to severe fluorosis.

Ceramic veneers can completely mask the discolored tooth with minimal reduction of sound tooth substance because they require a minimally invasive design preparation. In addition, advances in ceramic materials have facilitated this process. Ceramic veneers provide both predictable and long-lasting aesthetic rehabilitation [10, 11].

The durability and clinical success of porcelain veneers have been widely investigated in the literature. It has been reported that ceramic veneers provide durable and successful restoration with an estimated survival probability of 93.5% over 10 years [12]. Satisfactory results were obtained in a case of fluorosed teeth restored with porcelain laminate veneers over a 6-year follow-up [13]. Furthermore, numerous studies have demonstrated acceptable aesthetic outcomes in cases of moderate to severe fluorosis where restoration with porcelain veneers was performed [14].

4. Conclusion

Ceramic veneers are considered one of the most popular restorative materials in aesthetic dentistry. They provide

(a)

(b)

(c)

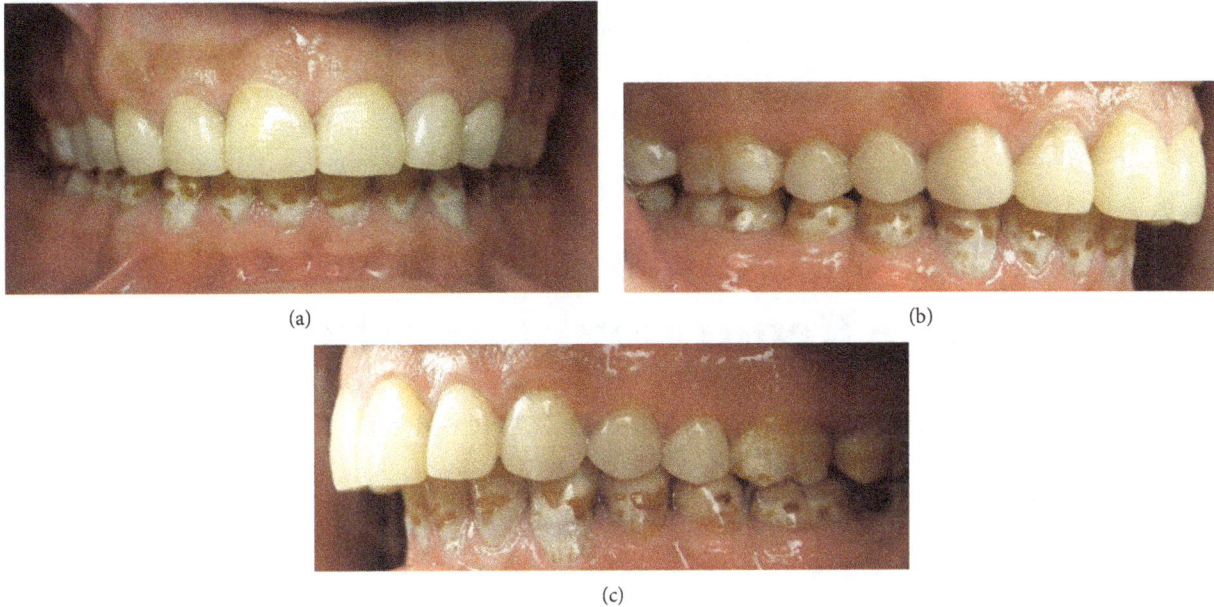

Figure 4: Postoperative clinical photographs: (a) frontal view, (b) lateral view: right side, and (c) lateral view: left side.

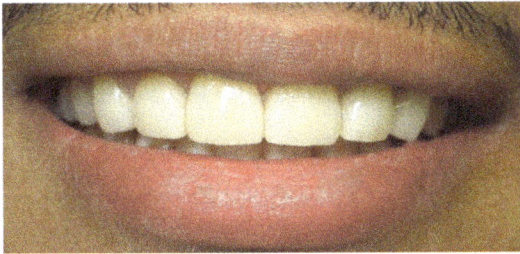

Figure 5: Final result.

excellent aesthetic results when an appropriate treatment plan and protocol are used during the clinical and laboratory fabrication stages. This case report describes the use of ceramic veneers to enhance the appearance of fluorosed teeth, thus improving the patient's smile and, consequently, self-esteem.

References

[1] P. K. Den Bestan, "Dental fluorosis: its use as a biomarker," *Advances in Dental Research*, vol. 8, no. 1, pp. 105–110, 1994.

[2] A. J. Spencer, G. D. Slade, and M. Davis, "Water fluoridation in Australia," *Community Dental Health*, vol. 13, pp. 27–37, 1996.

[3] M. S. Hopcraft, K. E. Yapp, G. Mahoney, and M. V. Morgan, "Dental caries experience in young Australian Army recruits 2008," *Australian Dental Journal*, vol. 54, no. 4, pp. 316–322, 2009.

[4] O. Fejerskov, M. J. Larsen, A. Richards, and V. Baelum, "Dental tissue effects of fluoride," *Advances in Dental Research*, vol. 8, no. 1, pp. 15–31, 1994.

[5] E. S. Akpata, "Occurrence and management of dental fluorosis," *International Dental Journal*, vol. 51, no. 5, pp. 325–333, 2001.

[6] P. Denbesten and W. Li, "Chronic fluoride toxicity: dental fluorosis," *Monographs in Oral Science*, vol. 22, pp. 81–96, 2011.

[7] B. T. Rotoli, "Porcelain veneers as an alternative for esthetic treatment: clinical report," *Operative Dentistry*, vol. 38, no. 5, pp. 459–466, 2013.

[8] A. Aqeel, A. Al-Amry, and O. Alharbi, "Assessment and geospatial distribution mapping of fluoride concentrations in the groundwater of Al-Howban Basin Taiz-Yemen," *Arabian Journal of Geosciences*, vol. 10, no. 14, p. 312, 2017.

[9] A. Thylstrup and O. Fejerskov, "Clinical appearance of dental fluorosis in permanent teeth in relation to histologic changes," *Community Dentistry and Oral Epidemiology*, vol. 6, no. 6, pp. 315–328, 1978.

[10] M. Peumans, B. Van Meerbeek, P. Lambrechts, and G. Vanherle, "Porcelain veneers: a review of the literature," *Journal of Dentistry*, vol. 28, no. 3, pp. 163–177, 2000.

[11] P. Magne and W. H. Douglas, "Porcelain veneers: dentin bonding optimization and biomimetic recovery of the crown," *The International Journal of Prosthodontics*, vol. 12, no. 2, pp. 111–121, 1999.

[12] U. S. Beier, I. Kapferer, D. Burtscher, and H. Dumfahrt, "Clinical performance of porcelain laminate veneers for up to 20 years," *The International Journal of Prosthodontics*, vol. 25, no. 1, pp. 79–85, 2012.

[13] Y. H. Aljazairy, "Management of fluorosed teeth using porcelain veneers: a six-year recall case report," *Saudi Dental Journal*, vol. 13, pp. 106–113, 2001.

[14] I. A. Sherwood, "Fluorosis varied treatment options," *Journal of Conservative Dentistry*, vol. 13, no. 1, pp. 47–53, 2010.

27

Oral Verruciform Xanthoma within Lichen Planus: A Case Report and Literature Review

Vasileios I. Theofilou,[1] **Alexandra Sklavounou,**[1] **Prokopios P. Argyris,**[2] **and Evanthia Chrysomali** ⓘ[1]

[1]Department of Oral Medicine and Pathology, School of Dentistry, National and Kapodistrian University of Athens, Athens, Greece
[2]Department of Diagnostic and Biological Sciences, School of Dentistry, University of Minnesota, Minneapolis, MN, USA

Correspondence should be addressed to Evanthia Chrysomali; echryso@dent.uoa.gr

Academic Editor: Pia L. Jornet

Background. Verruciform xanthoma is an uncommon benign tumor, which exhibits a wide range of clinical patterns. The occurrence of the lesion in patients with immune-mediated mucocutaneous diseases may suggest a role of localized epithelial cell damage and chronic inflammation in its pathogenesis. *Case Report*. A case of verruciform xanthoma on the tongue of a 56-year-old female with oral lichen planus is reported. An asymptomatic pink-white lesion with a granular surface was observed in the left lateral lingual border, which was closely associated with a white plaque and striae. An incisional biopsy was performed, and histologically, epithelial projections in a verrucous pattern were observed. In the subepithelial connective tissue, aggregates of foamy cells that exhibited immunoreactivity for CD68 were noted. The final diagnosis was verruciform xanthoma. The mucosa adjacent to the lesion demonstrated histopathological features consistent with lichen planus. *Conclusions*. A total of twelve cases of oral verruciform xanthomas in patients with oral lichen planus including the present case have been reported in the literature. The clinician should be aware that verruciform xanthoma may mimic malignancy, and therefore, biopsy is required for definitive diagnosis to be established, especially when this tumor develops within conditions that show potential for malignant transformation.

1. Introduction

Verruciform xanthoma (VX) is an uncommon benign tumor, which primarily affects the oral mucosa, with the anogenital area and the skin being the second sites affected. It occurs most commonly in white males between 40 and 70 years of age [1–3]. VX exhibits a wide spectrum of clinical presentation including a solitary, well-demarcated, asymptomatic lesion with variable color ranging from pink and red to white, yellowish, or brownish. The clinical features also encompass a papillary or granular roughened surface with a sessile or pedunculated base and delineated slightly raised margins. The center of the lesion may rarely appear crateriform and even ulcerated [3–5]. Microscopically, the hallmark of VX is the presence of foamy (xanthomatous) cells in the connective tissue papillae [1–5].

The pathogenesis of VX remains largely unknown, but the lesion appears to occur in the presence of a localized immune response or inflammation after a local injury [2–4, 6, 7]. Several VX cases have been reported in association with underlying immune-mediated or other conditions, such as pemphigus vulgaris [8], lupus erythematosus [9], dystrophic epidermolysis bullosa [10], graft-versus-host disease (GVHD) [11], epithelial dysplasia and squamous cell carcinoma [1, 12, 13], or congenital hemidysplasia with ichthyosiform erythroderma and limb defects (CHILD) syndrome [14]. The coexistence of VX with lichen sclerosus, lichen planus, or other conditions in the genitalia is well described in the dermatology literature [15], but only 11 cases have been reported in the oral mucosa of patients with the aforementioned disease [4, 7, 13, 16–21].

On the other hand, oral lichen planus (OLP) is a common inflammatory condition affecting 0.1–2.2% of the population, which has been associated with approximately 1% of OLP patients developing oral squamous cell carcinoma based on

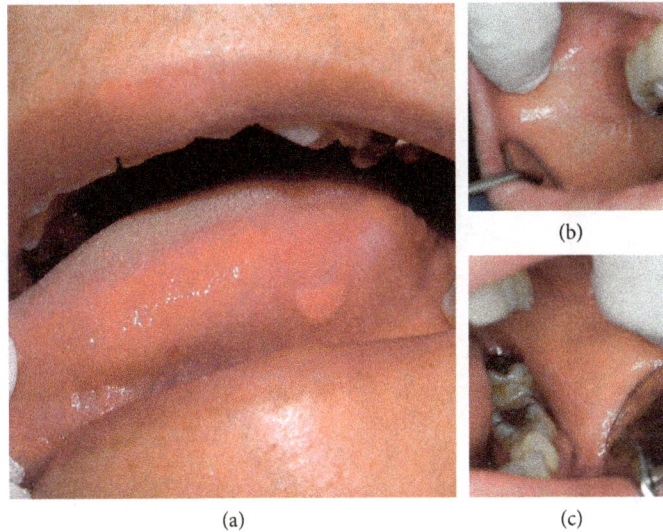

FIGURE 1: Lingual lesion with slightly raised margins and a granular surface closely associated with a white plaque and striae (a). Whitish striae located on the right (b) and left (c) buccal oral mucosa of the patient.

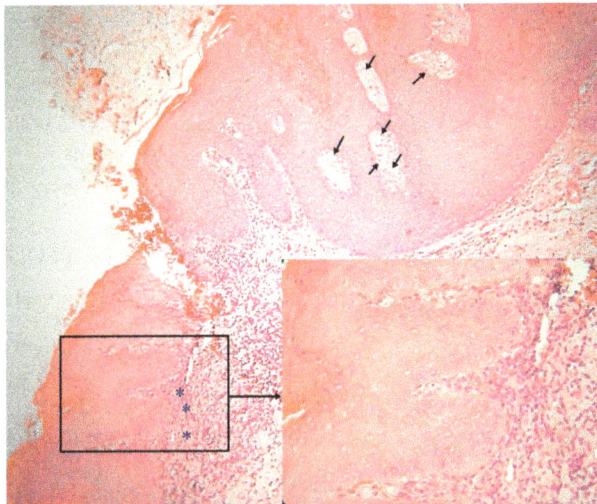

FIGURE 2: Photomicrograph of the VX that demonstrates hyperparakeratosis with keratin plugs, elongated, thickened epithelial rete ridges, and subepithelial connective tissue filled by foamy cells (arrows). The oral mucosa adjacent to the lesion shows a band-like (asterisks) dense inflammatory infiltrate (hematoxylin and eosin stain, ×150). A higher magnification (inset, ×400) showing epithelial parakeratosis, acanthosis, basal cell hydropic degeneration, and subepithelial predominant lymphocytic infiltrates.

a recent meta-analysis [22]. However, the potential of OLP malignant transformation is still controversial and yet to be completely clarified.

The clinical diagnosis of VX may be challenging, and the differential diagnosis should include benign lesions, such as squamous papilloma, condyloma acuminatum, and verruca vulgaris, potentially malignant disorders including leukoplakia and its subtypes and erythroplakia, and malignant epithelial tumors, such as verrucous carcinoma and invasive squamous cell carcinoma [1–4]. We report a case of VX occurring in proximity to OLP lesions that showed clinical features suspicious of malignancy.

2. Case Presentation

A 56-year-old female was referred for a painless tongue lesion of three-month duration. The patient had unremarkable medical history, was normolipemic, nonalcohol drinker, smoker (6–19 cigarettes/day) for 30 years, and was taking no medications. On clinical examination, an asymptomatic pink-white, well-demarcated, sessile lesion with a granular surface and slightly raised margins measuring $1 \times 0.5 \times 0.3$ cm was observed in the left lateral lingual border which extended to the ventral surface of the tongue. The lesion was soft in consistency on palpation and closely related to an area of combined white plaque and striae (Figure 1(a)). Similar white striae in a reticular pattern were also observed in the right and left buccal mucosa consistent with the clinical diagnosis of OLP (Figures 1(b) and 1(c)). There was no evidence of cervical lymph node enlargement. The extraoral examination performed by a dermatologist did not reveal any skin or genital lesions. Regarding the tongue lesion, the possibility of malignancy arising within OLP of the reticular/hypertrophic type was taken under consideration. An incisional biopsy was performed under local anesthesia from a region that included both the granular and the whitish tongue lesions.

Microscopic examination showed hyperparakeratosis and acanthosis with projections of the surface epithelium in a verrucous pattern, intense orange parakeratin plugs, and elongated thickened rete ridges (Figures 2 and 3(a)). Epithelial cell atypia was not evident. Accumulation of foamy cells in the subepithelial connective tissue confined in the lamina propria papillae was noted with sparse inflammatory infiltrates (Figures 2 and 3(b)). The oral mucosa adjacent to the lesion demonstrated histopathological features consistent with lichen planus. Specifically, the epithelial hyperplastic

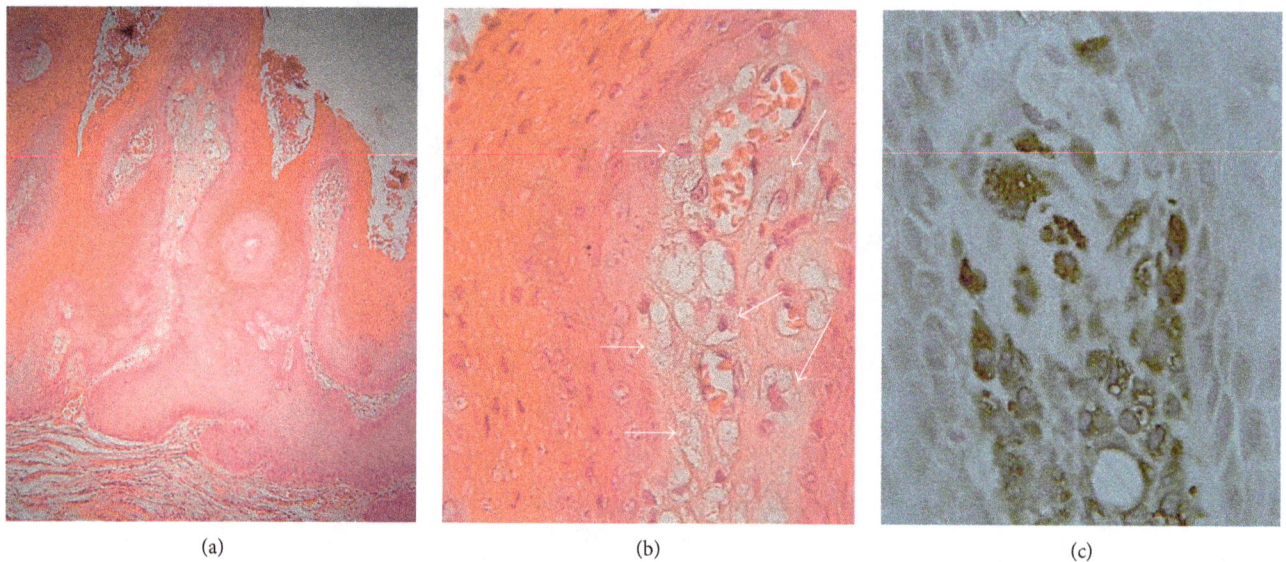

(a)   (b)   (c)

FIGURE 3: Low-power histologic aspect of the lesion (a) demonstrating exophytic growth in a verrucous/warty pattern with epithelial projections, hyperparakeratosis, orange keratin plugs, and elongated, thickened epithelial rete ridges (hematoxylin and eosin stain ×150). Higher magnification (b) shows aggregates of foamy cells (arrows) in the connective tissue between the rete ridges (hematoxylin and eosin stain ×400), which express (c) strong immunoreactivity for CD68 (immunohistochemical stain, ×400).

TABLE 1: Reports of verruciform xanthoma occurring in patients with diagnosis or clinical evidence of oral lichen planus in the literature.

Study	Cases	Age/sex	VX location	Size (cm)	Histological pattern	OLP type	Association of VX with OLP lesions
Neville and Weathers [16]	1	67/F	Base of the tongue	1.5	–	NS	Patient with a history of OLP
Hume et al. [17]	1	55/F	Buccal mucosa at the occlusal level	1	–	NS	Clinical evidence of OLP
Miyamoto et al. [18]	1	68/F	Lateral aspect of the tongue	1.3	Verrucous	Reticular-erosive	VX occurring within OLP lesion
Polonowita et al. [19]	3	65/M, 73/F, 42/F	Gingiva, alveolar mucosa, lateral aspect of the tongue	NS (3)	Flat (3)	Reticular (2) and reticular-hypertrophic (1)	VX occurring within OLP lesion (2) and VX at an independent oral site (1)
Anbinder et al. [20]	1	70/M	Labial mucosa	NS	Flat	Reticular	Clinical evidence of lichen planus
Stoopler et al. [21]	1	68/M	Lateral aspect of the tongue	0.5	Papillary	Reticular-atrophic	VX occurring in the site adjacent to OLP lesion
Present case	1	56/F	Lateral aspect of the tongue	1	Verrucous	Reticular-hypertrophic	VX occurring within OLP lesion

NS: not specified; the classification of VX into 3 patterns according to the histological architecture appearance of the lesion was made in 1981 [5].

pattern in a transitional manner changed into a relatively thinner squamous epithelium that exhibited parakeratosis, basal cell hydropic degeneration, and a band-like subepithelial dense chronic inflammatory infiltrate mainly by lymphocytes (Figure 2, inset). Based on the clinical and histopathological findings, a final diagnosis of VX with concomitant oral lichen planus features was rendered using the accepted diagnostic criteria for OLP [23].

Immunohistochemical evaluation on formalin-fixed paraffin-embedded tissue sections was performed using CD68 antibody (Dako, Glostrup, Denmark) on a Ventana NexES automated immunohistochemistry system (Ventana Medical Systems, Tucson, AZ). The foamy cells exhibited strong immunostaining for CD68 (Figure 3(c)).

The postsurgical healing was satisfactory, and complete removal was performed approximately two weeks after the incisional biopsy. Since OLP lesions remained unchanged and asymptomatic, no medications were prescribed, but follow-up was recommended. There was no evidence of recurrence after excision in a 7-year follow-up period, whereas the bilateral reticular OLP lesions on the buccal mucosa remained unchanged after the initial presentation.

3. Discussion

VX is a benign epithelial lesion that irrespective of intra- or extraoral development can simulate benign and malignant lesions causing diagnostic dilemmas [1–3]. The etiology remains obscure; the possibility of an association with lipid metabolism abnormalities was strongly speculated, but it has not been established [1–4, 13, 17]. The papillary morphology suggested the potential of HPV implication, but this was not confirmed by the results of several studies using immuno-histochemistry or in situ hybridization methods [6, 24].

The total number of oral verruciform xanthomas with concomitant lichen planus reported in the literature including the present case amounts to twelve. However, in the studies of Yu et al. [4], Ide et al. [7], and de Andrade et al. [13], there were no sufficient data about the demographic, clinical, or histologic characteristics of the OLP and VX. The above three cases [4, 7, 13] were omitted from Table 1. The patients' age ranged between 42 and 73 years, and females were more frequently affected (6/9). Hume [17] described the first case of VX in a patient with clinical OLP features. In a patient with neurofibromatosis reported by Anbinder et al. [20], VX was located in the labial mucosa, while the diagnosis of OLP was based on clinical criteria alone. Including our case, the histologically confirmed cases of VX adjacent to OLP lesions are 4 [18, 19], while in two patients, VX did not develop in proximity to OLP lesions [19, 21]. The reticular type of OLP was present in every single case, while erosions (erosive OLP) [18], white plaques (hypertrophic OLP) [19], or erythema (atrophic OLP) [21] were also present in three cases. In our case, both the reticular and the hypertrophic OLP types were present.

The masticatory mucosa (gingival and alveolar mucosae) is referred as the most common intraoral site for VX. Traumatic or other unknown local predisposing factors may account for the frequent occurrence of this lesion in the gingival tissues [1–5, 7, 13]. On the other hand, the literature data on VX cases associated with OLP (Table 1) disclosed that nonkeratinized mucosa sites (tongue, buccal, or labial mucosa) are most frequently involved. Given the fact that these oral sites are affected frequently by OLP, this could suggest that the inflammatory infiltration in OLP may play a pathogenic role in the development of VX. OLP is characterized by basal cell degeneration, apoptotic keratinocytes in association with a chronic T-cell-mediated infiltrate, which maintains a condition of repeated keratinocyte damage/destruction and a consequent change in epithelial turnover [18]. The epithelial cell membranes releasing lipids are taken up by macrophages in the connective tissue becoming foamy in appearance, which eventually leads to VX development [1, 3, 7, 11]. A causal relationship between OLP and VX seems unlikely [19], since OLP is a relatively common oral mucosal disease, in contrast to VX. An accidental coexistence of VX and OLP cannot be excluded, but the VX may also occur concomitantly with autoimmune diseases associated with the chronic inflammatory process and epithelial cell damage/destruction, such as pemphigus vulgaris [8], lupus erythematosus [9], or graft-versus-host disease (GVHD) [11]. VX may represent an atypical T-cell-mediated local reaction to different aetiological agents related to degenerative epithelial changes [7]; such a viewpoint may be supported by the immunologic mechanisms predominated by T lymphocytes, which have been shown to take place during the VX development [2, 25].

VX considered as a reactive process may be involved in other pathologic conditions, such as dystrophic epidermolysis bullosa, in which skin or mucosa blistering may occur after minor trauma [10], or neoplastic lesions (carcinoma), in which the epithelial turnover may be affected [12, 13]. In CHILD syndrome, the formation of lipid-laden cells in VX may be related to this genetic disorder of cholesterol metabolism [14].

VX demonstrates a pathognomonic histological profile consisting of abundant, lipoid-rich macrophages with foam cytoplasm between the elongated uniform depth rete ridges. These cells are characterized by PAS-positive, diastase-resistant granules in their cytoplasm and display positive immunoreaction for the monocyte-macrophage markers CD68 and cathepsin B [2–7, 13, 23]. Three different histological patterns have been described based on the histological architecture and morphology of the lesion: verrucous or warty (A), papillary or cauliflower (B), and flat (C) or slightly raised [5]. The papillary pattern shows a finger-like exophytic epithelial proliferation covering thin cores of connective tissue, whereas in the flat pattern, the lesion demonstrates "endophytic" (below the surface) growth. The number of the foamy cells (xanthoma cells) may be related to the VX pattern. For example, in the flat pattern, numerous foamy cells accumulation can be observed in the lamina propria, possibly leading to the rete ridge elongation and thinning of the covered oral epithelium through compression [2]. In our case, the diagnosis of VX was based on the histopathological features characterized by epithelial hyperplasia in a verrucous pattern and the acanthotic thickened rete ridges combined with the foamy cell aggregations that exhibited strong immunoreactivity for the macrophage marker CD68 [1, 3, 5]. According to the histopathological pattern classification [5], the oral VXs with concomitant OLP reported in the literature (Table 1) exhibited more frequently the flat pattern(4/7), followed by verrucous (2/7) and papillary (1/7).

A correlation between the three histological patterns and the location of the lesions, the patients' age, or the biologic behavior of VX has not been referred in the literature [4, 5, 13]. Oral VX has a benign course with excellent prognosis after complete surgical excision. Recurrences are rare [3, 20].

4. Conclusions

The clinicians should be aware that clinically, verruciform xanthoma may mimic malignancy. Biopsy is required for definitive diagnosis to be established especially when this benign tumor occurs in conjunction with lesions or conditions that may exhibit the potential of malignant transformation, such as oral lichen planus, or may occur at high-risk sites for squamous cell carcinoma development, such as the tongue.

References

[1] B. W. Neville, D. D. Damm, C. M. Allen, and A. C. Chi, "Epithelial pathology," in *Oral and Maxillofacial Pathology*, B. W. Neville, D. D. Damm, C. M. Allen, and A. C. Chi, Eds., pp. 331–421, Elsevier Saunders, St Louis, MO, USA, 4th edition, 2016.

[2] K. A. Mostafa, T. Takata, I. Ogawa, N. Ijuhin, and H. Nikai, "Verruciform xanthoma of the oral mucosa: a clinicopathological study with immunohistochemical findings relating to pathogenesis," *Virchows Archiv A Pathological Anatomy and Histopathology*, vol. 423, no. 4, pp. 243–248, 1993.

[3] H. P. Philipsen, P. A. Reichart, T. Takata, and I. Ogawa, "Verruciform xanthoma-biological profile of 282 oral lesions based on a literature survey with nine new cases from Japan," *Oral Oncology*, vol. 39, no. 4, pp. 325–336, 2003.

[4] C. H. Yu, T. C. Tsai, J. T. Wang et al., "Oral verruciform xanthoma: a clinicopathologic study of 15 cases," *Journal of the Formosan Medical Association*, vol. 106, no. 2, pp. 141–147, 2007.

[5] B. Nowparast, F. V. Howell, and G. M. Rick, "Verruciform xanthoma. A clinicopathologic review and report of fifty-four cases," *Oral Surgery, Oral Medicine, Oral Pathology*, vol. 51, no. 6, pp. 619–625, 1981.

[6] J. A. Hu, Y. Li, and S. Li, "Verruciform xanthoma of the oral cavity: clinicopathological study relating to pathogenesis," *APMIS*, vol. 113, no. 9, pp. 629–634, 2005.

[7] F. Ide, K. Obara, H. Yamada, K. Mishima, I. Saito, and K. Kusama, "Cellular basis of verruciform xanthoma: immunohistochemical and ultrastructural characterization," *Oral Diseases*, vol. 14, no. 2, pp. 150–157, 2008.

[8] R. D. Gehrig, R. A. Baughman, and J. F. Collins, "Verruciform xanthoma in a young male patient with a past history of pemphigus vulgaris," *Oral Surgery, Oral Medicine, Oral Pathology*, vol. 55, no. 1, pp. 58–61, 1983.

[9] A. K. Poulopoulos, A. Epivatianos, T. Zaraboukas, and D. Antoniades, "Verruciform xanthoma coexisting with oral discoid lupus erythematosus," *British Journal of Oral and Maxillofacial Surgery*, vol. 45, no. 2, pp. 159-160, 2007.

[10] S. Murat-Susić, Z. Pastar, I. Dobrić et al., "Verruciform xanthoma in recessive dystrophic epidermolysis bullosa Hallopeau-Siemens," *International Journal of Dermatology*, vol. 46, no. 9, pp. 955–959, 2007.

[11] S. Shahrabi Farahani, N. S. Treister, Z. Khan, and S. B. Woo, "Oral verruciform xanthoma associated with chronic graft-versus-host disease: a report of five cases and a review of the literature," *Head and Neck Pathology*, vol. 5, no. 2, pp. 193–198, 2011.

[12] J. F. Drummond, D. K. White, D. D. Damm, and J. R. Cramer, "Verruciform xanthoma within carcinoma in situ," *Journal of Oral and Maxillofacial Surgery*, vol. 47, no. 4, pp. 398–400, 1989.

[13] B. A. B. de Andrade, M. Agostini, F. R. Pires et al., "Oral verruciform xanthoma: a clinicopathologic and immunohistochemical study of 20 cases," *Journal of Cutaneous Pathology*, vol. 42, no. 7, pp. 489–495, 2015.

[14] M. Bittar and R. Happle, "CHILD syndrome avant la lettre," *Journal of the American Academy of Dermatology*, vol. 50, no. 2, pp. S34–S37, 2004.

[15] C. Fite, F. Plantier, N. Dupin, M. F. Avril, and M. Moyal-Barracc, "Vulvar verruciform xanthoma: ten cases associated with lichen sclerosus, lichen planus, or other conditions," *Archives of Dermatolog*, vol. 147, no. 9, pp. 1087–1092, 2011.

[16] B. W. Neville and D. R. Weathers, "Verruciform xanthoma," *Oral Surgery, Oral Medicine, Oral Pathology*, vol. 49, no. 5, pp. 429–434, 1980.

[17] W. J. Hume, C. J. Smith, and C. D. Franklin, "Verruciform xanthoma," *British Journal of Oral Surgery*, vol. 18, no. 2, pp. 157–161, 1980.

[18] Y. Miyamoto, M. Nagayama, and Y. Hayashi, "Verruciform xanthoma occurring within oral lichen planus," *Journal of Oral Pathology and Medicine*, vol. 25, no. 4, pp. 188–191, 1996.

[19] A. D. Polonowita, N. A. Firth, and A. M. Rich, "Verruciform xanthoma and concomitant lichen planus of the oral mucosa. A report of three cases," *International Journal of Oral and Maxillofacial Surgery*, vol. 28, no. 1, pp. 62–66, 1999.

[20] A. L. Anbinder, M. R. Quirino, and A. A. Brandao, "Verruciform xanthoma and neurofibromatosis: a case report," *British Journal of Oral and Maxillofacial Surgery*, vol. 49, no. 4, pp. e6–e7, 2011.

[21] E. T. Stoopler and B. Desai, "A tongue mass in a patient with oral lichen planus," *Journal-Canadian Dental Association*, vol. 78, p. c60, 2012.

[22] S. M. H. Aghbari, A. I. Abushouk, A. Attia et al., "Malignant transformation of oral lichen planus and oral lichenoid lesions: a meta-analysis of 20095 patient data," *Oral Oncology*, vol. 68, pp. 92–102, 2017.

[23] Y. S. Cheng, A. Gould, Z. Kurago, J. Fantasia, and S. Muller, "Diagnosis of oral lichen planus: a position paper of the American Academy of Oral and Maxillofacial Pathology," *Oral Surgery, Oral Medicine, Oral Pathology and Oral Radiology*, vol. 122, pp. 332–354, 2016.

[24] A. Iamaroon and R. A. Vickers, "Characterization of verruciform xanthoma by in situ hybridization and immunohistochemistry," *Journal of Oral Pathology and Medicine*, vol. 25, no. 7, pp. 395–400, 1996.

[25] P. T. Oliveira, R. G. Jaeger, L. A. Cabral, Y. R. Carvalho, A. L. Costa, and M. M. Jaeger, "Verruciform xanthoma of the oral mucosa. Report of four cases and a review of the literature," *Oral Oncology*, vol. 37, no. 3, pp. 326–331, 2001.

28

Lingual Leiomyomatous Hamartoma in an Adult Male

Amanda Phoon Nguyen ⓘ,[1] **Norman Firth,**[1] **Sophie Mougos,**[2] **and Omar Kujan**[1]

[1]*UWA Dental School, University of Western Australia, Nedlands, WA 6009, Australia*
[2]*Private Practice, OMFSurgery, Cambridge Street, Wembley, WA, Australia*

Correspondence should be addressed to Amanda Phoon Nguyen; phoonamanda@gmail.com

Academic Editor: Konstantinos Michalakis

An otherwise healthy 20-year-old male presented with an exophytic, polypoid, yellowish lesion involving the dorsal surface of his tongue, which he reported being present since birth and unchanged. This was removed by surgical excision and diagnosed as a leiomyomatous hamartoma. Histological examination revealed a combination of fibrovascular connective tissue, conspicuous smooth-muscle bundles, adipose tissue, minor salivary gland tissue, blood vessels, lymphoid tissue, peripheral nerves, and normal skeletal muscle. This case is exceptional due to the patient's age, as until now, lingual leiomyomatous hamartomas have been reported almost exclusively in a paediatric population. To our knowledge, this is the eldest age at which a LLH has been reported in the literature. This underscores the need for clinicians to consider this rarely reported entity when considering the radiographic and clinical differential diagnoses for these lesions, both in the paediatric and adult populations. We also present a review of the literature regarding lingual leiomyomatous hamartomas.

1. Introduction

The term *hamartoma* is used to describe a nonneoplastic, abnormal, and haphazard overgrowth of conglomerates of mature cells and tissues indigenous to the anatomic site from which it occurs, often with one predominating element [1, 2]. This tumor-like malformation is benign, and most hamartomas are located in the liver, spleen, pancreas, and kidneys [3]. Oral hamartomas are rare [3]. An oral leiomyomatous hamartoma, as the name suggests, is therefore a lesion composed mostly of smooth-muscle tissue. They typically present as smooth, soft, nodular lesions that are present at birth and further develop in the first decade of life [3]. They are usually painless masses without obvious symptoms [1]. In most of the published reports, manifestations have commonly been on the gingiva, tongue, and hard palate, specifically the dorsum of the tongue and the anterior maxillary gingiva or alveolar ridge in the incisive papilla region [1, 3]. Due to its low clinical morbidity and nonspecific symptoms, diagnosis and treatment remains a challenge [4].

Here, we report an unusual case of a lingual leiomyomatous hamartoma (LLH) occurring in a healthy 20-year-old male, treated successfully by surgical excision. We also present the histological and immunohistochemical features as well as a review of the literature. This case is exceptional due to the patient's age, as until now, LLHs have been reported almost exclusively in a paediatric population. To our knowledge, this is the eldest age at which a LLH has been reported in the literature.

2. Case Report

A 20-year-old medically fit and healthy male presented for an assessment in preparation for orthognathic surgery. On examination, a 1.5 cm diameter exophytic midline tongue lesion (Figure 1) was noted. This lesion was smooth, regular, and soft to palpation. He reported that this had been present since birth with no change since childhood. A magnetic resonance image (MRI) of his tongue was obtained (Figure 2).

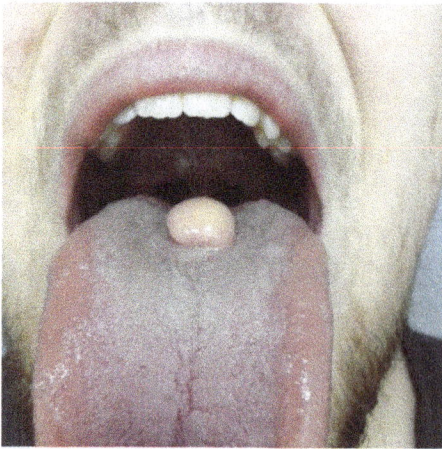

FIGURE 1: A midline lesion involving the dorsal surface of the patient's tongue.

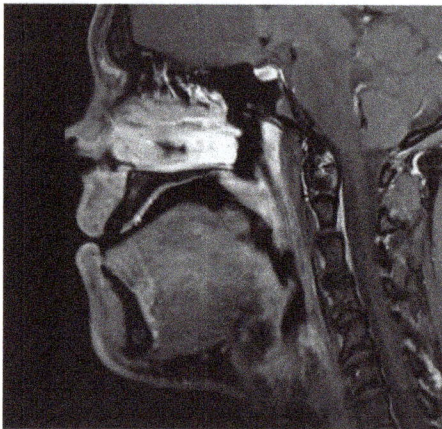

FIGURE 2: Lingual leiomyomatous hamartoma as seen on magnetic resonance imaging.

The MRI report described a 1.5 cm protuberant mass arising from the dorsal aspect of the tongue in the midline at the approximate junction of the oral component and base. The imaging suggested that this was in part fatty, probably arising from the submucosa, and is also seen to demonstrate very mild contrast enhancement. There appeared to be intact overlying mucosa and no apparent involvement of the intrinsic tongue muscles. The sublingual space and salivary glands appeared normal.

Thereafter, the mass was surgically excised and submitted for histological examination including haematoxylin and eosin staining and immunohistochemistry.

Histologically, a hamartoma is characterized by a combination of fibrovascular connective tissue, smooth-muscle bundles, skeletal muscle fibers, adipose tissue, salivary tissue, blood vessels, lymphoid tissue, peripheral nerves, and ganglion cells. One type of tissue is determinant in each lesion. In this specimen, microscopy revealed circumscribed nodules covered by stratified squamous epithelium, and interlacing cords of eosinophilic spindle-shaped cells consistent with the smooth muscle within the lamina propria (Figures 3(a)–3(c)). These mature spindle cells with the profile of smooth-muscle cells were determinant of a leiomyomatous hamartoma. Immunostaining for α-smooth-muscle actin demonstrated large concentrations of smooth-muscle bundles; however, S-100 was found only in peripheral nerve bundles intermingled with smooth-muscle fibers (Figures 4 and 5). No nuclear atypia, cellular pleomorphism, mitosis, or necrosis was noticed, consistent with the benign and developmental nature of these lesions. Based on these features, a histological diagnosis of a leiomyomatous hamartoma was made.

3. Discussion

Hamartomas are pathologically subclassified, depending on the relative abundance of a particular endogenous tissue, and the variants described include vascular, muscle-predominant, adipose tissue-predominant, and intramuscular capillary variants where numerous thin-walled mature capillaries are interspersed between and around muscle bundles [5]. Within the oral cavity, local tissues that might result in hamartomatous growths include odontogenic and nonodontogenic epithelial derivatives, smooth and skeletal muscle, bone, vasculature, nerve, and fat [2]. The borders with the surrounding tissues are typically ill-defined, merging with surrounding tissues [6]. Most hamartomas have been described as pink in colour, ranging in size from 0.1 cm to 2 cm, with a pedunculated, nodular, or polyploidy appearance [7]. These lesions are usually exophytic, although other unusual manifestations such as flat pigmented lesions have been described [6].

LLH most frequently occurs on the anterior palate in the region of the incisive papilla or gingiva and on the midline dorsal tongue, and this predilection may be due to the propensity to dysgenic events in the midline embryonic fusion regions [1]. The most important features of a LLH are its limited growth potential after adolescence and microscopic appearance of unencapsulated admixture of mature cells native to the anatomic location [2]. They are usually painless and relatively small lesions, and most of the published cases involve children (Table 1). They are known to occur most frequently in the first decade of life. In terms of gender, LLH has been reported to occur more frequently in females [3, 18], though the literature regarding this is controversial. In a study by Wushou et al. [4] on 194 cases of head and neck hamartomas, these were more common in males.

Microscopically, LLH should be differentiated from a solid oral leiomyoma and an angiomyoma (angioleiomyoma; vascular leiomyoma); the solid leiomyoma is a true neoplasm of smooth-muscle origin, which is rare in the oral cavity [1].

Clinically, an intraoral solid mass in or near the midline of the maxilla and the tongue, especially in children, should involve LLH as a differential diagnosis. Other lesions that have a similar clinical presentation such as a lipoma, granular cell tumor, choristoma, leiomyoma,

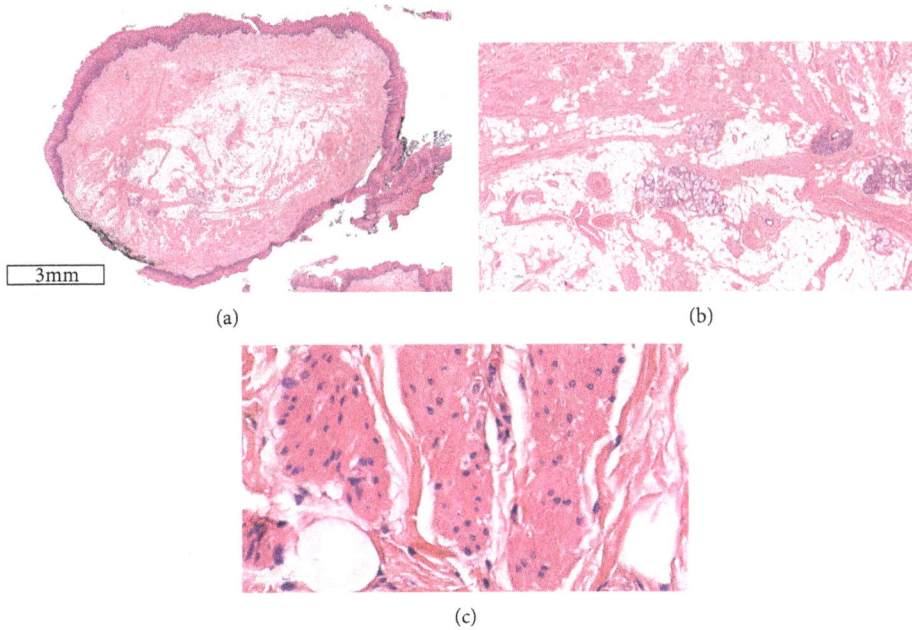

FIGURE 3: (a) Section of the hamartoma showing fascicles of smooth muscles, fat, and salivary glands, with normal covering epithelium (haematoxylin and eosin, original magnification ×10). (b) Section of the hamartoma showing blood vessels, fascicles of smooth muscles, fat, and salivary glands (haematoxylin and eosin, original magnification ×200). (c) High-power section of the hamartoma showing fascicles of smooth muscles and fat. (haematoxylin and eosin, original magnification ×400).

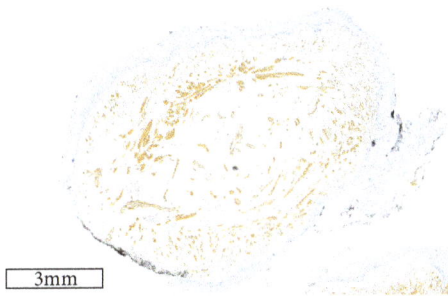

FIGURE 4: Immunohistochemical findings of a section of the hamartoma showing fascicles of smooth muscles with smooth-muscle actin immunoreactivity (original magnification ×100).

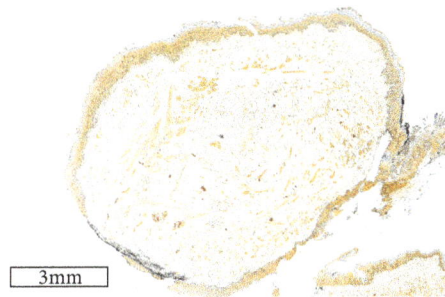

FIGURE 5: Immunohistochemical findings of a section of the hamartoma showing low S100 immunoreactivity (original magnification ×100).

fibrous epithelial polyp, and benign mesenchymoma should likewise be considered. As the appearance of LLH can be nonspecific, other lesions such as vascular or lymphatic lesions, mucus extravasation phenomena, reactive or traumatic lesions, benign or malignant neoplasm, and cystic lesions should not be neglected. Additionally, in a paediatric population, hamartomas should be differentiated from lingual thyroid thorough clinical examination, imaging, and histopathological examination.

Given the nonneoplastic nature of hamartomas, complete removal of the tumor mass by wide surgical excision is the accepted treatment of choice. Recurrences have been reported where surgical excision is incomplete. Wushou et al. [4] studied 194 cases of head and neck hamartoma and found that after following the patients for a median of 36 months, 6 patients developed a recurrence. They reported that lesions of less than 6 cm in diameter were well controlled; in contrast, all the recurrences were reported from the larger lesions, of more than 6 cm diameter, which could not be resected completely, especially multiple lesions involving bony tissue. Postoperative radiotherapy was used successfully in one of their recurrent cases [4].

This case is exceptional due to the patient's age, as until now, LLHs have been reported almost exclusively in a paediatric population. This underscores the need for clinicians to gain familiarity and consider this entity when considering the radiographic and clinical differential diagnoses for these lesions, both in the paediatric and adult populations.

TABLE 1: Clinical features of reported cases of lingual leiomyomatous hamartoma.

N	First authors	Location on tongue	Age	Sex	Hamartoma type	Congenital?	Associated syndromes
18 cases out of 135	Kreiger et al. [7]	16/18 were dorsal	8 d to 16 y	M = 6, F = 12	2/8 were neurovascular. 5/18 were SM dominant. 1/18 was fat dominant. 10/18 contained SM and fat.	8, One patient was both.	4
1	Fadzilah [8]	Midline posterior mass originating from the tongue base	2 months	M	SM predominant	Yes	No
1	Hanna et al. [9]	Left lateral tongue	3 months	F	SM dominant	Yes	Yes; ectrodactyly-ectodermal dysplasia-clefting syndrome
1	Stamm and Tauber [10]	Base of tongue	Newborn	F	SM dominant	Yes	No
1	Becker et al. [11]	Base of tongue	Newborn	M	SM dominant	Yes	No
1	Takimoto [12]	Base of tongue	6 years	F	SM dominant	Unsure	No
1	Ishii et al. [13]	Base and anterior tongue (4 masses)	4 months	F	SM dominant	Yes	No
1	Goold et al. [14]	Midline dorsum posterior	5 months	M	SM dominant	Yes	No
1	Goldsmith et al. [15]	Posterior tongue	16 months	M	SM dominant	Yes	No
1	Kobayshi et al. [16]	Antero dorsal tongue	3 month	M	SM dominant	Yes	No
1	De la Rosa García and Mosqueda-Taylor [17]	Anterior tongue	6 years	M	SM dominant	Yes	No

References

[1] D. M. Freitas da Silva, I. A. Fernandes, A. Wu, and B. W. Neville, "Oral leiomyomatous hamartoma of the anterior maxillary gingiva," *Clinical Advances in Periodontics*, vol. 6, no. 4, pp. 190–194, 2016.

[2] S. Patil, R. Rao, and B. Majumdar, "Hamartomas of the oral cavity," *Journal of International Society of Preventive & Community Dentistry*, vol. 5, no. 5, pp. 347–353, 2015.

[3] D. Al Qahtani and A. Qannam, "Oral leiomyomatous hamartoma of the median maxillary gingiva: a case report and review of the literature," *International Journal of Surgical Pathology*, vol. 21, no. 4, pp. 413–416, 2015.

[4] A. Wushou, W. Liu, X. Bai et al., "Clinical analysis of 194 cases of head and neck hamartoma," *Oral Surgery, Oral Medicine, Oral Pathology, Oral Radiology*, vol. 115, no. 3, pp. 299–303, 2013.

[5] S. Tandon, R. Meher, A. Raj, and C. Chitguppi, "Hamartoma of parapharyngeal space: a rare case report," *MAMC Journal of Medical Sciences*, vol. 2, no. 1, p. 51, 2016.

[6] I. Kaplan, I. Allon, B. Shlomi, V. Raiser, and D. Allon, "A comparative study of oral hamartoma and choristoma," *Journal of Interdisciplinary Histopathology*, vol. 3, no. 4, 2015.

[7] P. A. Kreiger, L. M. Ernst, L. M. Elden, K. Kazahaya, F. Alawi, and P. A. Russo, "Hamartomatous tongue lesions in children," *The American Journal of Surgical Pathology*, vol. 31, no. 8, pp. 1186–1190, 2007.

[8] N. Fadzilah, "Congenital midline tongue base mass in an infant: lingual hamartoma," *Journal of Clinical and Diagnostic Research*, vol. 10, no. 9, 2016.

[9] R. Hanna, Z. B. Argenyi, and J. A. Benda, "Hamartoma of the tongue in an infant with a primary diagnosis of ectrodactyly-ectodermal dysplasia-cleft lip and palate syndrome," *Journal of Cutaneous Pathology*, vol. 21, no. 2, pp. 173–178, 1994.

[10] C. Stamm and R. Tauber, "Hamartoma of tongue," *The Laryngoscope*, vol. 55, no. 3, pp. 140–146, 1945.

[11] G. D. Becker, R. Ridolfi, and C. Ingber, "Lingual hamartoma in a newborn," *Otolaryngology Head and Neck Surgery*, vol. 92, no. 3, pp. 357–359, 1984.

[12] T. Takimoto, "Hamartoma of the tongue base," *Practica oto-Rhino-Laryngologica*, vol. 83, no. 5, pp. 694-695, 1990.

[13] T. Ishii, S. Takemori, and J.-I. Suzuki, "Hamartoma of the tongue: report of a case," *Archives of Otolaryngology-Head and Neck Surgery*, vol. 88, no. 2, pp. 171–173, 1968.

[14] A. Goold, B. Koch, and J. Willging, "Lingual hamartoma in an infant: CT and MR imaging," *American Journal of Neuroradiology*, vol. 28, pp. 30-31, 2005.

[15] P. Goldsmith, J. V. Soames, and D. Meikle, "Leiomyomatous hamartoma of the posterior tongue: a case report," *The Journal of Laryngology and Otology*, vol. 109, no. 12, pp. 1190-1191, 1995.

[16] A. Kobayashi, T. Amagasa, and N. Okada, "Leiomyomatous hamartoma of the tongue: case report," *Journal of Oral and Maxillofacial Surgery*, vol. 59, no. 3, pp. 337–340, 2001.

[17] E. De La Rosa-García and A. Mosqueda-Taylor, "Leiomyomatous hamartoma of the anterior tongue: report of a case and review of the literature," *International Journal of Paediatric Dentistry*, vol. 9, no. 2, pp. 129–132, 1999.

[18] O. Kujan, S. Clark, and P. Sloan, "Leiomyomatous hamartoma presenting as a congenital epulis," *British Journal of Oral and Maxillofacial Surgery*, vol. 45, no. 3, pp. 228–230, 2007.

29

Clinical Application of the Socket-Shield Concept in Multiple Anterior Teeth

G. Esteve-Pardo ⓘ **and L. Esteve-Colomina** ⓘ

Private Practice at Clínica Dental Esteve SL, Group Aula Dental Avanzada, Alicante, Spain

Correspondence should be addressed to G. Esteve-Pardo; guillemjoes@hotmail.com

Academic Editor: Gavriel Chaushu

A case of rehabilitation of the upper front teeth is presented. To prevent bone resorption following extractions, a socket-shield technique on all the extracted teeth was performed. The combination of a staged extraction approach, the sequence of provisionals together with the minimal bone loss of vestibular volume, allowed solving this high aesthetic demanding case in a satisfactory way for the patient both in duration of the treatment and in its final outcome.

1. Introduction

The socket-shield technique (SST) was first described by Hürzeler et al. [1]. The procedure consists of leaving a root fragment when extracting the tooth, specifically the vestibular portion of the most coronal third of the root (Figures 1 and 2).

It is widely known that following the extraction of a tooth a dimensional modification of the ridge is going to happen. This unavoidable and irreversible shrinkage is very unfavorable from the restorative point of view, especially in the aesthetic area. After three months, horizontal and vertical contractions of the alveolar volume occur [2] and these changes affect both to the soft and hard tissues [3].

The SST is aimed at making up for this loss of the vestibular volume "misleading" the bundle bone since the periodontal ligament remains attached to the dentine and cement of the root fragment.

Various animal studies demonstrated that the postextraction loss of volume could be highly diminished when leaving a tooth fragment attached to the cortical bone in the vestibular part of the alveolus [1, 4, 5].

The SST is yet missing clinical long-term data to be recommended as a standard treatment. A recent systematic review showed that the documentation on SST is reduced to some short-term case reports and case series and only a case-control study [6]. For the moment, the clinician has only his or her individual expertise as a criterion to decide when and how to apply this technique. From 2010, several variations of the original technique have been proposed [7]. The SST is beginning to be considered as one type of partial extraction therapies (PET) [8], a concept derived from the root submergence technique (RST) initially proposed by Salama and coworkers for pontic site development [9].

The partial extraction of a tooth is a complex procedure since the tooth fragment to leave should not be luxated at all by the movements used to extract the rest of the root [10]. Otherwise, the following complications may occur: loss of the tooth fragment, resorption of vestibular bone, infection, exposure of implant threads, and even implant failure. All these could worsen the situation of having extracted the whole tooth completely [6].

The traditional way to try to compensate the loss of vestibular volume in an immediate postextraction implant has been hard and soft tissue grafting [3]. We should not see the SST as a substitute for it, but rather as a complement when it can be carried out. It seems to have advantages compared to the connective tissue graft (CTG), but this issue is beyond the scope of the article.

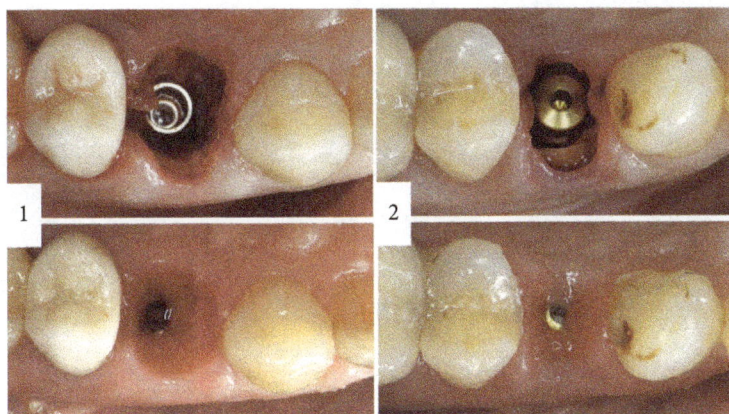

FIGURE 1: Two cases treated by immediate implant with SST and their occlusal view after three months of healing.

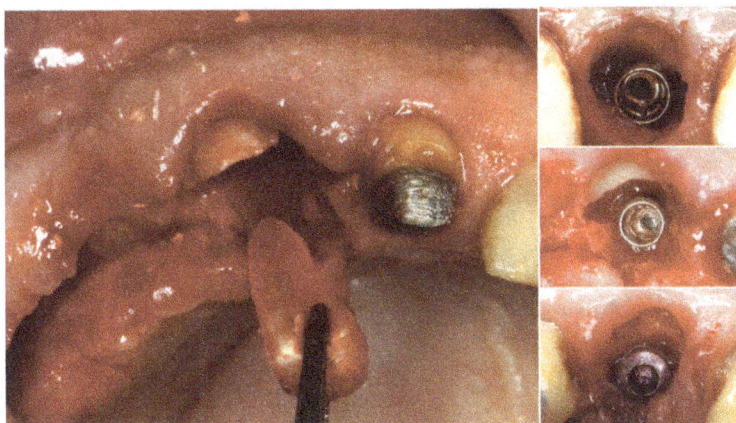

FIGURE 2: Different applications of the SST.

This case report will show a clinical case where immediate implant placement in the aesthetic area was performed using the SST. The sockets not to be implanted and receiving the pontics were treated by alveolar preservation with the SST. This way a successful aesthetic restoration was achieved as the tissue volume seems to be maintained.

2. Case Description

The patient was a 76-year-old man who came to the office in 2014 looking for possible treatments of his fractured central incisors. Nothing was found relevant about his medical condition. The patient shows a high risk for caries and also eccentric bruxism. He has partial edentulism in the superior left quadrant and multiple decay and fractured teeth. The initial approach was conservative aiming to keep the upper front by means of composite fillings (Figures 3(a) and 3(b)). Then, the posterior superior quadrants needed to be restored with implants.

Three years after, in 2017, the patient came back to the office referring pain of endodontic origin in the upper left canine. New and secondary subgingival caries were found in the six front teeth. The conservative prognosis was considered poor due to the subgingival depth and extent of decay

presented by the lesions from canine to canine. After having discussed the treatment options, especially the surgical lengthening of the front teeth or the orthodontic extrusion, the patient decides to replace the residual teeth with a new implant-supported bridge similar to the recently performed prostheses of the posterior areas that were judged by him as a highly satisfactory treatment. The patient preferred not to involve these restorations in the present anterior treatment and limited it to place only two implants in the lateral incisors' positions (Figure 4).

The treatment was carried out in a staged approach. Briefly, first, we extracted the lateral incisors, using the SST, and placed two immediate implants. The four residual teeth were then prepared to be used as abutments of a temporary bridge for the purpose of maintaining the aesthetics and function of the patient during the early osseointegration period. In a further step, the four remaining teeth were also extracted using the SST, and the initial provisional bridge was replaced by the second provisional screwed on the uncovered implants. Only one out of the four abutment teeth used for the temporization of root canal treatment was needed due to a periapical infection.

When placing the two immediate implants into the alveolus of the lateral incisors, a section of the buccal part of the

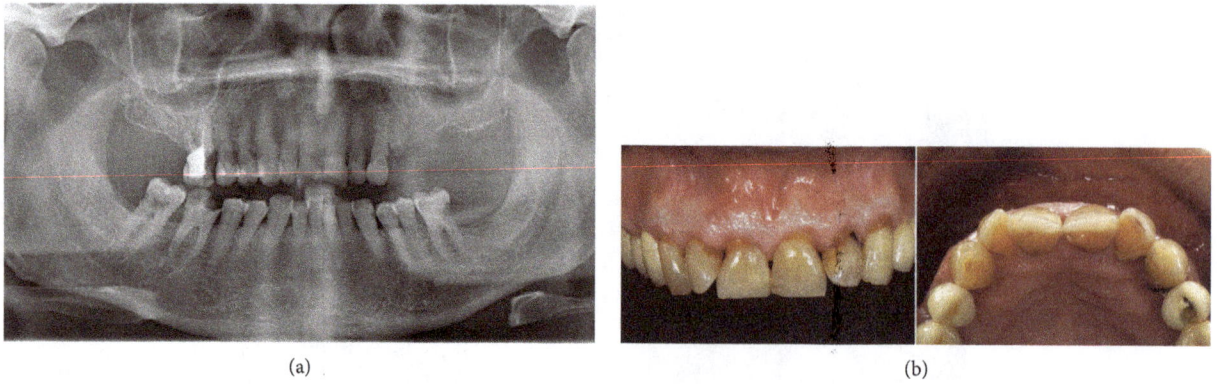

FIGURE 3: (a) Initial panoramic radiograph. (b) Clinical view of the anterior teeth. The roots are subgingivally and peripherally decayed.

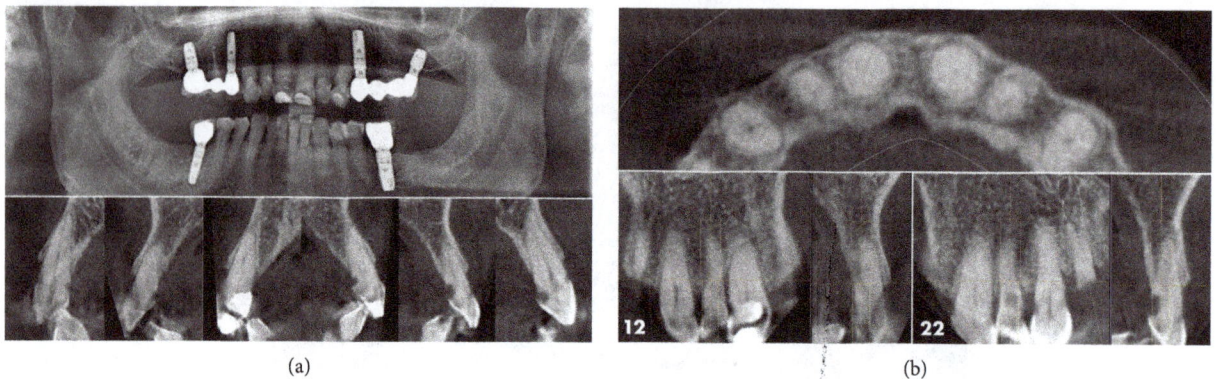

FIGURE 4: (a) Panoramic X-ray. (b) 3D slices showing the implant planning. The root caries can be seen.

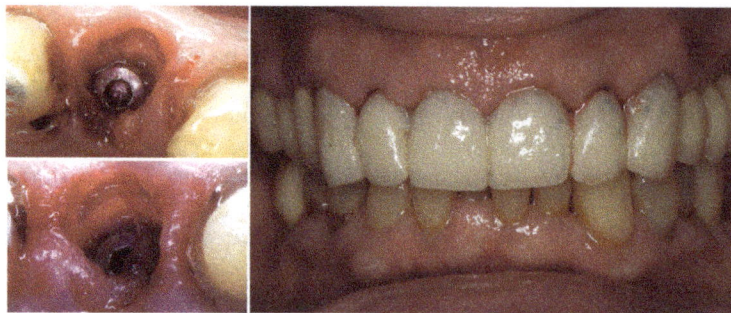

FIGURE 5: Stage one: implants placed with SST in the lateral incisors' sites and the immediate temporary bridge on the abutment teeth.

root (about the two middle thirds) was left in place and no biomaterial was used at all. An impression of the implants was taken to have the second temporary bridge available in the second surgery. Healing abutments were then attached with the proper height for the soft tissue to cover them but at the same time facilitating the uncovering. Finally, a temporary acrylic bridge was cemented onto the four abutment teeth 13-11 and 21-23 (Figure 5).

Three months later, the implants were uncovered, the four abutment teeth were extracted, again with the SST—partial extraction of the roots—but this time no more implants were placed in these sockets. The first provisional

cemented onto the teeth was then replaced by a second acrylic bridge screwed onto the implants though temporary abutments (Figure 6).

The partial extraction of the canines, aiming to leave a buccal slice of the root, was so hard to perform, and further instrumentation would lead to the socket destruction that a decision was intraoperatively made and a greater portion of the root, including the apex, was finally left. As the locations of the canines did not involve the implant sites, any potential complication could be addressed efficiently.

One month later, the prosthodontic phase was undertaken. Little if any differences in the buccal tissue volume

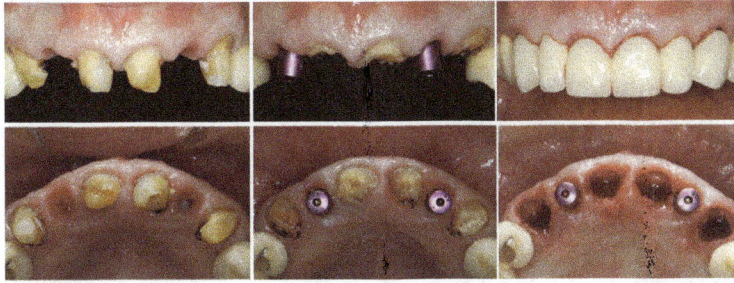

FIGURE 6: Stage two: partial extraction of the remaining teeth and placement of the second provisional onto the uncovered implants.

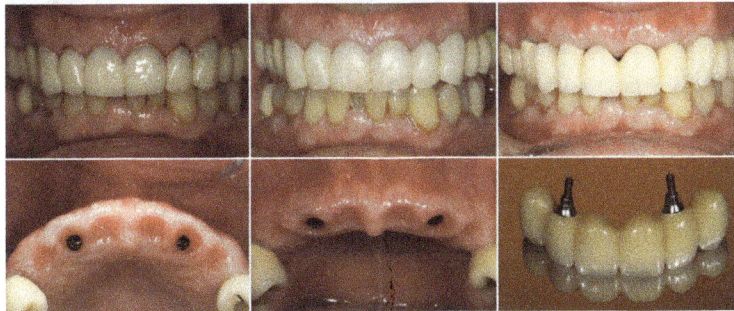

FIGURE 7: Frontal view of immediate provisional after implant placement, 3 months after healing and 1 month after 2nd implant provisional prosthesis. Soft tissue view before prosthodontic phase.

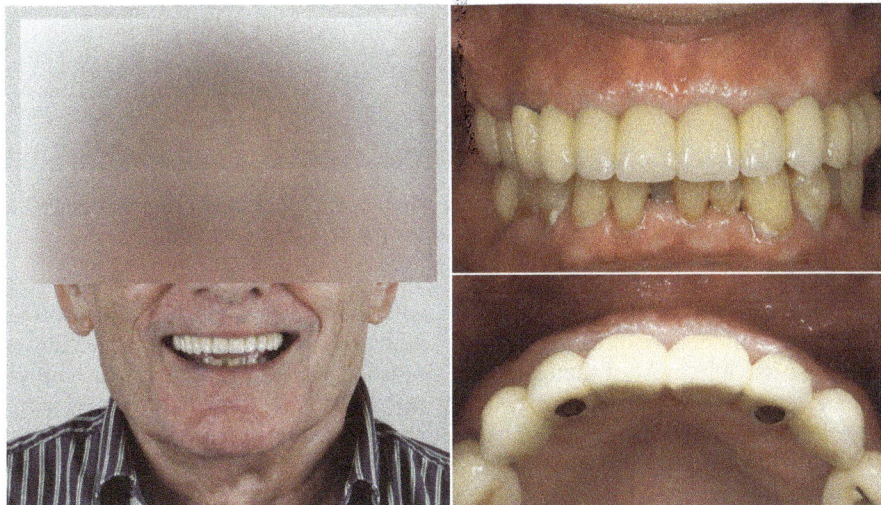

FIGURE 8: Final restoration in place and its integration on the patient smile.

and no noticeable aesthetic impact could be found after the multiple extractions (Figure 7). The desired position of the incisal border was determined by various try-ins, and five months after implant surgery, the definitive prosthesis was placed. The final clinical aspect can be appreciated in the pictures (Figures 8 and 9).

3. Discussion

There is still insufficient evidence to support the SST with simultaneous implantation. Only a few case reports are available showing variable data of bone loss. In a case-control study in 2014, a medium vertical bone loss of 0.8 mm was reported in 26 implants on 25 patients after 24 months of follow-up [11]. In a prospective clinical case series study, the marginal bone loss was reported to be 0.7 mm on average after 6 months [12]. In a retrospective study on 10 patients in 2017, a mean bone loss of 0.33 mm in mesial and 0.17 mm in distal were reported [7].

In a recent systematic review, the authors find a horizontal bone loss of 1.07 mm and 0.78 mm vertically after the immediate placement of implants [13]. Usually this horizontal bone loss has to be compensated by bone augmentation and/or a connective tissue graft [14].

Although the amount of marginal bone loss in the SST is still not conclusively proved, current clinical experiences

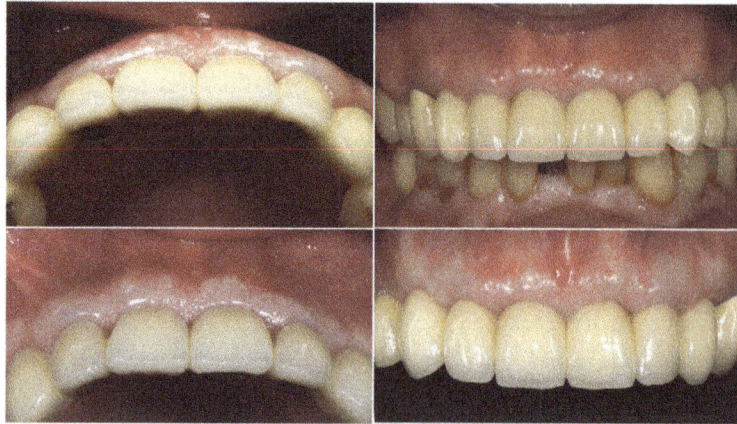

FIGURE 9: Aesthetic appearance after 6-month follow-up.

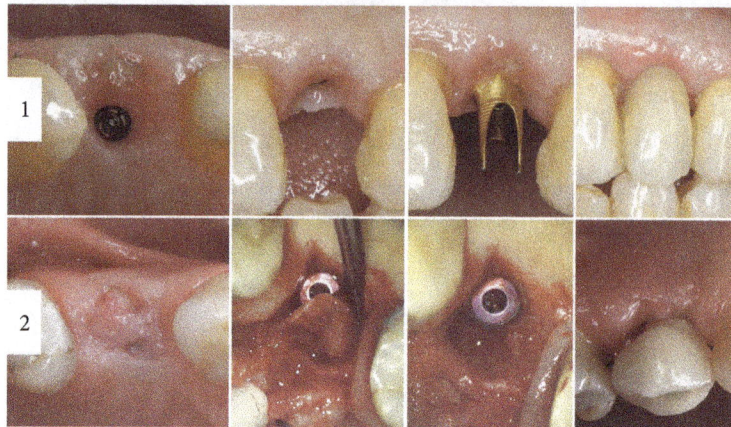

FIGURE 10: Two cases with SST complications. In 1, lateral incisor restoration with the shield communicated with oral cavity. In 2, first premolar with luxated shield on implant second stage. Implant failed at the last case after 4 months.

seem to point to a minimal, negligible, or even not existent bone loss after extraction. As a consequence of this, soft tissue grafting would not be necessary in most of the patients treated by this technique. In the aforementioned case-control study in 2014, the authors found a significant difference in aesthetic impact when comparing the socket shield to the conventional technique [11].

Needless to say that if grafting is not an aesthetic requirement to compensate the horizontal bone loss, the treatment becomes more patient-friendly with less duration and morbidity. Nevertheless, the SST is an operator-sensitive procedure, delicate to handle, and sometimes very hard to perform [15].

In this case, the first provisional bridge on abutment teeth allowed the patient to comfortably wear a fixed temporary prosthesis during the healing time of the immediately implanted sockets. This bridge was not used to shape the soft tissues. The staged extraction approach avoided a major tissue loss and contributed to maintain a more aesthetic tissue architecture [16].

To support, a 6-unit prosthesis by only two implants and with two cantilevers in the canine positions could also be a reason for discussion. Another option previously discussed

with the patient was a full-arch prosthesis splinting the two new implants to the four preexisting ones. The patient was satisfied with the recently restored posterior quadrants and rejected it. A three-fixed superior rehabilitation scheme allowed us to perform a simpler treatment with better acceptance by the patient. Given the evident bruxism, the number of implants could be considered low for the anterior bridge—six teeth on two implants—but there is a growing clinical evidence about lower number of implants to support a full arch. Should a proper occlusion is achieved and the patient wears an occlusal splint, the distal cantilevers seem not to be a problem [17].

Since decades, clinicians have been trying to avoid the loss of alveolar volume by leaving root remnants [18]. In an old study on 2000 patients, the authors reported that a 16.2% of the root remnants resulted in pathological condition signs especially when exposed to the oral environment [19]. Although numerous papers since the late seventies dealt with the so-called "root submergence technique," this still remains a controversial issue. The uneventful healing of sockets with root fragments has been well documented [20]. Both vital tooth retention [21, 22] and submergence of endodontically treated roots [23, 24] have been recommended to prevent excessive resorption of the residual ridge. This concept has been recently applied to teeth- or implant-supported fixed prostheses for pontic site development [9, 25–27]. Based on this background, a decision was made to leave the canine roots instead of performing a more invasive surgical procedure for extracting them. One of the main factors for the success of the SST is precisely that the root fragment does not come in contact with the external medium [7], something that could facilitate the infection and also be an aesthetic problem (Figure 10).

A human histologic study has been recently published demonstrating osseointegration between an implant surface and a dentin surface of a root fragment from a SST making the technique further promising [28].

4. Conclusion

The SST has currently not enough clinical evidence for being recommended as a routine option. It seems that if the proper clinical requirements are met and the technical handling of the operator is appropriate, the SST could minimize the resorption of the buccal tissues after the tooth extraction. In selected cases, the immediate placement of implants with the SST seems to be a useful tool for the replacement of the teeth lost, especially in the aesthetic area.

References

[1] M. B. Hürzeler, O. Zuhr, P. Schupbach, S. F. Rebele, N. Emmanouilidis, and S. Fickl, "The socket-shield technique: a proof-of-principle report," *Journal of Clinical Periodontology*, vol. 37, no. 9, pp. 855–862, 2010.

[2] M. G. Araújo and J. Lindhe, "Dimensional ridge alterations following tooth extraction. An experimental study in the dog," *Journal of Clinical Periodontology*, vol. 32, no. 2, pp. 212–218, 2005.

[3] S. T. Chen and D. Buser, "Esthetic outcomes following immediate and early implant placement in the anterior maxilla—a systematic review," *The International Journal of Oral & Maxillofacial Implants*, vol. 29, pp. 186–215, 2014.

[4] D. Bäumer, O. Zuhr, S. Rebele, D. Schneider, P. Schupbach, and M. Hürzeler, "The socket-shield technique: first histological, clinical, and volumetrical observations after separation of the buccal tooth segment – a pilot study," *Clinical Implant Dentistry and Related Research*, vol. 17, no. 1, pp. 71–82, 2015.

[5] J. L. Calvo-Guirado, M. Troiano, P. J. López-López et al., "Different configuration of socket shield technique in peri-implant bone preservation: an experimental study in dog mandible," *Annals of Anatomy - Anatomischer Anzeiger*, vol. 208, pp. 109–115, 2016.

[6] A. S. Gharpure and N. B. Bhatavadekar, "Current evidence on the socket-shield technique: a systematic review," *Journal of Oral Implantology*, vol. 43, no. 5, pp. 395–403, 2017.

[7] D. Bäumer, O. Zuhr, S. Rebele, and M. Hürzeler, "Socket shield technique for immediate implant placement - clinical, radiographic and volumetric data after 5 years," *Clinical Oral Implants Research*, vol. 28, no. 11, pp. 1450–1458, 2017.

[8] H. Gluckman, M. Salama, and J. Du Toit, "Partial extraction therapies (PET) part 1: maintaining alveolar ridge contour at pontic and immediate implant sites," *The International Journal of Periodontics & Restorative Dentistry*, vol. 36, no. 5, pp. 681–687, 2016.

[9] M. Salama, T. Ishikawa, H. Salama, A. Funato, and D. Garber, "Advantages of the root submergence technique for pontic site development in esthetic implant therapy," *International Journal of Periodontics & Restorative Dentistry*, vol. 27, no. 6, pp. 521–527, 2007.

[10] H. Gluckman, M. Salama, and J. Du Toit, "Partial extraction therapies (PET) part 2: procedures and technical aspects," *The International Journal of Periodontics & Restorative Dentistry*, vol. 37, no. 3, pp. 377–385, 2017.

[11] M. Abadzhiev, P. Nenkov, and P. Velcheva, "Conventional immediate implant placement and immediate placement with socket-shield technique – which is better," *International Journal of Clinical Medicine Research*, vol. 1, no. 5, pp. 176–180, 2014.

[12] M. Troiano, M. Benincasa, P. Sánchez, and J. L. Guirado, "Bundle bone preservation with Root-T-Belt: case study," *Annals of Oral Maxillofacial Surgery*, vol. 2, no. 1, p. 7, 2014.

[13] C. T. Lee, T. S. Chiu, S. K. Chuang, D. Tarnow, and J. Stoupel, "Alterations of the bone dimension following immediate implant placement into extraction socket: systematic review and meta-analysis," *Journal of Clinical Periodontology*, vol. 41, no. 9, pp. 914–926, 2014.

[14] D. Buser, V. Chappuis, U. C. Belser, and S. Chen, "Implant placement post extraction in esthetic single tooth sites: when immediate, when early, when late?," *Periodontology 2000*, vol. 73, no. 1, pp. 84–102, 2017.

[15] M. Glocker, T. Attin, and P. R. Schmidlin, "Ridge preservation with modified "socket-shield" technique: a methodological case series," *Dental Journal*, vol. 2, no. 1, pp. 11–21, 2014.

[16] E. Mijiritsky, Z. Mazor, A. Lorean, C. Mortellaro, O. Mardinger, and L. Levin, "Transition from hopeless dentition to full-arch fixed-implant-supported rehabilitation by a staged extraction approach: rationale and technique," *The Journal of Craniofacial Surgery*, vol. 25, no. 3, pp. 847–850, 2014.

[17] G. E. Romanos, B. Gupta, and S. E. Eckert, "Distal cantilevers and implant dentistry," *The International Journal of Oral & Maxillofacial Implants*, vol. 27, no. 5, pp. 1131–1136, 2012.

[18] D. M. Casey and F. R. Lauciello, "A review of the submerged-root concept," *The Journal of Prosthetic Dentistry*, vol. 43, no. 2, pp. 128–132, 1980.

[19] R. W. Helsham, "Some observations on the subject of roots of teeth retained in the jaws as a result of incomplete exodontia," *Australian Dental Journal*, vol. 5, no. 2, pp. 70–77, 1960.

[20] K. D. Siormpas, M. E. Mitsias, E. Kontsiotou-Siormpa, D. Garber, and G. A. Kotsakis, "Immediate implant placement in the esthetic zone utilizing the "root-membrane" technique: clinical results up to 5 years postloading," *The International Journal of Oral & Maxillofacial Implants*, vol. 29, no. 6, pp. 1397–1405, 2014.

[21] R. K. Gongloff, "Vital root retention: a 5-year experience," *International Journal of Oral and Maxillofacial Surgery*, vol. 15, no. 1, pp. 33–38, 1986.

[22] K. Fareed, R. Khayat, and P. Salins, "Vital root retention, a clinical procedure," *The Journal of Prosthetic Dentistry*, vol. 62, no. 4, pp. 430–434, 1989.

[23] R. B. O'Neal, T. Gound, M. P. Levin, and C. E. del Rio, "Submergence of roots for alveolar bone preservation: I. Endodontically treated roots," *Oral Surgery, Oral Medicine, Oral Pathology*, vol. 45, no. 5, pp. 803–810, 1978.

[24] W. A. Welker, G. J. Jividen, and D. C. Kramer, "Preventive prosthodontics—mucosal coverage of roots," *The Journal of Prosthetic Dentistry*, vol. 40, no. 6, pp. 619–621, 1978.

[25] K. M. Wong, C. M. Chneh, and C. W. Ang, "Modified root submergence technique for multiple implant-supported maxillary anterior restorations in a patient with thin gingival biotype: a clinical report," *The Journal of Prosthetic Dentistry*, vol. 107, no. 6, pp. 349–352, 2012.

[26] A. Çomut, M. Mehra, and H. Saito, "Pontic site development with a root submergence technique for a screw-retained prosthesis in the anterior maxilla," *The Journal of Prosthetic Dentistry*, vol. 110, no. 5, pp. 337–343, 2013.

[27] S. Choi, I. S. Yeo, S. H. Kim, J. B. Lee, C. W. Cheong, and J. S. Han, "A root submergence technique for pontic site development in fixed dental prostheses in the maxillary anterior esthetic zone," *Journal of Periodontal & Implant Science*, vol. 45, no. 4, pp. 152–155, 2015.

[28] C. Schwimer, G. A. Pette, H. Gluckman, M. Salama, and J. Du Toit, "Human histologic evidence of new bone formation and osseointegration between root dentin (unplanned socket-shield) and dental implant: case report," *The International Journal of Oral & Maxillofacial Implants*, vol. 33, no. 1, pp. e19–e23, 2018.

30

Rehabilitation of Posterior Maxilla with Obturator Supported by Zygomatic Implants

Sankalp Mittal,[1] **Manoj Agarwal,**[2] **and Debopriya Chatterjee** ⓘ[3]

[1]*Department of Oral and Maxillofacial Surgery, Government Dental College (RUHS-CODS), Jaipur, India*
[2]*Department of Conservative, Government Dental College (RUHS-CODS), Jaipur, India*
[3]*Department of Periodontics, Government Dental College (RUHS-CODS), Jaipur, India*

Correspondence should be addressed to Debopriya Chatterjee; banerjee.debo@gmail.com

Academic Editor: Gavriel Chaushu

Prosthetic rehabilitation of atrophic maxilla and large maxillary defects can be done successfully by zygomatic implant-supported prosthesis. Zygomatic implants are an avant-garde to complex and invasive-free vascularised osteocutaneous flaps, distraction osteogenesis, and the solution to flap failures. A treated case of tuberculous osteomyelitis, with a class II (Aramany's classification) maxillary defect, reported to oral maxillofacial department, Government Dental College (RUHS-CODS). The defect in this group was unilateral, retaining the anterior teeth. The patient was previously rehabilitated with a removable maxillary obturator. Inadequate retention affected essential functions like speaking, mastication, swallowing, esthetics, and so on due to lack of sufficient supporting tissues. A fixed prosthetic rehabilitation of posterior maxillary defect was done with obturator supported with two single-piece zygomatic implants. At 1-year follow-up, the patient was comfortable with the prosthesis, and no further complaints were recorded.

1. Introduction

Extensive maxillary defect and atrophic maxilla pose a challenge for prosthetic rehabilitation. Procedures for rehabilitation of large maxillary defect involve Le Fort I maxillary downfracture, onlay bone grafts, maxillary sinus graft procedures, and free osteocutaneous flaps. These procedures mostly require a second surgery at the donor site. Zygomatic implants provide an effective means to avoid the second surgical site and still rehabilitate the patient with a fixed prosthesis.

2. Case Presentation

A 42-year-male was referred to the oral maxillofacial department of Government Dental College and Hospital (RUHS-CODS), Jaipur with complaint of difficulty in speaking, swallowing, chewing, and visible appearance. There was a history of maxillectomy (class II defect according to Armany's classification of maxillectomy defect) of the right side posterior to the second premolar two years back

due to tuberculosis osteomylitis (Figure 1). The defect categorized in this group is unilateral, retaining the anterior teeth [1].

Six months after maxillectomy, the patient was rehabilitated with hollow bulb obturator. The maxillary obturator was not stable. The use of conventional dental implants was restricted as the defect size was large; adequate teeth for retention were not present, and underlying bone support was inadequate. The zygomatic implant was planned to address these issues and to rehabilitate the posterior maxillary defect.

A detailed case history was elicited with thorough extraoral and intraoral examination. Evaluation was done with respect to bone volume and density of the remaining zygomatic bone, intermaxillary relationship, occlusal relationship, and the condition of opposing dentition.

The 3-D computed tomography (CT) examination showed that the body of the maxilla on right side along with lateral border of pyriform aperture and medial infraorbital margin was missing (Figures 2 and 3). On clinical examination, 1.5×2.0 cm defect was present posterior to second premolar along with oroantral communication.

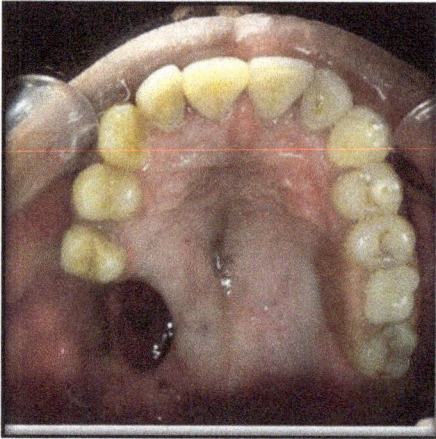

FIGURE 1: Preoperative intraoral view showing class II defect according to Armany's classification of maxillectomy defect.

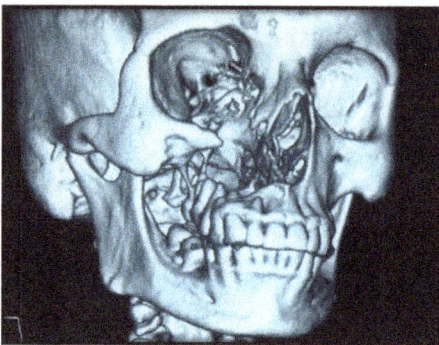

FIGURE 2: Preoperative 3-DCT view showing the missing body of the maxilla on the right side along with the lateral border of pyriform aperture and medial infraorbital margin.

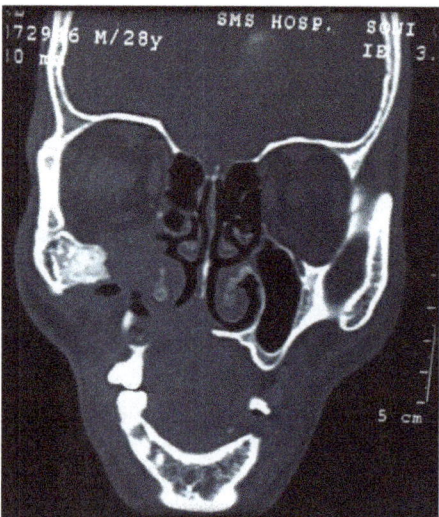

FIGURE 3: Axial CT view showing maxillectomy defect.

It was decided to use single-piece zygomatic implants (IHDE Dental, Sewden). The surgery was performed under general anesthesia. A modification of the traditional lefort 1 incision[9] was made, where in the incision was given in the

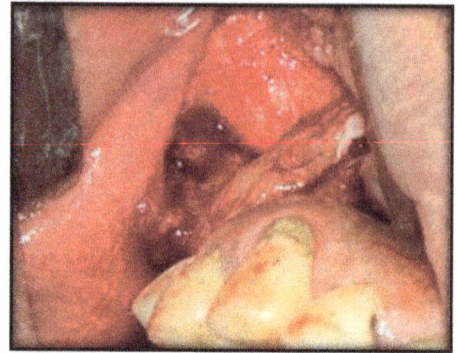

FIGURE 4: Mucoperiosteal flap elevated up to the zygomatic bone.

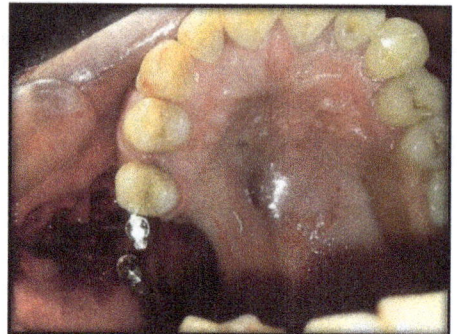

FIGURE 5: Intraoral view of two standard zygomatic single-piece implants placed in right zygomatic bone.

right lateral buccal mucosa in the zygomatic buttress region. Mucoperiosteal flap was elevated up to the zygomatic bone (Figure 4).

Two standard zygomatic single-piece implants were placed in the right zygomatic bone (Figure 5). The lengths were 47.5 and 45 mm. Horizontal mattress sutures were placed to close the mucoperiosteal flap. Silk sutures were used.

An antibiotic (amoxicillin and potassium clavulanate 625 mg TDS) was prescribed for 10 days postoperatively. Analgesic was prescribed. Sutures were removed after 15 days. A soft diet was advised for the first 2 weeks. Both the implants demonstrated good primary stability.

Postoperative CT showed that apical two-thirds of the zygomatic implant has engaged the medullary and cortical region of the zygomatic bone (Figure 6).

Zygomatic implant-supported prosthetic rehabilitation was initiated 3 weeks after placement of the implants. A wax pattern of the obturators was fabricated. Retention was mainly derived from the zygomatic implants, with support from the residual horizontal palatal bone.

The implant head copings were transferred to the obturator, and fit was checked on the master cast. The model was then mounted in an articulator to check for interarch occlusal relationship after arrangement of teeth. Trial insertion was done. The whole assembly was acrylised (Figure 7) and returned to the articulator for final occlusal equilibration.

Following insertion of the prosthesis (Figure 8), the obturator prosthesis demonstrated optimal retention and

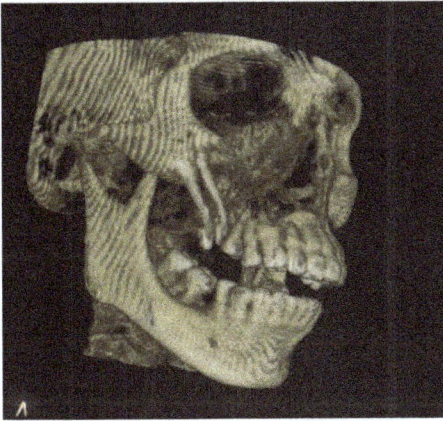

FIGURE 6: Postoperative CT shows apical two-thirds of zygomatic implant has engaged the medullary and cortical regions of the zygomatic bone.

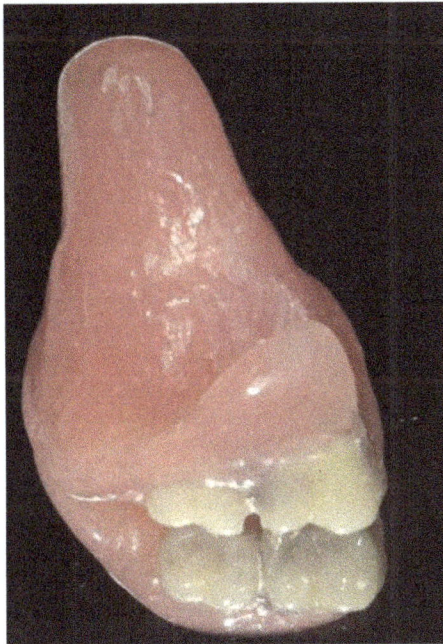

FIGURE 7: Acrylised obturator.

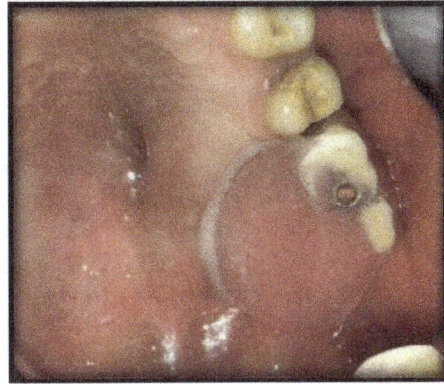

FIGURE 8: obturator supported by two zygomatic implants.

stability. Postinsertion instructions were given with focus on insertion, removal, and hygiene of the prosthesis. At 1-year follow-up, the patient confirmed his satisfaction and no significant complaints have been recorded. The patient's phonation, chewing, deglutition, and aesthetic improved.

3. Discussion

Maxillary posterior defects that occur due to tumor resection, trauma, or any pathologic lesion pose a challenge to reconstruct and rehabilitate. The aim of rehabilitation is to provide a cosmetically acceptable appearance and to restore functions [2].

Defects in posterior maxilla have been reconstructed with invasive and lengthy procedures such as onlay grafts, free or microvascular bone grafts, and transport distraction osteogenesis with or without a Le Fort I osteotomy with a success rates of 60–90% [3, 4].

Many factors affect the retention of the maxillary obturator example, size of the defect, the number of remaining teeth, the amount of the remaining bony structure, and the patient ability to adapt to the prosthesis [5].

Most of the cases with maxillectomy have limited bone support and large oral and facial soft tissue defects. Implant-supported or conventional obturator prosthesis is extremely complicated in these cases [6].

The introduction of dental implants in obturator brings wonderful improvement in the performance of obturator by exhibiting better mechanical qualities [7, 8].

Placement of the conventional endosteal implant would compromise long-term osseintegration. Limited support from the remaining anatomic structures results in placement of the endoosseous implant at an increased angle; hence, prosthetic rehabilitation becomes difficult [9].

Hence prosthetic rehabilitation of posterior maxillary defect with obturator supported with two single-piece zygomatic implants was done.

The zygomatic implant, first introduced by Brånemark in 1988, is especially for patients with atrophy of the maxilla or who suffer from a complication after bone grafting procedures [10].

Main indications of the zygomatic implant are significant sinus pneumatization and alveolar ridge resorption. Contraindications to the use of zygomatic implants include acute sinus infection, any kind of pathology of maxillary and zygomatic bone, and underlying uncontrolled or malignant systemic disease [11]. The zygomatic bone is pyramid in shape and contains dense cortical and trabecular bones. According to a cadaver study, the mean length of available bone in this region is about 14 mm. The bone length is sufficient for placement of the zygomatic implant in patients with severely resorbed posterior maxillary bone [12].

The original Branemark zygomatic implant was a self-tapping titanium implant with a treated surface, available in lengths of 30–52.5 mm. The diameter at the threaded apical part was 4 mm and 4.5 mm at the crestal part. The implant head was provided with an inner thread for connection of standard abutments.

At present, there are three different companies that offer zygomatic implants with an oxidized rough surface, a smooth midimplant body, a wider neck at the alveolar crest, and a 55° angulation of the implant head [12].

The zygomatic bone has thick cortical layer that offers a solid and extended anchorage that can bear the vertical masticatory forces. The tricortical anchorage increases the success and survival of the zygomatic implant [13].

In the present case, two zygomatic implants provided sufficient retention and support for the obturator.

The greatest advantage of the zygomatic implant is the elimination of donor site morbidity and infection in graft material.

There is literature available on zygomatic implant, but till date, no randomized controlled trials comparing the clinical outcomes of zygomatic implants with alternative means for rehabilitating patients with atrophic edentulous maxilla are available [14].

Although limited clinical data are available on the long-term clinical performance of zygomatic implants, the present case report provides evidence that the zygomatic implant is an adaptable option to rehabilitate wide maxillary defects.

References

[1] Z. Durrani, S. G. Hussain, and S. A. Alam, "A study of classification systems for maxillectomy defects," *Journal of Photochemistry and Photobiology A: Chemistry*, vol. 1, no. 2, pp. 117–124, 2013.

[2] L. Vrielinck, C. Politis, S. Schepers, M. Pauwels, and I. Naert, "Image-based planning and clinical validation of zygoma and pterygoid implant placement in patients with severe bone, atrophy using customized drill guides: preliminary results from a prospective clinical follow-up study," *International Journal of Oral and Maxillofacial Surgery*, vol. 32, no. 1, pp. 7–14, 2003.

[3] J. Clavero and S. Lundgren, "Ramus or chin grafts for maxillary sinus inlay and local onlay augmentation: comparison of donor site morbidity and complications," *Clinical Implant Dentistry and Related Research*, vol. 5, no. 3, pp. 154–160, 2003.

[4] M. J. Yaremchuk, "Vascularized bone grafts for maxillofacial reconstruction," *Clinics in Plastic Surgery*, vol. 16, no. 1, pp. 29–39, 1989.

[5] M. Fukuda, T. Takahashi, H. Nagai, and M. Iino, "Implant-supported edentulous maxillary obturators with milled bar attachments after maxillectomy," *Journal of Oral and Maxillofacial Surgery*, vol. 62, no. 7, pp. 799–805, 2004.

[6] C. R. Leles, J. L. R. Leles, C. de Paula Souza, R. R. Martins, and E. F. Mendonça, "Implant-supported obturator overdenture for extensive maxillary resection patient: a clinical report," *Journal of Prosthodontics*, vol. 18, no. 3, pp. 240–244, 2009.

[7] K. E. Kahnberg, P. Nilsson, and L. Rasmusson, "Le Fort I osteotomy with interpositional bone grafts and implants for rehabilitation of the severely resorbed maxilla: a 2-stage procedure," *International Journal of Oral and Maxillofacial Implants*, vol. 14, no. 4, pp. 571–578, 1999.

[8] E. E. Keller, D. E. Tolman, and S. Eckert, "Surgical-prosthodontic reconstruction of advanced maxillary bone compromise with autogenous onlay block bone grafts and osseointegrated endosseous implants: a 12-year study of 32 consecutive patients," *International Journal of Oral and Maxillofacial Implants*, vol. 14, no. 2, pp. 197–209, 1999.

[9] T. Weischer, D. Schettler, and C. Mohr, "Titanium implants in the zygoma as retaining elements after hemimaxillectomy," *International Journal of Oral and Maxillofacial Implants*, vol. 12, no. 2, pp. 211–214, 1997.

[10] C. Aparicio, P. I. Branemark, E. E. Keller, and J. Olive, "Reconstruction of the premaxilla with autogenous iliac bone in combination with osseointegrated implants," *International Journal of Oral and Maxillofacial Implants*, vol. 8, pp. 61–67, 1993.

[11] C. Aparicio, C. Manresa, K. Francisco et al., "Zygomatic implants: indications, techniques and outcomes, and the Zygomatic Success Code," *Periodontology 2000*, vol. 66, no. 1, pp. 41–58, 2014.

[12] M. Olsson, G. Urde, J. B. Andersen, and L. Sennerby, "Early loading of maxillary fixed cross-arch dental prostheses supported by six or eight oxidized titanium implants: results after 1 year of loading, case series," *Clinical Implant Dentistry and Related Research*, vol. 5, no. 1, pp. 81–87, 2003.

[13] P. Maló, M. de Araujo Nobre, and I. Lopes, "A new approach to rehabilitate the severely atrophic maxilla using extramaxillary anchored implants in immediate function: a pilot study," *Journal of Prosthetic Dentistry*, vol. 100, no. 5, pp. 354–366, 2008.

[14] M. Esposito, H. V. Worthington, and P. Coulthard, "Interventions for replacing missing teeth: dental implants in zygomatic bone for the rehabilitation of the severely deficient edentulous maxilla," *Cochrane Database of Systematic Reviews*, no. 4, p. CD004151, 2005.

31

Intraoral Sebaceous Carcinoma: Case Report of a Rare Tumor Emphasizing the Histopathological Differential Diagnosis

Manveen Kaur Jawanda,[1] **R. V. Subramanyam** ⓘ,[2] **Harshaminder Grewal** ⓘ,[3] **Chitra Anandani** ⓘ,[1] **and Ravi Narula**[4]

[1]Department of Oral Pathology, Luxmi Bai Institute of Dental Sciences, Patiala, Punjab, India
[2]Department of OMFS and Diagnostic Sciences, College of Dentistry, King Faisal University, Al-Ahasa 31982, Saudi Arabia
[3]Department of Oral Pathology, Desh Bhagat Dental College, Mandi Gobindgarh, Punjab, India
[4]Department of Oral and Maxillofacial Surgery, Guru Nanak Dev Dental College, Sunam, Punjab, India

Correspondence should be addressed to R. V. Subramanyam; subrarv@gmail.com

Academic Editor: Giuseppe Alessandro Scardina

Background. Sebaceous carcinoma (SC) is an uncommon cutaneous malignancy, usually occurring predominantly in the eyelids and only occasionally involving the oral cavity. Sebaceous carcinoma (SC) is a rare malignancy. Only 10 cases of sebaceous carcinoma of the oral cavity have been reported so far. *Case Presentation.* A 40-year-old female presented with a mass on the left side of the middle third of the face. Radiographic findings were inconclusive. Resection of the mass was consistent with the diagnosis of primary sebaceous carcinoma. *Conclusion.* Intraoral sebaceous carcinoma is uncommon. Due to its varied clinical appearance and presence of a diverse histopathologic appearance, the diagnosis is quite often confounding and elusive. Hence, it is imperative to familiarize oneself about various aspects of this rare tumor for earlier diagnosis, to improve the chances of patient's survival.

1. Introduction

Sebaceous carcinoma has been defined by the WHO as "a malignant tumor composed of sebaceous cells of varying maturity that are arranged in sheets and/or nests with different degrees of pleomorphism, nuclear atypia, and invasiveness" [1].

Sebaceous carcinoma is an aggressive, uncommon, cutaneous tumor first described by Allaire in 1891. This tumor is thought to arise from sebaceous glands in the skin and thus may arise anywhere on the body where these glands exist [2]. Sebaceous carcinoma predominantly occurs in the skin of the eyelid, face, neck, and scalp [3]. Extraocular noncutaneous sebaceous carcinoma mainly involves the major salivary glands. Primary sebaceous carcinoma of oral cavity is rare [4]. It is thought to arise from Fordyce granules or salivary gland elements [5]. Oral sebaceous carcinoma can be a

diagnostic challenge for the clinicians as well as the pathologist. Because oral sebaceous carcinoma presents most commonly as an asymptomatic nonencapsulated nodule, diagnosis and treatment therapy tend to be delayed because it is frequently mistaken for more common benign entities. In addition to its varied clinical appearance, the presence of a diverse histologic appearance may delay the diagnosis or result in a misdiagnosis. To our knowledge, only ten cases of intraoral sebaceous carcinoma have been reported in the literature [6]. The current report describes another case of oral sebaceous carcinoma, indicating the need for comprehensive histopathological differential diagnosis.

2. Case Presentation

A 40-year female reported with a swelling on the right side, involving the middle third of the face, since 1 year. The

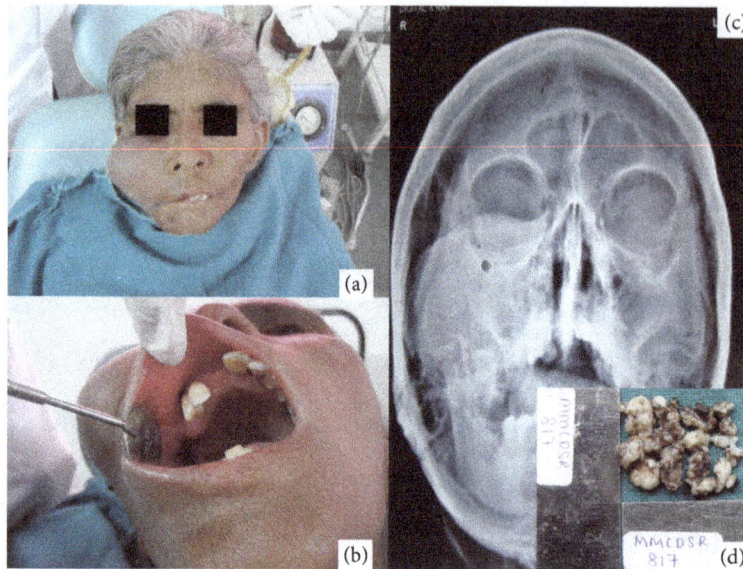

FIGURE 1: (a) Clinical and (b) intraoral picture showing an intact buccal mucosa. (c) Water's view radiograph of the patient. (d) Gross incisional tissue.

swelling was firm in consistency, nontender, and of approximately 5 × 4 cm, extending superoinferiorly from the infraorbital ridge to 2 cm above the inferior border of the mandible and anteroposteriorly from the right corner of the mouth to 1.5 cm anterior to the tragus (Figure 1(a)). The borders of the swelling were diffuse, and the skin overlying the swelling was normal in color. The swelling was mobile with no ulceration of the overlying skin. Intraoral examination revealed no obvious swelling with intact oral mucosa, and scattered foci of Fordyce's spots were seen on the buccal mucosa (Figure 1(b)). Water's view of the skull showed impression of the soft tissue swelling in the right cheek area (Figure 1(c)). The hemoglobin level was 7.5 gm/dl (anemic), and other routine hematological findings were within normal limits. Chest radiograph showed no abnormality. No palpable lymph nodes were found. A definite clinical diagnosis was not possible, and an incisional biopsy (Figure 1(d)) was taken from the buccal mucosa and subjected to histopathological examination.

Microscopically, the tumor mass appeared to be located in the deeper mucosa with pushing margins of tumor nests (Figure 2). The tumor was composed of large nests of neoplastic cells with squamous appearance, separated by scanty stroma (Figure 3). The neoplastic cells had large vesicular nuclei with prominent nucleoli. Cellular and nuclear pleomorphism with few nuclei showing multilobation was seen, along with typical and atypical mitotic figures (Figures 4 and 5). The sebaceous nests were composed of clear tumor cells with foamy cytoplasm exhibiting absence of mucin on periodic acid-Schiff (PAS) stain (Figure 6). In contrast, a variable number of smaller, darkly staining basaloid cells with oval-shaped nuclei and scant cytoplasm were also seen (Figure 7). A final diagnosis of sebaceous carcinoma was accorded based on the histopathological features. The patient was further advised for a full body scan and referred to an oncologist for further treatment.

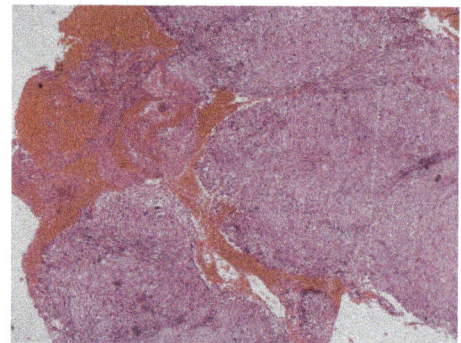

FIGURE 2: Pattern of asymmetry, a lack of circumscription with pushing or locally infiltrating margins (H and E stain; original magnification, 4x).

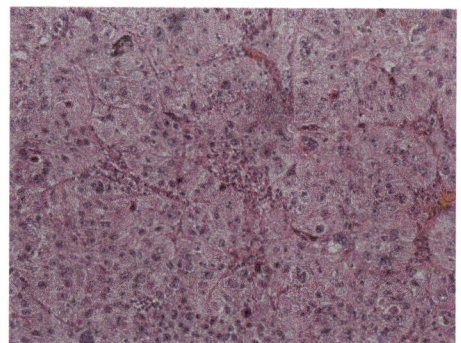

FIGURE 3: Large nests or lobules of neoplastic cells with squamous appearance, separated by scant stroma (H and E stain; original magnification, 10x).

3. Discussion

The diagnosis of oral sebaceous carcinoma, "a benign-appearing" malignant neoplasm, remains challenging both

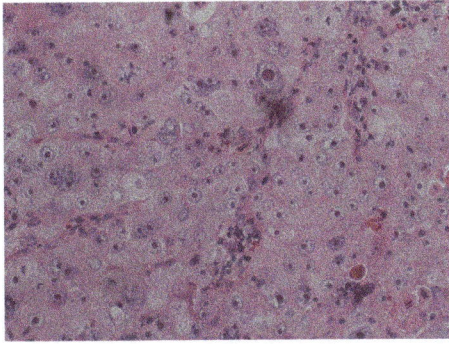

FIGURE 4: Neoplastic cells had large vesicular nuclei with prominent nucleoli. Cellular and nuclear pleomorphism with few nuclei showing multilobation. Scattered typical and atypical mitotic figures seen (H and E stain; original magnification, 20x).

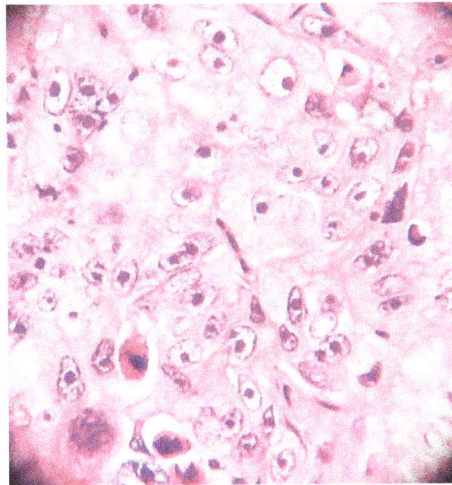

FIGURE 5: Sheets of multivacuolated/vesiculated cells having squamoid appearance, multilobation of some nuclei, high mitotic rate with abnormal mitosis (H and E stain; original magnification, 100x).

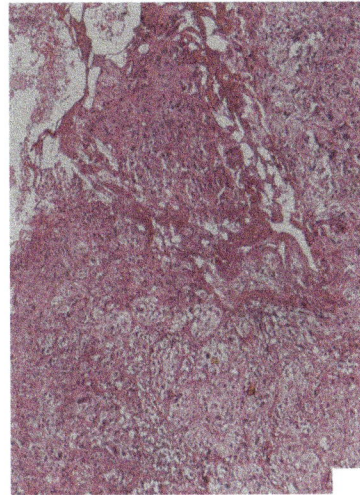

(a)

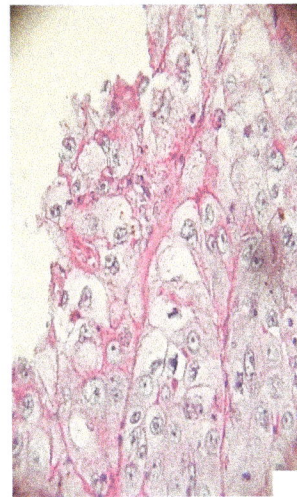

(b)

FIGURE 6: Photomicrograph showing lobules composed of clear tumor cells with foamy cytoplasm exhibiting absence of any mucin on PAS stain. (a) H and E stain; original magnification, 10x. (b) PAS stain; original magnification, 40x.

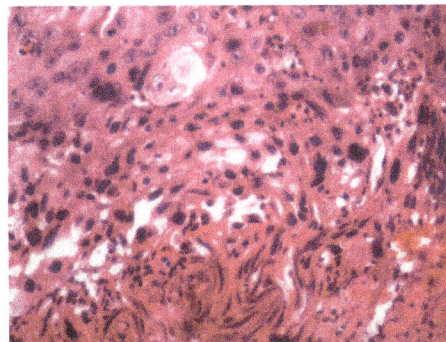

FIGURE 7: Variable number of smaller, darkly staining basaloid cells with oval-shaped nuclei and scant cytoplasm (H and E stain; original magnification, 40X).

clinically and histopathologically. Any anatomic site that contains sebaceous glands may potentially give rise to neoplasms exhibiting sebaceous differentiation. Fordyce's spots represent ectopic sebaceous glands in the oral cavity and are commonly found in the buccal mucosa, upper lip, retromolar trigone, anterior tonsillar pillar, soft palate, and gingiva [7]. Although approximately 80% of the adult populations have clinically evident sebaceous glands in the oral mucosa, only ten cases of sebaceous carcinoma have been documented until now. Intraoral sebaceous carcinoma was first reported by Damm et al. in 1991 (Table 1, case 1) [4]. Since then, another 9 cases were reported in the literature (Table 1) [4–6, 8–14].

The origin of sebaceous carcinoma in the oral cavity is still unclear. It may arise from intraoral minor salivary glands, parotid duct, or Fordyce granules [4, 5]. In the current case, there was confusion about the possible origin of the neoplasm. Several possible origins were thought on the basis of close association of various structures with the

TABLE 1: Clinical findings of reported cases of intraoral sebaceous carcinoma.

	Reference	Age/sex	Anatomic site	Size (cm)
1.	Damm et al. [4]	53/M	Left buccal mucosa	3
2.	Abuzeid et al. [8]	11/F	Left buccal mucosa	3
3.	Liu et al. [5]	68/M	Right buccal mucosa	2.5
4.	Li et al. [9]	78/M	Left buccal mucosa	3.5
5.	Handschel et al. [10]	80/F	Anterior floor of the mouth	1.5
6.	Alawi and Siddiqui [11]	66/M	Left upper labial mucosa	1.5
7.	Gomes et al. [12]	55/M	Right floor of the mouth	Not known
8.	Wang et al. [6]	50/M	Left buccal mucosa	4.6
9.	Oshiro et al. [13]	66/M	Dorsum of tongue	2.5
10.	Rowe et al. [14]	76/M	Gingival mucosa, with metastasis to the lung and subcutis	3
11.	Present case (2017)	40/F	Right buccal mucosa	5

tumor. As the tumor presented as a swelling on the middle third of the face with normal overlying skin and an intact buccal mucosa intraorally, with scattered foci of Fordyce's spots, there was a confusion regarding the primary site. On the basis of close association of the swelling to the eye and ear, the lower eyelid, external auditory canal, preauricular lymph nodes, and parotid gland were thought to be the primary sites. The patient was therefore submitted to instrumental examination (eye, ear) to evaluate the possible origin, all with a negative result. No preauricular lymph node enlargement was found; furthermore, no evidence of appendageal structures within the biopsy specimen was seen, thus ruling out the possibility that the tumor originated from the skin of the cheek or lymph node. Therefore, based on these observations, it was concluded that the primary site of the tumor was the buccal mucosa. The presence of Fordyce granules in the area of involvement suggests that the tumor may have arisen from the malignant transformation of these ectopic sebaceous glands [11]. Alternatively, sebaceous differentiation of Stensen's duct could also be considered a probable etiology due to the inclination towards the buccal region [14].

Histologically, sebaceous carcinoma shows quite a range of differentiation, ranging from obviously multivacuolated epithelium to basaloid or squamoid populations of cells with more occult cytoplasmic lipid content [15]. Hence, it is imperative to differentiate an intraoral sebaceous carcinoma from basal cell carcinoma with sebaceous differentiation, clear cell as well as basaloid squamous cell carcinoma with hydrophilic swelling, metastatic clear cell renal carcinoma, and salivary gland malignancies such as mucoepidermoid carcinoma, solid-type adenoid cystic carcinoma, basal cell adenocarcinoma, and salivary duct carcinoma [4, 13].

According to Plaza et al. [16], histology remains the gold standard for the diagnosis of SC, and they suggested that the immunohistochemical assessment for epithelial markers and lipid droplet-associated proteins is a helpful diagnostic adjunct and that immunostaining for epithelial markers should be performed once careful standard microscopic evaluation has taken place. If these results are nonconclusive for SC, the prospective diagnosis can be confirmed

by a lipid droplet-associated protein, such as adipophilin (Figure 8) [16].

We did not perform IHC in our case because the diagnosis was quite obvious. Periodic acid-Schiff (PAS) stain was negative, confirming that the vacuolated clear cells were neither mucus cells nor glycogen-rich squamous cells, thus ruling out the possibility of a carcinoma arising from oral epithelium or salivary epithelium. Moreover, clear cell squamous cell carcinoma is characterized by areas of squamous differentiation with foci of keratinization and keratin pearls, which were absent in our case. In addition, basaloid squamous cell carcinoma was also excluded due to the absence of comedonecrosis, hyalinization of the stroma, or microcyst formation.

Furthermore, we observed a variable number of smaller, darkly staining, basaloid cells with oval-shaped nuclei and prominent nucleoli. These cells are thought to represent undifferentiated sebaceous cells [17], thus giving a basaloid cytological appearance; however, peripheral palisading pattern of the basaloid cells and retraction artifacts between the mucinous stroma and the tumor nests, characteristic of basal cell carcinoma, were absent. Also, clear cells with foamy-bubbly cytoplasm or starry nuclei, typical of sebaceous cells, were seen in our case. A diagnosis of intraoral basal cell carcinoma (with sebaceous differentiation) was, therefore, excluded.

In the current case, due to the presence of large nests of polygonal tumor cells with an optically clear cytoplasm, metastatic clear cell renal carcinoma was also thought as one of the differential diagnoses. This tumor is characterized by tumor cells arranged in nests and separated from each other by extensive rich network of delicate sinusoidal vascular channels. The tumor cells are generally large and polygonal, having a distinct cell membrane as if drawn by a "pencil" and an optically clear cytoplasm. This clear appearance of the cytoplasm of clear cell renal carcinoma is due to the presence of abundant glycogen and neutral lipids but not mucin [18]. However, PAS negativity in our case excludes the possibility of this neoplasm.

Besides, benign tumors, including sebaceous adenoma, could not be considered in the histological differential

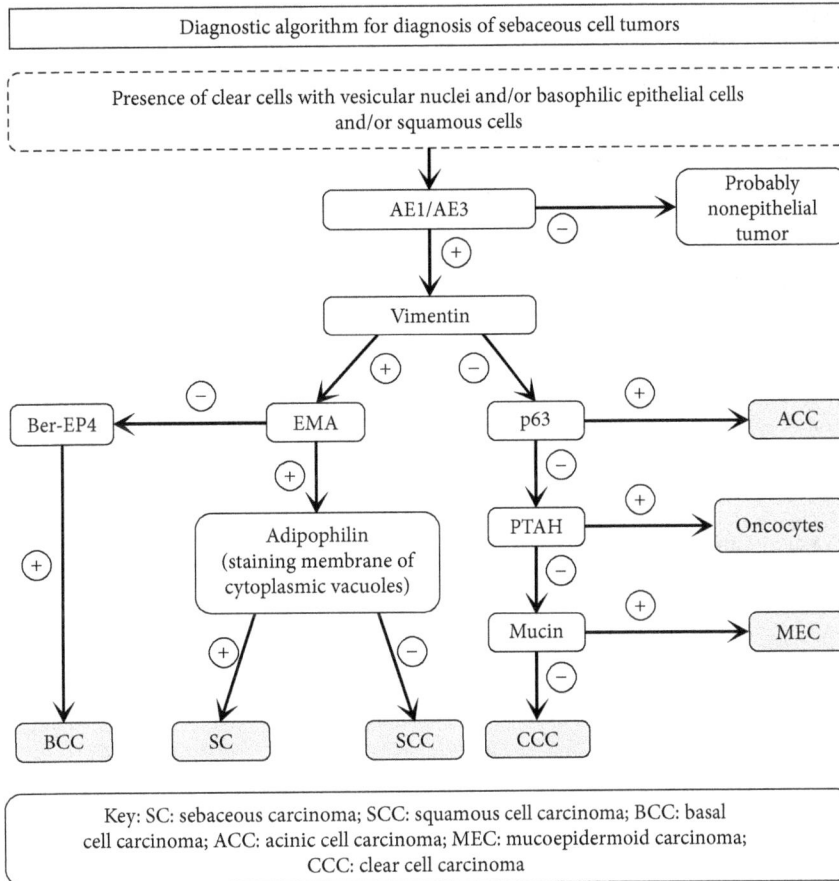

FIGURE 8: Diagnostic algorithm depicting the use of immunohistochemistry (IHC) to logically arrive to the diagnosis of sebaceous carcinoma (SC).

diagnosis due to the infiltrative pattern and cytological features associated with sebaceous carcinoma. The presence of foci of cells with cytoplasmic microvacuoles and atypical scalloped nuclei confirmed the diagnosis of sebaceous carcinoma and ruled out the abovesaid malignant neoplasms.

The treatment of choice for sebaceous carcinoma is surgery, with complete excision verified by negative margins. Radiotherapy is used if metastatic disease and/or a high risk of recurrence are present. Multiagent chemotherapy has been used to treat recurrent disease [19]. Nevertheless, an increased proclivity for local recurrence and metastasis calls for a long-term follow-up of the affected patients [11].

4. Conclusion

Sebaceous carcinoma is a very aggressive, rare tumor which is generally not considered in the differential diagnosis of tumors arising from a site such as the buccal mucosa. This often leads to a delay in treatment. We emphasize the need to generate awareness about this rare entity occurring at unusual sites to expedite the patient's survival.

References

[1] L. Barnes, J. W. Eveson, P. Reichart, and D. Sidransky, *WHO Classification of Tumours, Pathology and Genetics, Head and Neck Tumours*, IARC Press, Lyon, 2005.

[2] L. G. Kass and A. Hornblass, "Sebaceous carcinoma of the ocular adnexa," *Survey of Ophthalmology*, vol. 33, no. 6, pp. 477–490, 1989.

[3] T. Das Gupta, L. D. Wilson, and L. B. Yu, "A retrospective review of 1349 cases of sebaceous carcinoma," *Cancer*, vol. 115, no. 1, pp. 158–165, 2009.

[4] D. D. Damm, W. N. O'Connor, D. K. White, J. F. Drummond, L. W. Morrow, and D. E. Kenady, "Intraoral sebaceous carcinoma," *Oral Surgery, Oral Medicine, Oral Pathology*, vol. 72, no. 6, pp. 709–711, 1991.

[5] C. Liu, K. Chang, and R. C. S. Chang, "Sebaceous carcinoma of buccal mucosa: report of a case," *International Journal of Oral and Maxillofacial Surgery*, vol. 26, no. 4, pp. 293-294, 1997.

[6] H. Wang, J. Yao, M. Solomon, and C. A. Axiolis, "Sebaceous carcinoma of the oral cavity: a case report and review of the literature," *Oral Surgery, Oral Medicine, Oral Pathology, Oral Radiology, and Endodontology*, vol. 110, no. 2, pp. e37–e40, 2010.

[7] C. Lipani, J. J. Woytash, and G. GW, "Sebaceous adenoma of the oral cavity," *Journal of Oral and Maxillofacial Surgery*, vol. 41, no. 1, pp. 56–60, 1983.

[8] M. Abuzeid, K. Gangopadhyay, C. S. Rayappa, and J. I. Antonios, "Intraoral sebaceous carcinoma," *The Journal of Laryngology & Otology*, vol. 110, no. 05, pp. 500–502, 1996.

[9] T. J. Li, M. Kitano, H. Mukai, and S. Yamashita, "Oral sebaceous carcinoma: report of a case," *Journal of Oral and Maxillofacial Surgery*, vol. 55, no. 7, pp. 751–754, 1997.

[10] J. Handschel, H. Herbst, B. Brand, U. Meyer, and J. Piffko, "Intraoral sebaceous carcinoma," *Journal of Oral and Maxillofacial Surgery*, vol. 41, no. 2, pp. 84–87, 2003.

[11] F. Alawi and A. Siddiqui, "Sebaceous carcinoma of the oral mucosa: case report and review of the literature," *Oral Surgery Oral Medicine Oral Pathology Oral Radiology and Endodontology*, vol. 99, no. 1, pp. 79–84, 2005.

[12] C. C. Gomes, L. JCT, F. J. Pimenta, M. A. V. do Carmo, and R. S. Gomez, "Intraoral sebaceous carcinoma," *European Archives of Oto-Rhino-Laryngology*, vol. 264, no. 7, pp. 829–832, 2007.

[13] H. Oshiro, T. Iwai, M. Hirota et al., "Primary sebaceous carcinoma of the tongue," *Medical Molecular Morphology*, vol. 43, no. 4, pp. 246–252, 2010.

[14] M. E. Rowe, A. S. Khorsandi, G. R. R. Urken, and B. M. Wenig, "Intraoral sebaceous carcinoma metastatic to the lung and subcutis: case report and discussion of the literature," *Head & Neck*, vol. 38, no. 1, pp. E20–E24, 2016.

[15] GneppDR, *Diagnostic Surgical Pathology of the Head and Neck*, Saunders Elsevier, 2nd edition, 2009.

[16] J. A. Plaza, A. Mackinnon, L. Carrillo, V. G. Prieto, M. Sangueza, and S. Suster, "Role of immunohistochemistry in the diagnosis of sebaceous carcinoma: a clinicopathologic and immunohistochemical study," *The American Journal of Dermatopathology*, vol. 37, no. 11, pp. 809–821, 2015.

[17] D. Weedon, *Skin Pathology*, Churchill Livingstone, London, 2nd edition, 2002.

[18] R. Audisio, D. Lodeville, V. Quagliuolo, and C. Clemente, "Sebaceous carcinoma arising from the eyelid and from extra-ocular sites," *Tumori*, vol. 73, no. 5, pp. 531–535, 1987.

[19] K. A. Arndt, P. E. Leboit, J. K. Robinson, and B. Wintroub, *Cutaneous Medicine and Surgery*, Saunders, Philadelphia, PA, USA, 1996.

32

Restorative Management of Severe Localized Tooth Wear Using a Supraoccluding Appliance: A 5-Year Follow-Up

Tsz Leung Wong(iD) **and Michael George Botelho**(iD)

Prosthodontics, Faculty of Dentistry, The University of Hong Kong, Sai Ying Pun, Hong Kong

Correspondence should be addressed to Michael George Botelho; botelho@hku.hk

Academic Editor: Tatiana Pereira-Cenci

This case report illustrates a novel conservative restorative management of a patient with bulimia nervosa who presented with severe localized upper palatal tooth wear and an anterior reverse overjet. This was achieved by using a localized bite raising or supraoccluding appliance, cemented on the lingual side of the lower anterior teeth to create interocclusal space, obviating the need for tooth reduction of the eroded upper palatal and incisal tooth surfaces. Surgical crown lengthening was performed to create a better aesthetic gingival architecture. All-ceramic restorations were provided on the upper anterior teeth to restore the tooth surface loss and provide a positive overbite and overjet. There was no complication or other observable biological change detected at the 5-year follow-up. The use of an appliance applying the supraoccluding technique, or Dahl concept, is a safe, conservative, and useful treatment option in the management of localized tooth wear.

1. Introduction

Restoration of the localized worn dentition, especially in the aesthetic zone, is often challenging, as the localized tooth loss can be accompanied by compensatory tooth eruption and alveolar bone growth such that the worn surface will maintain contact with the opposing dentition [1, 2]. This may lead to an irregular gingival contour or level and may result in compromised aesthetics. Also, tooth preparation of such worn teeth to create interocclusal space for the planned restorations may endanger pulp vitality. In addition, tooth wear from erosion may reduce the crown height which in turn reduces the resistance and retention form which may warrant surgical crown lengthening to overcome this. Elective devitalization and the use of postcore crowns may solve the retention problem; however, this may significantly affect the long-term prognosis of these teeth. Orthodontic intrusion can be considered to create space; however, treatment cost, time duration, or patient's preference may exclude this treatment. Increasing the occlusal vertical dimension (OVD) in a full mouth rehabilitation is an alternative to create the necessary space. However, this is usually considered when the tooth surface loss is generalized and the whole arch needs restoring which makes this cost prohibitive to many patients. Space for restoration can also be created by occlusal adjustment of the anteroposterior discrepancy between the centric occlusion and centric relation. However, such discrepancies are not always present and can still involve multiple restorations.

An alternative approach described by Dahl is a technique where interocclusal space is created using an anterior bite platform [3, 4]. The platform was designed to disclude the posterior teeth with subsequent reestablishment of the posterior occlusion from a combination of intrusion of the anterior teeth and overeruption of the posterior teeth [5, 6]. This takes an average of about 6 months to occur [7, 8]. This technique was shown to be safe and can be a conservative and useful option in the management of the localized worn dentition [7–9]. The original Dahl appliance was a removable one covering the palatal surface of the upper anterior teeth [3, 4]. However, this is not applicable to patients with reverse overjet, as extension of the metal coverage beyond the incisolabial

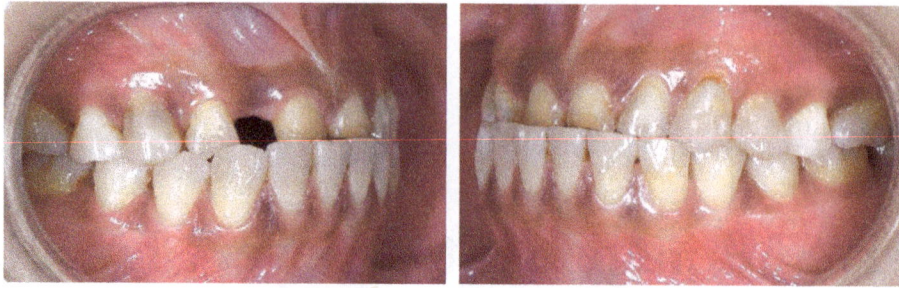

FIGURE 1: Preoperative lateral views with teeth in centric occlusion.

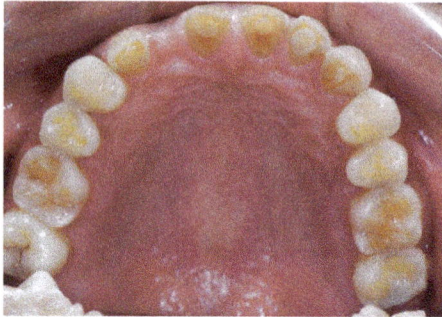

FIGURE 2: Preoperative upper occlusal view.

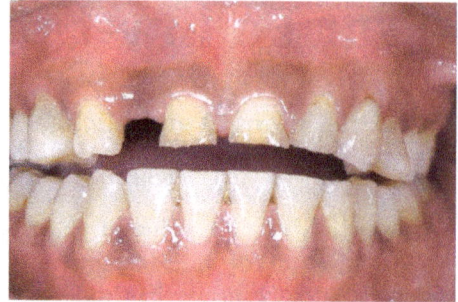

FIGURE 3: Preoperative frontal view with teeth apart.

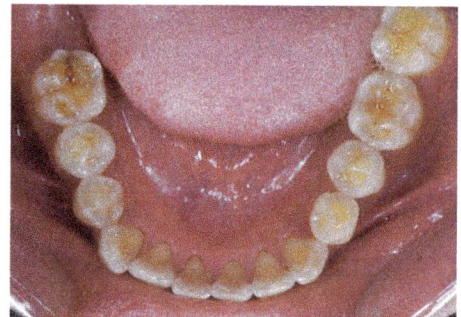

FIGURE 4: Preoperative lower occlusal view.

and in supraocclusion with the opposing would create an aesthetic problem and a high dislodging force when biting. In this case report, a novel appliance applying the Dahl concept was designed in the localized management of worn anterior teeth. There appears to have been no previous report of the use of a similar lower bite platform in the creation of interocclusal space.

2. Case Presentation

2.1. History and Chief Complaint. A 33-year-old Chinese female presented with concerns about the appearance of her anterior teeth and was referred by a private dental practitioner to the Prince Philip Dental Hospital (PPDH) for aesthetic management of her upper worn anterior teeth. History revealed that she had endodontic treatment on her two upper central incisors because of pain. She also had some tenderness on her lower right molar when chewing. She reported gastric regurgitation after eating but denied self-induced purging at that time.

2.2. Clinical Findings. This patient presented with competent lips, average lip line, normal TMJ's, and class III incisor relation (Figure 1) on a skeletal class 3 base. The patient had good oral hygiene and a healthy periodontal condition. Tooth 13 was missing and 12 had drifted to the 13 position (Figure 2). There was severe erosive tooth surface loss on the palatal and incisal surfaces of teeth 11, 21, and 22 with exposure of dentine over the whole palatal surface. The crown height of the two upper central incisors was reduced to 5 mm. This gave rise to a reduced visible crown height and a reverse smile line (Figure 3). The gingival level of the upper central incisors was level with the lateral incisors and

below that of the canine teeth. A crack line was detected at 46 distoocclusal area (Figure 4) with no periapical radiolucency (Figure 5), and a diagnosis of crack tooth syndrome was suspected. Teeth 12, 22, 23, and 46 were judged vital with the use of electric pulp testing.

2.3. Diagnosis and Treatment Plan. This patient was advised to seek medical consultation and management concerning her gastric regurgitation. She received conservative medical counseling for approximately one year, and her gastrointestinal disturbance improved. To prevent further symptoms and crack propagation, an orthodontic band was cemented on 46 after which no pain during chewing was reported. Upper and lower impressions were recorded using irreversible hydrocolloid (Aroma Fine Plus, GC Corporation, Tokyo, Japan). A facebow record was taken, and the casts were hand articulated and mounted in maximum intercuspal position. After analysis of the study models, it was decided to perform localized "intrusion" of the anterior teeth using a lower supraoccluding appliance and to build up the correct contour

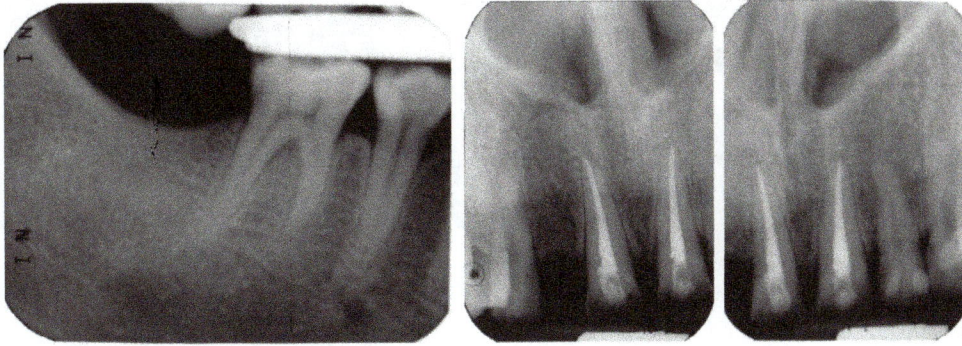

FIGURE 5: Preoperative periapical of 46 and upper anterior teeth showing no periapical radiolucency with good alveolar bone level.

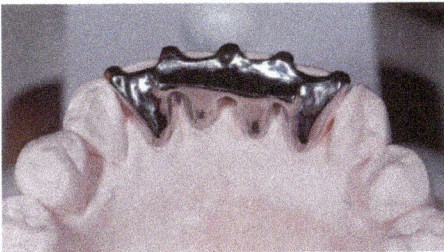

FIGURE 6: Lingual view of the bite platform on working model.

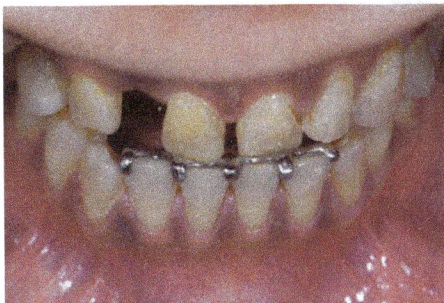

FIGURE 7: Stable occlusion of numbers 11 and 21 on the lingual bite platform.

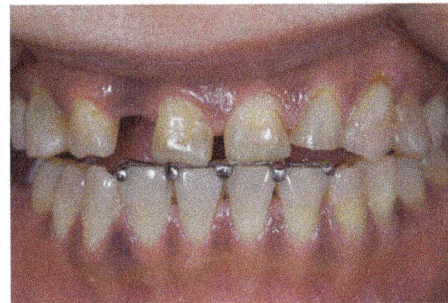

FIGURE 8: The appliance in situ with composite build-up in supraocclusion on numbers 11 and 21 incisal to separate all other teeth by 1.5 mm. The design of using incisal hooks on the lower teeth helps improve the resistance to dislodgement of the appliance.

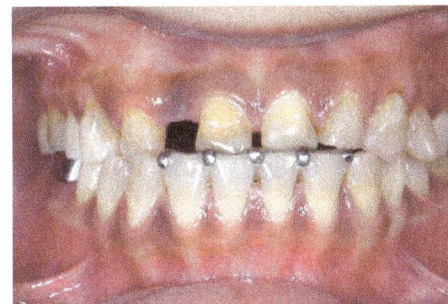

FIGURE 9: Complete reestablishment of the occlusal contacts 2 months after appliance cementation.

of upper incisors to facilitate the restorative rehabilitation. It was determined that an increase in the OVD by 1.5 mm would provide sufficient space for restoration. To control the anticipated increased OVD for the composite build-up, a silicone putty (Exafine Putty, GC Corporation, Tokyo, Japan) jaw record was performed on the posterior teeth of the articulated study models as a reference jig.

The supraoccluding appliance was waxed up on the lingual surface of the lower incisors with a bite platform designed to load the opposing incisor axially. Incisal hooks were included to give the appliance resistance form. This was then cast in cobalt-chromium (CoCr) (Remanium® GM 800+, DENTAURUM GmbH & Co., Ispringen, Germany) (Figure 6). The appliance was then cemented on lower incisors with glass ionomer cement (Ketac Cem, ESPE-Premier Sales Corp., Norristown, PA, USA). At the same visit, composite resin (Aeliteflo™, Bisco Inc., Schaumburg, IL, U.S.A) was directly added to restore the incisal edges of 11 and 21 and facilitate occlusion on the opposing bite platform

at the increased OVD of 1.5 mm (Figures 7 and 8) using a silicone putty jaw record as a jig.

The patient was informed of possible transitory problems with this supraoccluding technique, including thermal sensitivity; difficulty in eating, speaking, or sleeping; and temporomandibular joint (TMJ) pain [10]. This patient was reviewed at one week and then at monthly intervals. She reported only some reduced chewing efficiency at the first review and no other symptoms. In order to determine whether tooth movement had occurred, an interocclusal record using Protemp (Protemp II, ESPE, Seefeld, Germany) was taken and it was then inserted at the next review appointment. If tooth movement had occurred, there would be interocclusal separation of the upper anterior teeth with the bite platform of the appliance.

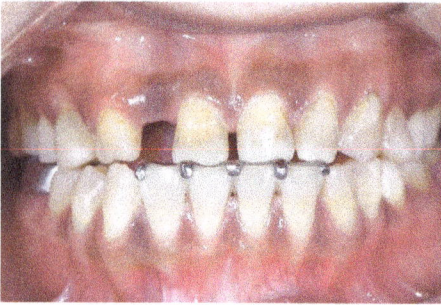

FIGURE 10: Further composite build-up on numbers 11, 21, and 22 incisal to separate all other teeth by 1.5 mm.

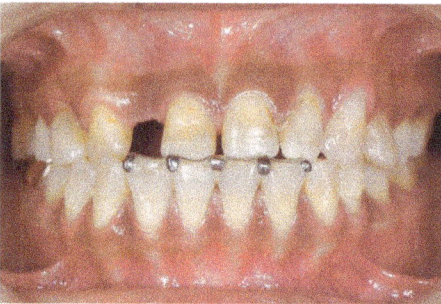

FIGURE 11: The occlusion reestablished full arch contacts over 9 months after appliance insertion, with crown heights of numbers 11 and 21 increased from 5 to 8 mm and number 22 from 5 to 7 mm.

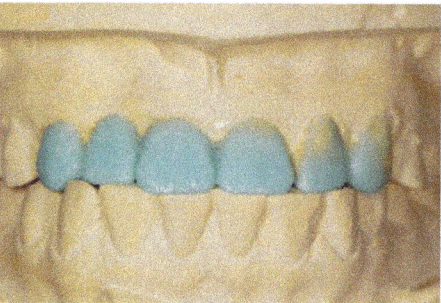

FIGURE 12: Diagnostic wax-up on number 13 to number 23 new study casts.

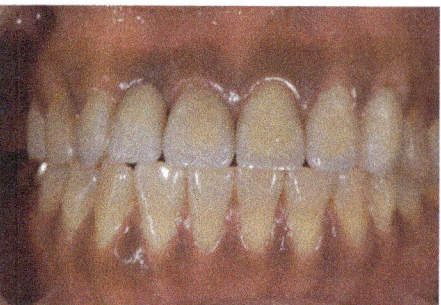

FIGURE 13: Temporary crowns in situ, which were designed to provide positive overjet. However, the crown height of numbers 11 and 21 looked short, and the tooth number 12 at 13 region did not look like a canine.

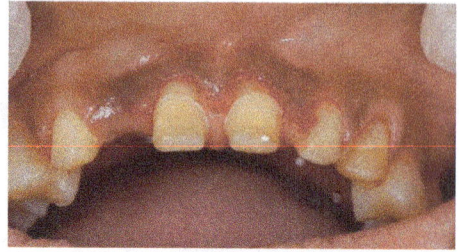

FIGURE 14: Surgical crown lengthening.

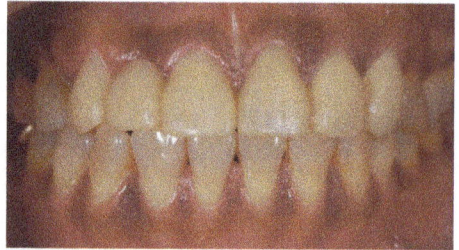

FIGURE 15: Temporary restorations numbers 13–23 in situ 1 month after crown lengthening on numbers 12, 11, and 21.

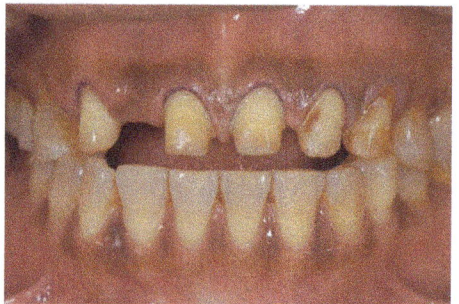

FIGURE 16: Tooth preparation on numbers 12 to 23.

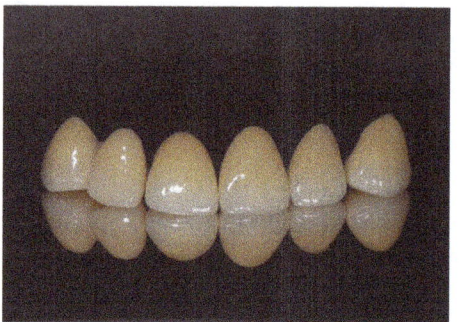

FIGURE 17: Empress crowns and bridge.

After 2 months, the posterior teeth were found to be in occlusion (Figure 9). At this time, further "intrusion" of the upper incisors was judged to be necessary if the incisal overjet was to be changed from reverse to positive. Therefore, further composite build-up was performed on the incisal edges of 11, 21, and 22 to again create supraoccluding restorations on the lower appliance (Figure 10). The OVD was raised by another

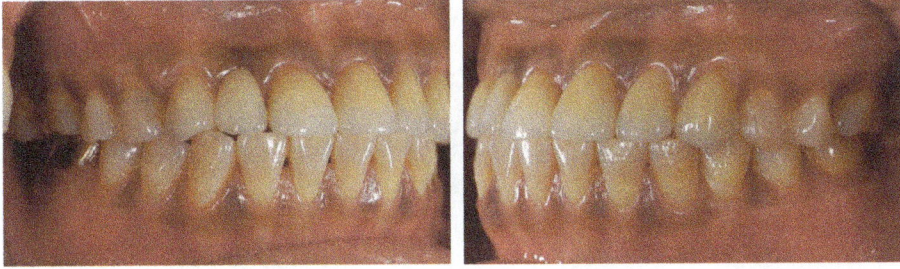

FIGURE 18: Postoperative lateral views showing successful reestablishment of the occlusion.

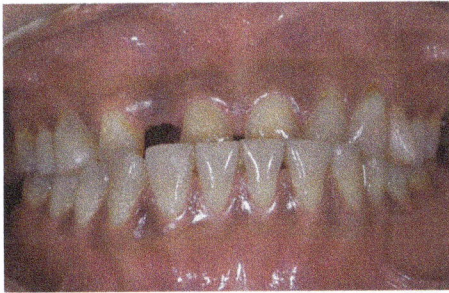

FIGURE 19: Preoperative frontal view.

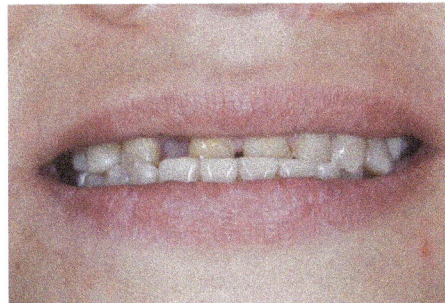

FIGURE 21: Preoperative smile line.

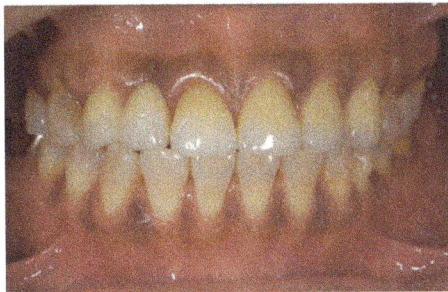

FIGURE 20: Postoperative frontal view.

1.5 mm which was measured between the midlabial gingival margins of 21 and 32. Complete reestablishment of all occlusal contacts was achieved after another seven months (Figure 11). Therefore, at this time, the lower supraoccluding appliance was removed by cutting off the incisal hooks and tapping off the prosthesis.

The 46 remained symptomless, and a full gold crown restoration was provided for cuspal protection. To allow tooth preparation of sufficient resistance form for the future crowns, it was decided to cement glass fibre posts on 11 and 21 with composite core build-up to restore the palatal tooth surface loss. Teeth 12 to 23 were prepared and provisional restorations made according to the diagnostic wax-up of the study casts which were taken at the new OVD and after complete reestablishment of occlusal contacts (Figure 12). With the temporary restorations in the mouth, the aesthetic outcome as well as patient's expectations were assessed (Figure 13). It was determined that lengthening the 13 to 23 incisally by 1 mm would improve the crown proportions, and crown lengthening was proposed to the patient. The soft tissue requirement was guided by a stent showing

the expected final crown contour and margins. Surgical crown lengthening was performed (Figure 14) with alveolar bone being removed by approximately 1.5 mm limited to the midlabial of 12, 11, and 21. Tooth preparation margins were refined, and new temporary restorations using Protemp were made chairside using an index of the diagnostic wax-up of the expected final restorations (Figure 15).

The intrusion of the incisors now permitted the incisal edges to be positioned with a positive overjet and overbite. A period of six months was allowed for the healing and stabilization of the soft tissues, and the patient was satisfied with the aesthetics with diagnostic restorations following review after 6 months. The form and contour of these diagnostic restorations were recorded and copied in the final restorations. Definitive restorations were provided in Empress II (Ivoclar Vivadent, Amherst, NY, USA) and cemented with an adhesive resin cement (Calibra, Dentsply, Konstanz, Germany) (Figures 16, 17, and 18).

The patient achieved good oral hygiene and maintained periodontal health during the follow-up period (Figures 19, 20, 21, 22, 23, and 24). No radiographic periapical change of the crowned teeth or resorption of the roots was observed at 5 years follow-up (Figure 25).

3. Discussion

Eating disorders and the associated regurgitation is not uncommon, and young women seem to be more at risk [11]. Because of the characteristic dental manifestations, dentists are often the first healthcare professionals to encounter patients with undiagnosed eating disorders. Although the main concern of this patient was to improve the appearance of her upper worn anterior teeth, identification and control of

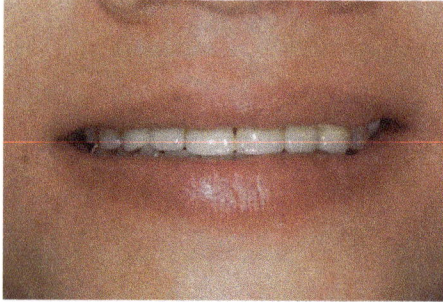

FIGURE 22: Postoperative smile line.

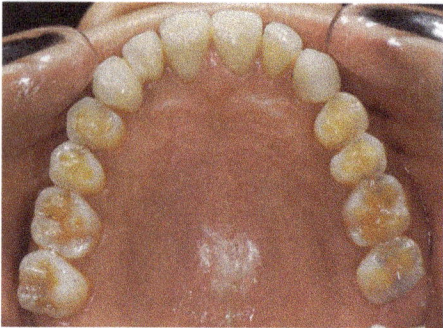

FIGURE 23: Upper occlusal view 5 years postoperatively.

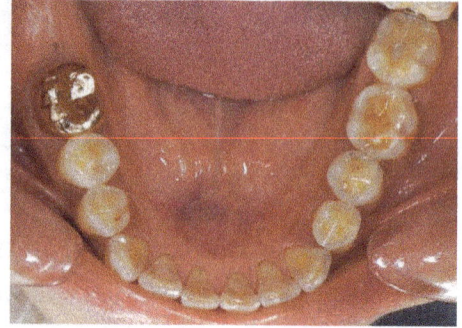

FIGURE 24: Lower occlusal view 5 years postoperatively.

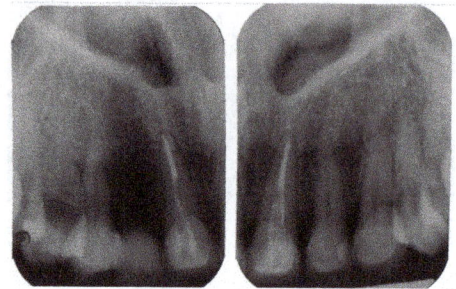

FIGURE 25: Periapical radiographs of the upper anterior teeth at review visits showing no periapical change or sign of root resorption.

the etiological factors are essential before any definitive extensive restorative work [9]. This patient followed the advice to seek medical management and her gastric disturbance was controlled. There had been no more reported regurgitation or discomfort on chewing or thermal sensitivity reported. The success of the gastric reflux management may be indirectly observed by the apparent absence of observed tooth wear in the clinical photographs at the initial and subsequent treatment and review appointments.

Compliance of the patient to wear a removable appliance is also essential for treatment success, and for this reason, a fixed approach is preferred [12, 13]. Due to the reverse overjet, a novel lower bite platform was designed to disclude the posterior teeth. Because of the increased interincisal angle with the lower incisors, it may be anticipated that higher shear stresses may occur on the cement interface under occlusal loading. For this reason, incisal hooks were included to the framework to improve the resistance form. Instead of using an adhesive resin cement, a glass ionomer cement was used, and this has the advantage that the appliance could ultimately be more easily removed by tapping at the cement interface with a chisel after cutting the hooks due to the lower tensile strength.

While traditionally concern may be expressed about possible overloading of "high" crowns that may become symptomatic, studies appear to show little if any signs or symptoms being reported in supraoccluding restorations [8, 10]. There was no dental, muscle, or TMJ discomfort experienced by this patient, other than some reduced chewing efficiency initially. Follow-up periapical radiographs were taken, and there were no signs of root resorption or

periapical change of the teeth concerned (Figure 25). There were no other complications, biological as well as mechanical, reported in this case during treatment and the 5-year follow-up period.

The rate of space closure to reestablish tooth contacts appears to vary among individuals and differs among different reports [5–8]. In this case, 3 mm of interocclusal space, more than enough clearance for the restorative material, was created in 9 months, within the range being reported [3–5]. The creation of the initial 1.5 mm interocclusal space occurred within 2 months, which is considered quite favorable to the literature [5–8]. However, the rate slowed down, and further intrusion (and eruption of posterior teeth) by the same amount, i.e., 1.5 mm, took a much longer period of time (7 months). The limit of the space that can be created with the Dahl concept is not known, although up to 4.7 mm has been reported [4]. Moreover, there is no mention in the literature whether vitality of the teeth, when applying this supraoccluding technique, has an effect on the tooth movement. Yet, it seems it makes no difference for the two root-treated upper central incisors.

4. Conclusion

This case report documents localized management of advanced erosive tooth wear in a patient with a negative overjet. A conservative and novel lower bite raising appliance was used to improve the anterior incisal relations both from a functional and aesthetic point of view. A satisfactory 5-year result is presented.

References

[1] D. C. Berry and D. F. G. Poole, "Attrition: possible mechanisms of compensation," *Journal of Oral Rehabilitation*, vol. 3, no. 3, pp. 201–206, 1976.

[2] B. Loomans and N. Opdam, "A guide to managing tooth wear: the Radboud philosophy," *British Dental Journal*, vol. 224, no. 5, pp. 348–356, 2018.

[3] B. J. R. N. L. Dahl, O. Krogstad, and K. Karlsen, "An alternative treatment in cases with advanced localized attrition," *Journal of Oral Rehabilitation*, vol. 2, no. 3, pp. 209–214, 1975.

[4] D. Dietschi and A. Argente, "A comprehensive and conservative approach for the restoration of abrasion and erosion. Part II: clinical procedures and case report," *European Journal of Esthetic Dentistry*, vol. 6, no. 2, pp. 142–159, 2011.

[5] B. L. Dahl and O. Krogstad, "Long-term observations of an increased occlusal face height obtained by a combined orthodontic/prosthetic approach," *Journal of Oral Rehabilitation*, vol. 12, no. 2, pp. 173–176, 1985.

[6] S. B. Mehta, S. Banerji, B. J. Millar, and J. M. Suarez-Feito, "Current concepts on the management of tooth wear: part 2. Active restorative care 1: the management of localised tooth wear," *British Dental Journal*, vol. 212, no. 2, pp. 73–82, 2012.

[7] N. J. Poyser, R. W. J. Porter, P. F. A. Briggs, H. S. Chana, and M. G. D. Kelleher, "The Dahl concept: past, present and future," *British Dental Journal*, vol. 198, no. 11, pp. 669–676, 2005.

[8] M. B. Gough and D. J. Setchell, "A retrospective study of 50 treatments using an appliance to produce localised occlusal space by relative axial tooth movement," *British Dental Journal*, vol. 187, no. 3, pp. 134–139, 1999.

[9] S. B. Mehta, S. Banerji, B. J. Millar, and J. M. Suarez-Feito, "Current concepts on the management of tooth wear: part 1. Assessment, treatment planning and strategies for the prevention and the passive management of tooth wear," *British Dental Journal*, vol. 212, no. 1, pp. 17–27, 2012.

[10] M. G. Botelho, "Retrospective patient evaluation of supraoccluding cast restorations," *Journal of Dental Research*, vol. 78, no. 5, p. 1163, 1999.

[11] R. E. Kreipe and S. A. Birndorf, "Eating disorders in adolescents and young adults," *Medical Clinics of North America*, vol. 84, no. 4, pp. 1027–1049, 2000.

[12] R. Ibbetson and D. Setchell, "Treatment of the worn dentition: 2," *Dental Update*, vol. 16, no. 7, pp. 300–307, 1989.

[13] K. E. Ahmed and S. Murbay, "Survival rates of anterior composites in managing tooth wear: systematic review," *Journal of Oral Rehabilitation*, vol. 43, no. 2, pp. 145–153, 2016.

33

Endocrown: An Alternative Approach for Restoring Endodontically Treated Molars with Large Coronal Destruction

Houda Dogui [iD],[1,2,3] **Feriel Abdelmalek,**[1,2,3] **Adel Amor,**[1,2,3] **and Nabiha Douki** [iD][1,2,3]

[1]*Department of Dental Medicine, Hospital Sahloul, Sousse, Faculty of Dental Medicine, Monastir, Tunisia*
[2]*Laboratory of Research in Oral Health and Maxillo Facial Rehabilitation (LR12ES11), University of Monastir, Monastir, Tunisia*
[3]*Faculty of Dental Medicine, University of Monastir, Monastir, Tunisia*

Correspondence should be addressed to Houda Dogui; houdadogui@gmail.com

Academic Editor: Tatiana Pereira-Cenci

Rehabilitation of endodontically treated molar still remains a challenge. After endodontic treatment, molars lost their mechanical characteristics. In fact, they became fragile and that is in relation with the removal of pulp and surrounding dentin tissues. Endocrown which is a single partial restoration could be considered as a good alternative for restoring molars having large coronal destruction and presenting endodontic treatment difficulties. Through this work, we discuss the indication and use of endocrown to replace single crowns with intraradicular retention and to present a clinical case report of an endocrown-type restoration, fabricated from lithium disilicate ceramic (IPS e.Max CAD) in a mandibular first molar with extensive coronal destruction.

1. Introduction

There is still an important challenge for most dentists before being optimistic about the rehabilitation of endodontically treated teeth with extensive coronal destruction. The biomechanical principles of retention and resistance are deteriorating [1]. The existing biomechanical changes due to root canal therapy and the degree of lost dental tissue lead clinicians to restorative treatment planning [2].

For the case of teeth heavily damaged by dental caries or fractures, a treatment with a total crown supported by a cast metal core has been suggested [3]. Yet, a root perforation and thinning of the root canal walls due to over preparation might happen after using intraradicular posts [4].

Moreover, the limitations to the use of intraradicular posts, such as calcified root canals, narrow canals, or a fracture of an instrument, have led dentists to think of other alternatives, as the use of endocrowns, an adhesive endodontic crown [5, 6].

This complete glass ceramic crown restoration was proposed in 1999 by Bindl and Mörmann as a substitute to the full post-and-core-supported crown; "endocrown" is a one-piece ceramic construction. This crown would be fixed to the internal walls of the pulp chamber and on the cavity margins to improve macromechanical retention and the use of adhesive cementation would also improve microretention [7].

The purpose of the present paper is to present a clinical case, in which an esthetic and conservative posterior endocrown was used to restore a mandibular molar that presented endodontic treatment and extensive coronal destruction. We will discuss through this work the indication and the use of endocrown.

2. Case Report

A 23-year-old female was referred to our medicine dental department in UHC Sahloul, Sousse, for treatment of tooth #46. She suffered from major coronal destruction and needed to have her first molar restored. The medical history was noncontributory. Radiographic and clinical examinations were performed initially, and an extensive glass ionomer cement restoration of a nonvital tooth (46) was identified (Figures 1 and 2). The tooth was treated endodontically. The patient had an acceptable oral hygiene and a favorable occlusion. After removing the restoration, an endocrown restoration was recommended because of the amount of remaining

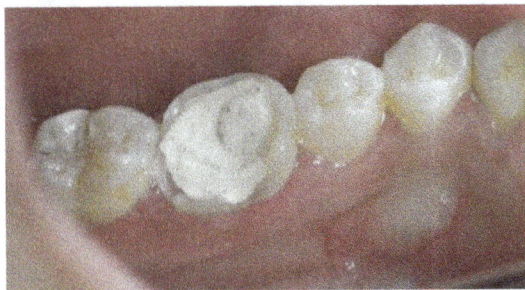

FIGURE 1: Clinical condition of tooth #46 with extensive glass ionomer cement restoration.

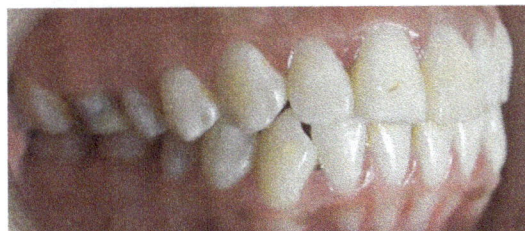

FIGURE 2: Relationship of crown height in occlusion with the antagonist tooth (side view).

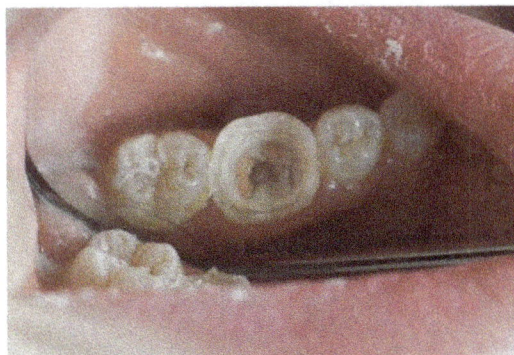

FIGURE 3: The molar after removal of the restoration.

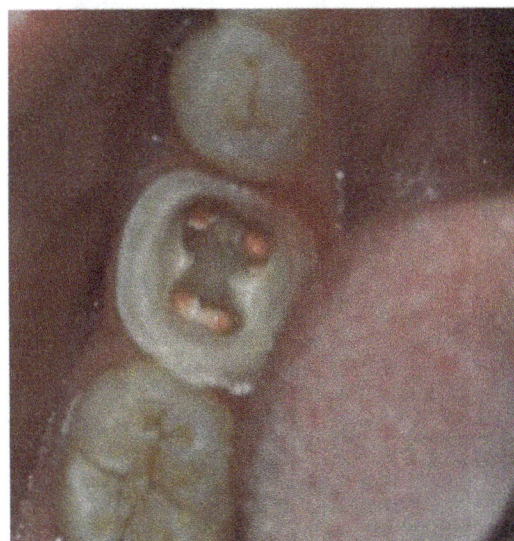

FIGURE 4: Removing Gutta-percha to a depth not exceeding 2 mm.

tooth structure and the thickness of the walls (Figure 3). The prosthetic decision was to restore tooth (46) with an endocrown fabricated from lithium disilicate ceramic (IPS e.Max CAD). The preparation for the endocrown is different from the conventional complete crown. This monolithic, ceramic adhesive restoration requires specific preparation techniques to be suitable for especial biomechanical needs.

This is aimed at achieving achieve an overall reduction in the height of the occlusal surface of at least 2 mm in the axial direction and to get a cervical margin or "cervical sidewalk" in the form of a butt joint. The cervical margin has to be supragingival and enamel walls less than 2 mm have to be eliminated.

Differences in levels between the various parts of the cervical margin should be linked by a slope of no more than 60° to escape a staircase effect. We used a cylindrical-conical diamond bur held parallel to the occlusal plane, to reduce the occlusal surface. Then we used a diamond wheel bur to control the orientation of the reduction and to guarantee a flat surface thanks to its shape.

We used a cylindrical-conical diamond bur with a total occlusal convergence of 7° to create continuity between the coronal pulp chamber and endodontic access cavity. The bur was orientated along the long axis of the tooth; the preparation was done without too much pressure and without touching the pulpal floor.

Removing too much tissue from the pulp chamber walls will reduce their thickness and the width strip of enamel. The depth of the cavity must be at least 3 mm.

The entrance to the pulpal canal was opened. Gutta-percha was removed to a depth not exceeding 2 mm to profit from the saddle-like anatomy of the cavity floor. Nonabrasive instrument was required to maintain the integrity of the

canal entrance. No drilling of dentin was carried out. The remaining tooth structure was still strong (Figure 4).

We ended the preparation with lining the root canal entrances with glass ionomer cement to protect the orifice of the canal (Figure 5).

After evaluating the entire cavity and the interocclusal space, the impression of the tooth was taken by double impression technique using additional silicone. After visualization and analysis of the quality of the impression, we selected the ceramic shade and sent the impression to the laboratory.

A provisional acrylic resin restoration was made by using block technic and cemented with eugenol-free temporary cement (Figure 6). The endocrown was fabricated in the laboratory using CAD-CAM technology and was positioned on the master cast (Figure 7).

Then we made a try-in of the endocrown and tested occlusion, internal, and proximal adjustments. Right after this, we sent it back to the laboratory for application of the colorant and glaze. In the following session, the internal surface of the endocrown was etched with hydrofluoric acid, rinsed with water, and dried with an air syringe. Next, a coat of a silane coupling agent was applied for 1 minute and dried.

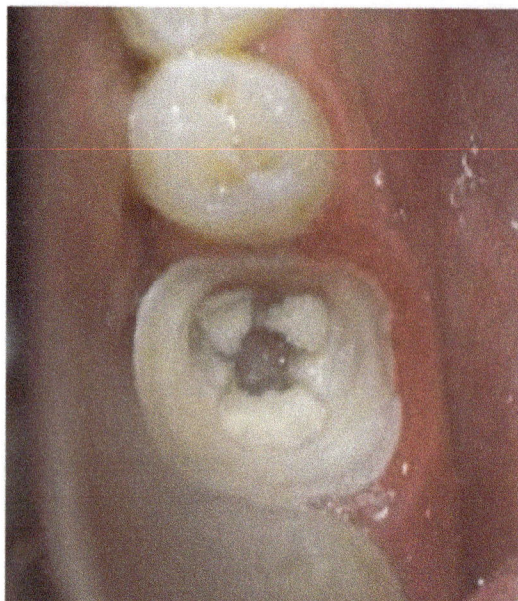

FIGURE 5: Lining the root canal entrances with glass ionomer cement.

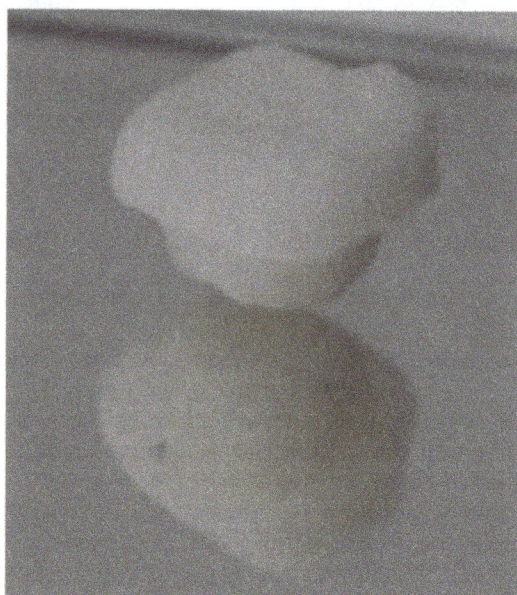

FIGURE 6: Aspect of the provisional restoration.

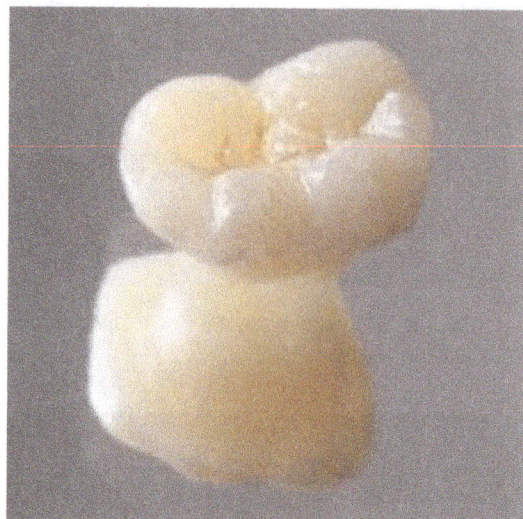

FIGURE 7: Aspect of the endocrown.

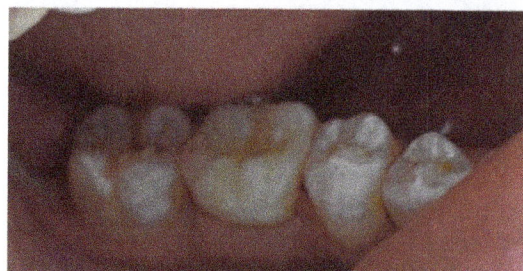

FIGURES 8: Try-in of the occlusion.

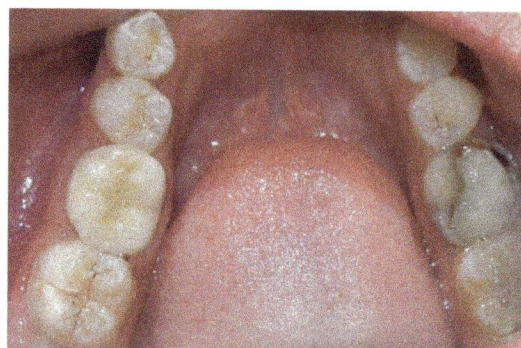

FIGURE 9: Final occlusal view after bonding the endocrown.

Rubber dam was used to achieve proper isolation, and then phosphoric acid was applied onto the tooth surface for 15 sec on dentin and 30 sec on enamel, then abundantly washed and dried, applied with adhesive, and polymerized for 20 sec with light curing.

A thin layer of a dual polymerizing resin was applied to the prosthetic endocrown and then was inserted into the tooth and polymerized at intervals of 5 seconds, making it easy to remove cement excesses. After that, it was polymerized for 60 seconds on all surfaces. The restoration was examined for any occlusal interference using ceramic finishing instruments (Figure 8). The final restoration is shown in Figure 9.

3. Discussion

The project of the restorative treatment of molars with a large coronal destruction, a clinical challenge, requires careful planning. That is why the dentist has to decide for the best treatment option to ensure an efficient treatment providing clinical longevity of molars.

The endocrown is convenient for all molars, particularly those with clinically low crowns, calcified root canals, or narrow canals [8]. But it is not recommended if adhesion cannot be assured, if the pulpal chamber is less than 3 mm deep, or if the cervical margin is less than 2 mm wide for most of its circumference [9].

This has been shown to be an advantageous technique as the procedure is easy; it facilitates the steps of impression taking and protects the periodontium [8, 10]. Also, the use of ceramic has the advantages of biocompatibility and biomimicry and its wear coefficient is close to that of the natural tooth. Furthermore, the single interface of a 1-piece restoration makes cohesion look better [11, 12].

The objective of the preparation is to get a wide and stable surface resisting the compressive stresses that are frequent in molars [13]. The prepared surface is parallel to the occlusal plane to provide stress resistance along the major axis of the tooth [14]. The stress levels in teeth with endocrowns were lower than in teeth with prosthetic crowns [11, 15].

Due to the development of adhesive cementation systems, the need for macroretentive preparation for crowns has decreased [16].

The pulpal chamber cavity provides also retention and stability. Its trapezoidal shape in mandibular molars and triangular shape in maxillary molars increase the restoration's stability, and additional preparation is not needed. The saddle form of the pulpal floor increases stability. This anatomy, along with the adhesive qualities of the bonding material, makes it unessential to attempt further use of post-involving root canals [14]. In fact, the root canals do not need any specific shape; therefore, they are not fragilized by the drilling and they will not receive the stresses associated with the use of post [17]. The compressive stresses are reduced, being distributed over the cervical butt joint and the walls of the pulp chamber [8, 14, 18, 19].

In 2018, Dartora et al. have evaluated the biomechanical behavior of endodontically treated teeth restored using different extensions of endocrowns inside the pulp chamber; it has concluded that the greater extension of endocrowns provided better mechanical performance. A 5 mm extension presented lower intensity and a better stress distribution pattern than a 1 mm extension which presented a low fracture resistance and a high possibility of rotating the piece when in function [20, 21].

An in vitro study performed by Taha et al. was done to assess the effect of varying the margin designs on the fracture resistance of endodontically treated teeth restored with polymer-infiltrated ceramic endocrown restorations. The results showed that endocrowns with axial reduction and a shoulder finish line had higher mean fracture resistance values than endocrowns with butt margin design.

It has been also shown that butt joint designs provided a stable surface that resists the compressive stresses because it is prepared parallel to the occlusal plane [22].

In 2012, Biacchi and Basting compared the fracture strength of 2 types of full ceramic crowns: indirect conventional crowns retained by glass fibre posts and endocrowns. They came to the conclusion that endocrowns were more resistant to compressive forces than the first ones. More recently, finite element analysis highlighted the role of endocrowns in stress distribution [7].

According to Schultheis et al., endocrown seems to be a more reliable alternative for posterior loadbearing teeth,

whereas a bilayer configuration is more susceptible to reduce load fracture failure [23].

As stated by Biacchi et al., endocrowns procure adequate function and esthetics and preserve the biomechanical integrity of nonvital posterior teeth. The restoration is reported to be less exposed to the adverse effects of degradation of the hybrid layer [24].

A research comparing equivalent stresses in molars restored with endocrowns as well as posts and cores during masticatory simulation using finite element analysis revealed that teeth restored by endocrowns are potentially more resistant to failure than those with FRC posts. This study also showed that under physiological loads, ceramic endocrowns ideally cemented in molars should not be damaged or debonded [15].

A systematic review achieved by Sedrez-Porto et al. has evaluated clinical (survival) and in vitro (fracture-strength) studies of endocrown restorations compared to conventional treatments using intraradicular posts, direct composite resin, or inlay/onlay restorations; it has been shown that endocrowns may perform similarly or better than the conventional treatments [25].

Altier et al. compared the fracture resistance of three different endocrowns made of lithium disilicate ceramic and two different indirect resin composites (Solidex composite and Gradia composite) and determined that lithium disilicate ceramic endocrowns exhibited higher fracture strength than the indirect composite groups [26].

It has been shown that endocrowns made of lithium disilicate-based ceramics are considered among the best restorative materials because of their adhesive properties; also, they promoted micromechanical interlocking with resin cement [7, 27].

An in vitro study accomplished by Gresnigt et al. evaluated the effect of axial and lateral forces on the strength of endocrowns made of $Li_2Si_2O_5$ and multiphase resin composite. It has been concluded that under axial loading, both $Li_2Si_2O_5$ and multiphase resin composite used as endocrown material presented similar fracture strength but under lateral forces, the latter exhibited significantly lower results [27].

In 2018, Tribst et al. evaluated the influence of a restorative material type on the biomechanical behavior of endocrown restorations and concluded that Leucite presents a better stress distribution and it can be a promising alternative to lithium disilicate for the manufacture of endocrown restorations [28].

Another research achieved by Skalskyi et al. compared the fracture resistance of different restorative materials used in dental endocrown restorations. It has demonstrated that the mechanical behavior of the restorative materials in the tooth restorations changed. The zirconium dioxide endocrowns cracked resulting to crack propagation in the tooth. It has been also shown that the use of metal ceramic as endocrown material may provide the lowest risk of failure during clinical use and had the highest fracture strength [29].

An investigation made by Darwish et al. showed that endodontically treated maxillary premolars restored with resin nanoceramic endocrowns presented better internal adaptation compared to those restored with lithium disilicate endocrowns and that endocrown preparation with smaller axial wall divergence ("6"degree) provided better internal fit [30].

In a recent study, Zoidis et al. proposed polyetheretherketone (PEEK) as an alternative framework material for endocrown restorations. They demonstrated that the elastic modulus of the polyetheretherketone framework (4 GPa) veneered with indirect composite resin could dampen the occlusal forces protecting tooth structures better than ceramic materials. But further long-term clinical evidence is required [31].

CAD-CAM system, with an estimated success of 90.5% for molars and 75% for premolars in 55 patients [1, 32].

According to Belleflamme et al., even in the presence of extensive coronal tissue loss or occlusal risk factors, such as bruxism or unfavorable occlusal relationships, endocrowns could be a reliable approach to restore severely damaged molars and premolars [33].

4. Conclusion

The preparation for endocrowns is simple and can be achieved quickly. Root canals are not engaged in the process, and the procedure is less traumatic than others. The supragingival position of the cervical margin protects the marginal periodontium, facilitates impression taking, and preserves the solid substance of the remaining tooth. Forces are dispersed over the cervical butt joint (compression) and axial walls (shear force), thus moderating the load on the pulpal floor.

The endocrown represents a very hopeful treatment alternative for endodontically treated molars, it allows maintaining of tooth structure, it is compatible with goal minimally invasive dentistry, and it is adequate for the concept of biointegration. It is a conservative approach for mechanical and aesthetic restoration of nonvital posterior teeth.

This type of reconstruction, which is still uncommon, should be more widely known and practised.

References

[1] A. Ploumaki, A. Bilkhair, T. Tuna, S. Stampf, and J. R. Strub, "Success rates of prosthetic restorations on endodontically treated teeth; a systematic review after 6 years," *Journal of Oral Rehabilitation*, vol. 40, no. 8, pp. 618–630, 2013.

[2] A. Polesel, "Restoration of the endodontically treated posterior tooth," *Giornale Italiano di Endodonzia*, vol. 28, no. 1, pp. 2–16, 2014.

[3] N. Stern and Z. Hirshfeld, "Principles of preparing endodontically treated teeth for dowel and core restorations," *The Journal of Prosthetic Dentistry*, vol. 30, no. 2, pp. 162–165, 1973.

[4] E. Asmussen, A. Peutzfeldt, and A. Sahafi, "Finite element analysis of stresses in endodontically treated, dowel-restored teeth," *The Journal of Prosthetic Dentistry*, vol. 94, no. 4, pp. 321–329, 2005.

[5] A. Bindl and W. H. Mörmann, "Clinical evaluation of adhesively placed cerec endo-crowns after 2 years: preliminary results," *The Journal of Adhesive Dentistry*, vol. 1, no. 3, pp. 255–265, 1999.

[6] T. N. Göhring and O. A. Peters, "Restoration of endodontically treated teeth without posts," *American Journal of Dentistry*, vol. 16, no. 5, pp. 313–317, 2003.

[7] G. R. Biacchi and R. T. Basting, "Comparison of fracture strength of endocrowns and glass fiber post-retained conventional crowns," *Operative Dentistry*, vol. 37, no. 2, pp. 130–136, 2012.

[8] R. Menezes-Silva, C. A. V. Espinoza, M. T. Atta, M. F. L. Navarro, S. K. Ishikiriama, and R. F. L. Mondelli, "Endocrown: a conservative approach," *Brazilian Dental Science*, vol. 19, no. 2, 2016.

[9] M. Fages and B. Bennaser, "The endocrown: a different type of all-ceramic reconstruction of molars," *Journal of the Canadian Dental Association*, vol. 29, no. 79, article d140, 2013.

[10] R. B. Carlos, M. Thomas Nainan, S. Pradhan, R. Sharma, S. Benjamin, and R. Rose, "Restoration of endodontically treated molars using all ceramic endocrowns," *Case Reports in Dentistry*, vol. 2013, Article ID 210763, 5 pages, 2013.

[11] C. L. Lin, Y. H. Chang, C. Y. Chang, C. A. Pai, and S. F. Huang, "Finite element and Weibull analyses to estimate failure risks in the ceramic endocrown and classical crown for endodontically treated maxillary premolar," *European Journal of Oral Sciences*, vol. 118, no. 1, pp. 87–93, 2010.

[12] F. Zarone, R. Sorrentino, D. Apicella et al., "Evaluation of the biomechanical behavior of maxillary central incisors restored by means of endocrowns compared to a natural tooth: a 3D static linear finite elements analysis," *Dental Materials*, vol. 22, no. 11, pp. 1035–1044, 2006.

[13] L. V. Zogheib, G. de Siqueira Ferreira Anzaloni Saavedra, P. E. Cardoso, M. C. Valera, and M. A. M. Araújo, "Resistance to compression of weakened roots subjected to different root reconstruction protocols," *Journal of Applied Oral Science*, vol. 19, no. 6, pp. 648–654, 2011.

[14] M. Fages and B. Bennasar, "The endocrown: a different type of all-ceramic reconstruction for molars," *Journal Canadian Dental Association*, vol. 79, article d140, 2013.

[15] B. Dejak and A. Młotkowski, "3D-finite element analysis of molars restored with endocrowns and posts during masticatory simulation," *Dental Materials*, vol. 29, no. 12, pp. e309–e317, 2013.

[16] E. Lander and D. Dietschi, "Endocrowns: a clinical report," *Quintessence International*, vol. 39, no. 2, pp. 99–106, 2008.

[17] A. S. Fernandes and G. S. Dessai, "Factors affecting the fracture resistance of post-core reconstructed teeth: a review," *The International Journal of Prosthodontics*, vol. 14, no. 4, pp. 355–363, 2001.

[18] G. T. Rocca, R. Daher, C. M. Saratti et al., "Restoration of severely damaged endodontically treated premolars: the influence of the endo-core length on marginal integrity and fatigue resistance of lithium disilicate CAD-CAM ceramic endocrowns," *Journal of Dentistry*, vol. 68, pp. 41–50, 2018.

[19] L. Fernandes da Cunha, J. Mondelli, C. M. Auersvald et al., "Endocrown with leucite-reinforced ceramic: case of restoration of endodontically treated teeth," *Case Reports in Dentistry*, vol. 2015, Article ID 750313, 4 pages, 2015.

[20] N. R. Dartora, M. B. de Conto Ferreira, I. C. M. Moris et al., "Effect of intracoronal depth of teeth restored with

endocrowns on fracture resistance: in vitro and 3-dimensional finite element analysis," *Journal of Endodontia*, vol. 44, no. 7, pp. 1179–1185, 2018.

[21] Y. Silva-Sousa, E. A. Gomes, N. R. Dartora et al., "Mechanical behavior of endodontically treated teeth with different endocrowns extensions," *Dental Materials*, vol. 33, no. 1, pp. e73–e74, 2017.

[22] D. Taha, S. Spintzyk, C. Schille et al., "Fracture resistance and failure modes of polymer infiltrated ceramic endocrown restorations with variations in margin design and occlusal thickness," *Journal of Prosthodontic Research*, vol. 62, no. 3, pp. 293–297, 2018.

[23] S. Schultheis, J. R. Strub, T. A. Gerds, and P. C. Guess, "Monolithic and bi-layer CAD/CAM lithium–disilicate versus metal–ceramic fixed dental prostheses: comparison of fracture loads and failure modes after fatigue," *Clinical Oral Investigations*, vol. 17, no. 5, pp. 1407–1413, 2013.

[24] G. R. Biacchi, B. Mello, and R. T. Basting, "The endocrown: an alternative approach for restoring extensively damaged molars," *Journal of Esthetic and Restorative Dentistry*, vol. 25, no. 6, pp. 383–390, 2013.

[25] J. A. Sedrez-Porto, W. L. de Oliveira da Rosa, A. F. da Silva, E. A. Münchow, and T. Pereira-Cenci, "Endocrown restorations: a systematic review and meta-analysis," *Journal of Dentistry*, vol. 52, pp. 8–14, 2016.

[26] M. Altier, F. Erol, G. Yildirim, and E. E. Dalkilic, "Fracture resistance and failure modes of lithium disilicate or composite endocrowns," *Nigerian Journal of Clinical Practice*, vol. 21, no. 7, pp. 821–826, 2018.

[27] M. M. M. Gresnigt, M. Özcan, M. L. A. van den Houten, L. Schipper, and M. S. Cune, "Fracture strength, failure type and Weibull characteristics of lithium disilicate and multiphase resin composite endocrowns under axial and lateral forces," *Dental Materials*, vol. 32, no. 5, pp. 607–614, 2016.

[28] J. P. M. Tribst, A. M. de Oliveira Dal Piva, C. F. L. Madruga et al., "Endocrown restorations: influence of dental remnant and restorative material on stress distribution," *Dental Materials*, 2018.

[29] V. Skalskyi, V. Makeev, O. Stankevych, and R. Pavlychko, "Features of fracture of prosthetic toothendocrown constructions by means of acoustic emission analysis," *Dental Materials*, vol. 34, no. 3, pp. e46–e55, 2018.

[30] H. A. Darwish, T. S. Morsi, and A. G. El Dimeery, "Internal fit of lithium disilicate and resin nanoceramic endocrowns with different preparation designs," *Future Dental Journal*, vol. 3, no. 2, pp. 67–72, 2017.

[31] P. Zoidis, E. Bakiri, and G. Polyzois, "Using modified polyetheretherketone (PEEK) as an alternative material for endocrown restorations: a short-term clinical report," *The Journal of Prosthetic Dentistry*, vol. 117, no. 3, pp. 335–339, 2017.

[32] T. Otto and W. H. Mörmann, "Clinical performance of chairside CAD/CAM feldspathic ceramic posterior shoulder crowns and endocrowns up to 12 years," *International Journal of Computerized Dentistry*, vol. 18, no. 2, pp. 147–161, 2015.

[33] M. M. Belleflamme, S. O. Geerts, M. M. Louwette, C. F. Grenade, A. J. Vanheusden, and A. K. Mainjot, "No post-no core approach to restore severely damaged posterior teeth: an up to 10-year retrospective study of documented endocrown cases," *Journal of Dentistry*, vol. 63, pp. 1–7, 2017.

34

Oral Rehabilitation of Oral Cancer Patients Using Zygomatic Implant-Supported Maxillary Prostheses with Magnetic Attachment: Three Case Reports

Hisashi Ozaki [iD],[1,2] Hiromasa Sakurai,[3] Yukie Yoshida,[2] Hideyuki Yamanouchi,[2] and Mitsuyoshi Iino[2]

[1]Department of Dentistry, Oral and Maxillofacial Surgery, Yamagata Prefectural Central Hospital, Yamagata, Japan
[2]Department of Dentistry, Oral and Maxillofacial-Plastic and Reconstructive Surgery, Faculty of Medicine, Yamagata University, Yamagata, Japan
[3]Department of Dentistry, Oral and Maxillofacial Surgery, Nihonkai General Hospital, Yamagata Prefectural and Sakata Municipal Hospital Organization, Sakata, Japan

Correspondence should be addressed to Hisashi Ozaki; ozahisa19@yahoo.co.jp

Academic Editor: Maria Beatriz Duarte Gavião

Maxillectomy for malignant tumor often results in a maxillary defect and serious oral dysfunction. A prosthesis is usually provided for postoperative oral rehabilitation of such patients with maxillary defects. However, the further the resected region extends, the less stable the prosthesis becomes, due to insufficient bone and tooth support. Therefore, in many cases, conventional resection dentures may not be adequate to restore the oral function. Effective utilization of dental and zygomatic implants may help to restore oral function in patients with severe maxillary defects. This clinical report describes the management of three patients with severe maxillary defects following cancer ablative surgery who were rehabilitated using maxillary prostheses with magnetic attachments supported by dental and zygomatic implants. Occlusal reconstruction was performed with removable prostheses supported with two or four implants and magnetic attachment. The oral function was evaluated before and after prosthodontic treatment with implants using the Oral Health Impact Profile (OHIP-14) and functional chewing score. Results indicated improvement in all cases. These findings show that quality of life (QOL) and oral function were improved.

1. Introduction

Maxillectomy is performed for radical treatment of maxillary malignant tumors leading to serious problems in mastication, swallowing, speech, and facial esthetics. Reconstruction is of paramount importance for these individuals but is often a major challenge. There are several reconstructive techniques that involve the use of vascularized or nonvascularized autogenous material or prosthetic devices with dental and/or zygomatic implants. Conventional dental implants have been used to improve the stability and retention of maxillary prosthetic obturators and to restore oral function [1, 2]. However, dental implant placement is often difficult following resection of maxillary malignant tumor because of inadequate amount of bone tissue for anchorage of the implants. As an alternative procedure, the use of zygomatic implants is effective for prosthetic rehabilitation [3–5]. The effective utilization of dental and zygomatic implants may help to restore oral function in patients with severe maxillary defects.

Here, we describe the management of three patients who underwent extensive maxillary resection resulting in huge maxillary defects, followed by the introduction of maxillary prostheses with magnetic attachment using dental and zygomatic implants.

2. Case Presentation

Between October 2012 and November 2013, three patients with maxillary defects following resection of malignant

TABLE 1: Detailed information on the patients.

	Case 1	Case 2	Case 3
Age/gender	76/F	81/M	83/F
Type of cancer	Malignant melanoma	Squamous cell carcinoma	Malignant melanoma
Defect	Class IIc	Class Ia	Class IIc
Location	Bilateral buccal bone	Buccal bone and anterior region	Bilateral buccal bone
Number of implants	Dental implant: 2	Dental implant: 2	Dental implant: 2
	Zygomatic implant: 2	Zygomatic implant: 1	Zygomatic implant: 2
Length and width	Dental implant: 10 mm, 3.5 mm	Dental implant: 10 mm, 3.5 mm	Dental implant: 18 mm, 4 mm
	Zygomatic implant: 40 mm, 4 mm	Zygomatic implant: 30 mm, 4 mm	Zygomatic implant: 30 mm, 4 mm
Healing period	8 months	6 months	6 months
Period of loading	3 years	1 year and 6 months	2 years
Radiation	None	None	50 Gy

tumor were recruited. The clinical findings of these patients are presented in Table 1. Type of maxillary defect was defined based on the classification by Brown et al. [6]. The implant systems used were Brånemark System® MK-III and Zygoma TiUnite (Nobel Biocare, Zurich, Switzerland). The mean healing period until second surgery was 6.7 months (range: 6–8 months). Conventional resection dentures were initially fabricated, followed by implant-supported overdentures with magnetic attachments.

2.1. Case 1. A 76-year-old woman with malignant melanoma of the upper gingiva underwent subtotal maxillectomy and neck dissection of the right side. Six months after tumor resection, two zygomatic implants were inserted into bilateral zygomatic bones. After another 6 months, second-stage surgery was performed and two dental implants were placed in the anterior region of the maxilla. However, the position and depth of the dental implants were inappropriate for the final prosthesis. Therefore, the two anterior implants could not be used for support. The zygomatic implants and prosthesis have remained stable for 3 years since functional loading (Figures 1(a)–1(c)).

2.2. Case 2. An 81-year-old man was diagnosed with squamous cell carcinoma of the left maxillary gingiva and underwent partial maxillectomy. Two years after tumor resection, two dental implants in the anterior maxillary region and one zygomatic implant into the right side zygomatic bone were placed. After another 6 months, second-stage surgery was performed; however, one dental implant in the anterior region had to be explanted due to loss of osseointegration. Subsequently, the implants and prosthesis have remained stable for 1 year and 6 months since functional loading (Figures 2(a)–2(c)).

2.3. Case 3. An 83-year-old woman had a chief complaint of difficulty in eating due to severe instability of her upper removable denture. Fifteen years ago, she had been diagnosed with malignant melanoma of the maxillary gingiva. After preoperative superselective arterial injection chemotherapy, bilateral partial maxillectomy and postoperative concurrent chemoradiotherapy were performed. Thirteen

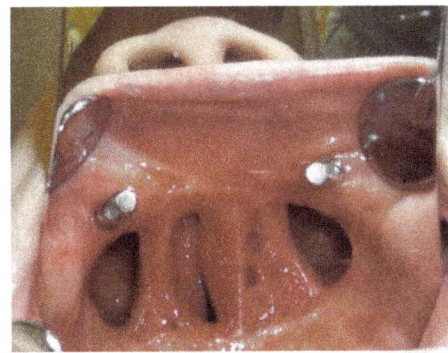

(a)

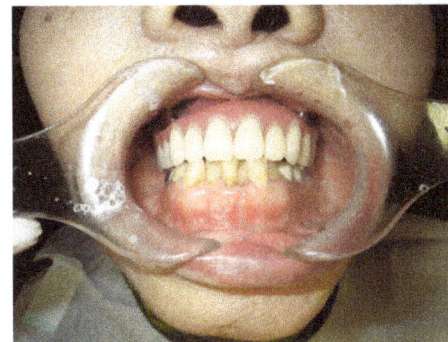

(b)

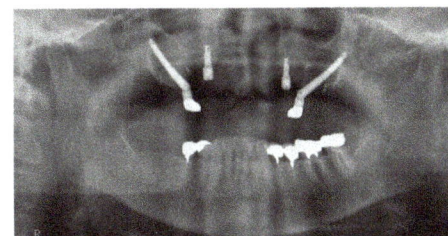

(c)

FIGURE 1: (a) Postoperative intraoral photograph (mirror image). (b) Intraoral view with the prosthesis in place. (c) Postoperative radiograph.

years after tumor resection, two dental implants and two zygomatic implants were placed on each side of the zygomatic bones. Two years after functional loading, the left

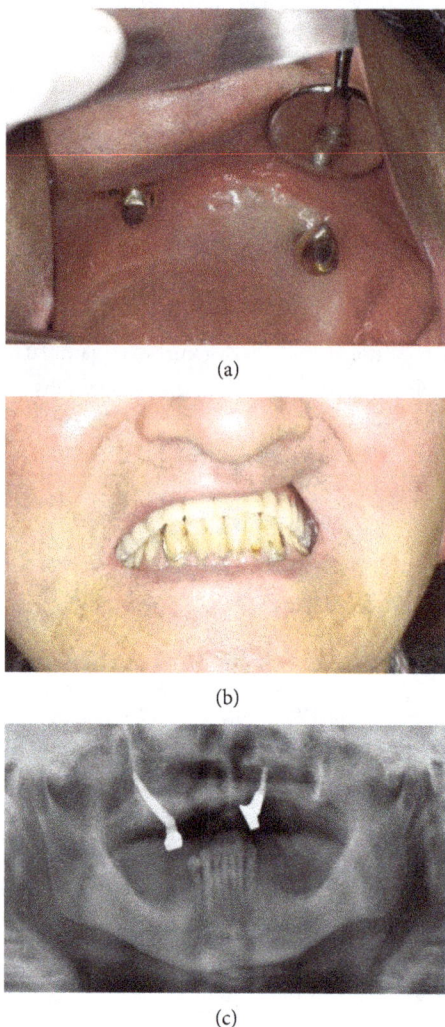

(a)

(b)

(c)

FIGURE 2: (a) Postoperative intraoral photograph (mirror image). (b) Intraoral view with the prosthesis in place. (c) Postoperative radiograph.

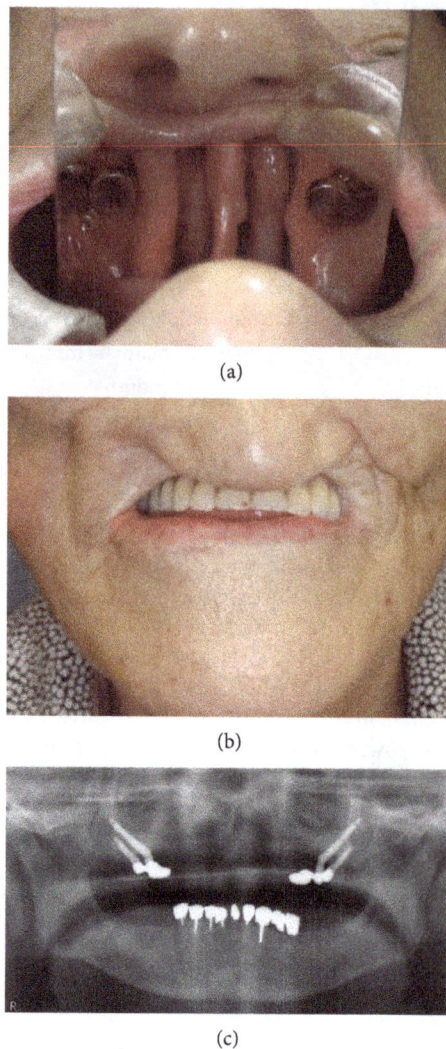

(a)

(b)

(c)

FIGURE 3: (a) Postoperative intraoral photograph (mirror image). (b) Intraoral view with the prosthesis in place. (c) Postoperative radiograph.

abutment with magnetic attachments was fractured. A new abutment with magnetic attachments was fabricated, and the prosthesis is currently being used without any complications (Figures 3(a)–3(c)).

2.4. Evaluation of OHRQoL and Masticatory Function. Oral health-related quality of life (OHRQoL) was measured using the Oral Health Impact Profile [7] (OHIP-14) before and after prosthodontic treatment with implants. Higher scores in OHIP-14 indicate worse result. Masticatory function was assessed using an evaluation sheet for chewing function [8]. In all cases, the numerical value decreased in OHRQoL and the chewing function scores increased after prosthodontic treatment with implants (Table 2).

3. Discussion

Maxillary defects caused by cancer ablative surgery are commonly reconstructed with prostheses. Good functional results are reportedly attained with obturator prostheses

TABLE 2: Evaluation on OHIP-14 and functional chewing score.

Questionnaire	OHIP-14		Functional chewing score	
	Pre	Post	Pre	Post
Case 1	45	12	20	50
Case 2	16	6	30	35
Case 3	31	18	45	65

[9–12]. However, the further the resected region extends, the less stable the prosthesis becomes because of insufficient bone and tooth support for the denture. The use of dental implants is effective in such cases. In the present study, it is obvious that the maxillary prosthesis with magnetic attachment supported by dental and zygomatic implants was effective as shown on OHRQoL. With regard to masticatory function, in Cases 1 and 3, the chewing function scores with the conventional resection denture were 20 and 45, respectively. In contrast, the scores with the maxillary prosthesis supported by the implants were 50 and 65, respectively.

Sato et al. reported that the mean score of complete denture wearers with "satisfied" was 58.7, "partly satisfied" 48.5, and "not satisfied" 32.4. These scores offer a ready explanation that the chewing function score corresponds closely to chewing satisfaction [8]. Therefore, in Case 1 and Case 3, it is thought that the chewing function is not inferior to the function of complete denture wearers. This treatment could provide the recovery of chewing function in consideration of poor environment in the oral cavity. However, in Case 2, the chewing function score showed only a slight increase, probably because there were only few remaining teeth in the mandible and the mandibular partial denture did not fit well. The limitation of the present treatment is incomplete closure of the resulting maxillary defect, such as Cases 1 and 3. For this problem, Butterworth et al. suggested a new surgical technique with the zygomatic implant perforated flap. The technique involves the use of a zygomatic implant perforated microvascular soft tissue flap (ZIP flap) for the primary management of maxillary malignancy with surgical closure of the resultant maxillary defect and the installation of osseointegrated support for a zygomatic implant-supported maxillary fixed dental prosthesis [13]. In the report, this treatment demonstrated good result for the case of the maxillary malignant. However, the treatment with free tissue transfer is very invasive. Moreover, the application of the treatment is a low-level Brown class 2b maxillectomy and limited [14]. Our cases are all very elderly people, and Cases 1 and 3 are Brown class 2d. Therefore, the ZIP flap technique is not suitable in our cases.

Various attachment systems have been successfully used with implant-supported overdentures in recent years. These systems include telescopic crowns, bars, locators, balls, and magnets. Dental practitioners and technicians generally select attachment systems based on their experience and training [15]. We selected the magnet attachment system to reduce the load to the implants. Depending on the extent of the maxillary defect, the denture tends to become larger and wider. Therefore, it was assumed that the load to the prosthesis, including implant and abutment, may increase during occlusion, compared to conventional implant-supported overdentures without the maxillary defect. Rigid retention between the denture and implant may increase the risk of prosthodontic complications, including fracture of denture, abutment, and implant. As magnetic attachments resist only vertical force and do not resist lateral force, it is thought that retention is low against lateral force compared to the other attachment. Consequently, the abutment and implant body appear to be better protected. However, in Case 3, the abutment with magnet attachment was fractured. This fracture could have occurred because the abutment was too long. Therefore, a favorable position and angle of placement of the implant are important for the prosthesis.

There is no clear consensus on the appropriate number of dental and zygomatic implants required for the implant-supported maxillary prosthesis in patients with maxillary defects. Schmidt et al. [4] presented a review of patients who underwent reconstruction using zygomatic implants after maxillectomy and found that four zygomatic implants or a combination of two dental implants and zygomatic implants were used for functional and aesthetic rehabilitation after maxillectomy. The prognosis of such treatment was acceptable. In the present study, the oral functions of 2 cases were restored by a two-implant-supported overdenture in short term. This approach will offer several advantages [3]. First, additional procedures for reconstruction of the maxilla will not be necessary in many cases. Second, the placement of implants and fabrication of the prosthesis become simple. Finally, the time required for surgery is reduced and the reduced number of implants reduces the cost [3].

These cases demonstrated that a maxillary prosthesis with magnetic attachment supported by dental and zygomatic implants is effective for patients with maxillary defects.

Consent

Informed consent was obtained from the patient for publication of this case report and any accompanying images.

References

[1] Z. H. Baqain, M. Anabtawi, A. A. Karaky, and Z. Malkawi, "Morbidity from anterior iliac crest bone harvesting for secondary alveolar bone grafting: an outcome assessment study," *Journal of Oral and Maxillofacial Surgery*, vol. 67, no. 3, pp. 570–575, 2009.

[2] M. Chiapasco, F. Biglioli, L. Autelitano, E. Romeo, and R. Brusati, "Clinical outcome of dental implants placed in fibula-free flaps used for the reconstruction of maxillo-mandibular defects following ablation for tumors or osteoradionecrosis," *Clinical Oral Implants Research*, vol. 17, no. 2, pp. 220–228, 2006.

[3] H. Ozaki, S. Ishikawa, K. Kitabatake, K. Yusa, H. Sakurai, and M. Iino, "Functional and aesthetic rehabilitation with maxillary prosthesis supported by two zygomatic implants for maxillary defect resulting from cancer ablative surgery: a case report/technique article," *Odontology*, vol. 104, no. 2, pp. 233–238, 2016.

[4] B. L. Schmidt, M. A. Pogrel, C. W. Young, and A. Sharma, "Reconstruction of extensive maxillary defects using zygomaticus implants," *Journal of Oral and Maxillofacial Surgery*, vol. 62, 9 Suppl 2, pp. 82–89, 2004.

[5] Y. J. Hu, A. Hardianto, S. Y. Li, Z. Y. Zhang, and C. P. Zhang, "Reconstruction of a palatomaxillary defect with vascularized iliac bone combined with a superficial inferior epigastric artery flap and zygomatic implants as anchorage," *International Journal of Oral and Maxillofacial Surgery*, vol. 36, no. 9, pp. 854–857, 2007.

[6] J. S. Brown, S. N. Rogers, D. N. McNally, and M. Boyle, "A modified classification for the maxillectomy defect," *Head & Neck*, vol. 22, no. 1, pp. 17–26, 2000.

[7] G. D. Slade, "Derivation and validation of a short-form oral health impact profile," *Community Dentistry and Oral Epidemiology*, vol. 25, no. 4, pp. 284–290, 1997.

[8] Y. Sato, S. Minagi, Y. Akagawa, and T. Nagasawa, "An evaluation of chewing function of complete denture wearers," *The Journal of Prosthetic Dentistry*, vol. 62, no. 1, pp. 50–53, 1989.

[9] J. Irish, N. Sandhu, C. Simpson et al., "Quality of life in patients with maxillectomy prostheses," *Head & Neck*, vol. 31, no. 6, pp. 813–821, 2009.

[10] J. M. Rieger, J. F. Wolfaardt, N. Jha, and H. Seikaly, "Maxillary obturators: the relationship between patient satisfaction and speech outcome," *Head & Neck*, vol. 25, no. 11, pp. 895–903, 2003.

[11] A. B. Kornblith, I. M. Zlotolow, J. Gooen et al., "Quality of life of maxillectomy patients using an obturator prosthesis," *Head & Neck*, vol. 18, no. 4, pp. 323–334, 1996.

[12] G. Tirelli, R. Rizzo, M. Biasotto et al., "Obturator prostheses following palatal resection: clinical cases," *Acta Otorhinolaryngologica Italica*, vol. 30, no. 1, pp. 33–39, 2010.

[13] C. J. Butterworth and S. N. Rogers, "The zygomatic implant perforated (ZIP) flap: a new technique for combined surgical reconstruction and rapid fixed dental rehabilitation following low-level maxillectomy," *International Journal of Implant Dentistry*, vol. 3, no. 1, p. 37, 2017.

[14] J. S. Brown and R. J. Shaw, "Reconstruction of the maxilla and midface: introducing a new classification," *The Lancet Oncology*, vol. 11, no. 10, pp. 1001–1008, 2010.

[15] O. Savabi, F. Nejatidanesh, and F. Yordshahian, "Retention of implant-supported overdenture with bar/clip and stud attachment designs," *The Journal of Oral Implantology*, vol. 39, no. 2, pp. 140–147, 2013.

35

Correction of Deep Overbite by Using a Modified Nance Appliance in an Adult Class II Division 2 Patient with Dehiscence Defect

Zhujun Li[ID],[1] Zhengxi Chen[ID],[1] Jian Sun,[2] Li'an Yang,[3] and Zhenqi Chen[ID][1]

[1]*Department of Orthodontics, Shanghai Ninth People's Hospital, School of Stomatology, Shanghai Key Laboratory of Stomatology, Shanghai Jiao Tong University, Shanghai, China*
[2]*Department of Stomatology, Shanghai East Hospital, Tongji University School of Medicine, Shanghai, China*
[3]*Department of Stomatology, Xin Hua Hospital Affiliated to Shanghai Jiao Tong University School of Medicine, Shanghai Jiao Tong University, Shanghai, China*

Correspondence should be addressed to Zhenqi Chen; zqchen@shsmu.edu.cn

Academic Editor: Khalid H. Zawawi

A modified Nance Appliance (MNA) is introduced as a treatment option for an adult class II division 2 malocclusion (CII/2) patient with deep overbite and dehiscence on the facial root surface of retroclined upper incisors through the cone-beam computed tomography (CBCT). Indications for this modified MNA as well as a brief description of fabrication procedure and biomechanical analysis of the treatment effects are shown in detail. Root control and absolute intrusion without enlarging the bony defect were achieved. The treatment results were satisfying and favorable.

1. Introduction

The management of alveolar defects, namely, dehiscence and fenestration in orthodontic patients, remains a tricky task for orthodontists to accomplish. Dehiscence could be presented with the lack of the facial or lingual cortical plate, which has a tendency of exposing the cervical root surface and affecting the marginal bone [1]. Bone dehiscences are common in the mandibular symphysis region before orthodontic treatment, especially among adults [2]. To avoid further risks, the alveolar morphology should be determined before orthodontic treatment. Currently, cone-beam computed tomography (CBCT) is an ideal option chosen in such a clinical dental situation for its ability to provide accurate images of the entire bone structure and visualizing these defects three dimensionally [3, 4]. According to the research of Fuhrmann [5], 80% of defects identifiable on CT scan images were not readily visible on the lateral cephalograms.

Clinically, patients with characteristic angle class II division 2 malocclusion (CII/2) always have manifestations including a prognathic maxilla, retroclined maxillary central incisors with alveolar bone defect on the cervical root surface, a retrusive mandible, upright mandibular incisors, a deep overbite, and a deep curve of Spee. The updated study suggested that early intervention should be taken to intercept, disrupt, and diminish the effects of malocclusions [6]. Coskuner and Ciger [7] indicated that in patients with class II/2 malocclusion, the elimination of maxillary interferences may lead to a greater increase in the mandibular dimensions. After eliminating the factors restricting mandibular movement in the transverse and sagittal planes, changes in the mandible and temporomandibular joints were observed. Patients in the pubertal growth period determined using the cervical vertebral maturation method who exhibited class II division 2 malocclusion deficiency were considered eligible for early intervention [8, 9]. For adult class II/2 patients who have no growth potential, a possible dental compensation or surgical-orthodontic treatment might be considered a favorable choice; many patients were still expecting an invasive method of treatment. According to the literature research,

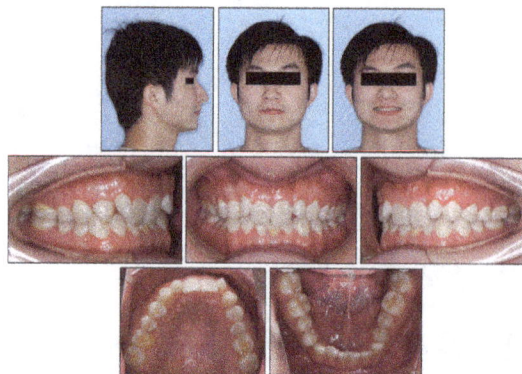

FIGURE 1: Pretreatment facial and intraoral photographs.

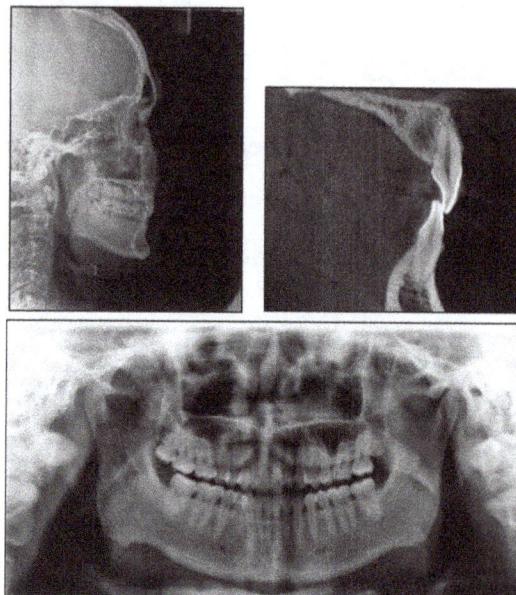

FIGURE 2: Pretreatment dental casts.

the class II group has a greater prevalence of dehiscences and fenestration than the class I and class III groups. Fenestrations has greater prevalence in the maxilla, but more dehiscences were found in the mandible [10]. Although the limitation of alveolar bone modeling and remodeling during intrusion of maxillary incisors existed [2, 5] and the alveolar bone dehiscence might get worse after treatment [11], good alveolar bone adaptation could still be achieved with care. Decker and Chen [12] demonstrated good upper alveolar bone adaptation after 32 years of follow-up by a case report.

In this case, we describe our treatment of an adult male patient diagnosed as class II/2 malocclusion with undersized lateral incisors and a dehiscence defect through the bone extending from the buccal root surface of upper retroclined incisors using a modified Nance Appliance (MNA).

2. Diagnosis and Etiology

A 27 years and two months old male patient who had a chief complaint of upper front teeth lingually tipped came to our department of orthodontics for further treatment. He pointed out that his mother shared the similar malocclusion.

The clinical examination showed a mild convex profile, a decreased anterior lower facial height, a prominent chin button, and a symmetrical face in frontal view (Figure 1). No significant temporomandibular joint discomfort was found. He was healthy, with no specific medical problems. Intraoral examination and dental casts showed that the patient was in the permanent dentition. He had an overjet of 3 mm, an overbite of 6 mm, retroinclined upper incisors, two undersized upper lateral incisors, and mild crowding in both dental arches. Class II canine and molar relationship were shown on the right side while class I canine and molar relationship was shown on the left side. Clinical periodontal examinations were evaluated at 6 sites on the number of teeth, which showed the means of probing depth (PD: 2.7 mm), gingival index score (GI: 1.5), and bleeding on probing (BOP) positive percentage (16.7%). In addition, his oral hygiene was unsatisfactory and needed periodontal scaling before fixed orthodontic treatment (Figures 1 and 2).

The panoramic radiograph showed missing third molars. The condyles appeared normal in size and form. Normal root length and bone height were present, with no caries or other pathology noted (Figure 3). Dehiscence was found on the

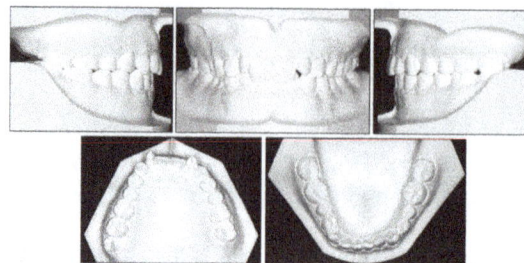

FIGURE 3: Pretreatment cephalography, panoramic radiograph, and pretreatment image of maxillary left central incisor from CBCT.

facial root surface of upper central incisor through the CBCT (Figure 3). The lateral cephalometric analysis indicated a skeletal class II pattern (ANB, 5.2°; wits appraisal, −1.4 mm) with a decreased lower anterior facial height (FMA, 23.7°; face height ratio, 51.7%). The maxillary incisors and the mandibular incisors were retroclined (U1-SN, 76.8°; IMPA, 79.7°). As a result, the interincisal angle was increased (U1/L1, 172.7°) (Figure 3 and Table 1). Cephalogram suggested that he had a class II skeletal pattern, hypodivergent growth, and decreased lower anterior facial height.

According to the examination above, the patient was diagnosed of CII/2 subdivision malocclusion with retroinclined upper incisors, undersized lateral incisors, dehiscence defect in the maxillary anterior alveolar bone, and deep overbite.

3. Treatment Objectives

The treatment objectives were to establish ideal overbite, overjet, and class I molar relationship on both sides, obtain favorable inclination of the maxillary and mandibular incisors, correct the maxillary and mandibular dental midline, relieve crowding, align the lower arch, provide proper space for the prosthesis of the undersized lateral incisor, maintain

TABLE 1: Skeletal and dental changes indicated by the cephalometric measurements.

| Variables | Norm | | Pretreatment | Posttreatment | Difference |
	Mean	SD			
Angular (°)					
SNA	82.3	3.5	84.2	81.7	−2.5
SNB	77.6	2.9	79	79.2	0.2
ANB	4.7	1.4	5.2	2.5	−2.7
U1-SN	104.8	5.3	76.8	102.4	25.6
U1/L1	122	6	172.7	141	−31.7
FMA	31.8	4.4	23.7	25.9	2.2
L1/MP	94.7	5.2	79.7	89.5	9.8
Linear (mm)					
Wits appraisal	−1.4	2.6	−1.4	−2.7	−1.3
N-ANS	49	2.2	51.9	51.9	0
ANS-Me	60.8	4.9	55.5	56.9	1.4
L1-Apo	3.9	1.5	−4	0.2	−3.8
Low lip to E-line	3	1.8	−4.7	−4	0.7
Face height ratio (%)	55.4	1.3	51.7	52.3	1.6

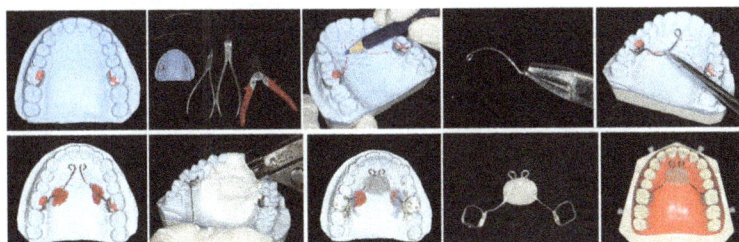

FIGURE 4: Fabrication of the MNA.

the profile, and avoid excessive lip protrusion, further dehiscence defect, and gingival recession as well.

4. Treatment Alternatives

The following two treatment alternatives were considered.

(i) Option 1: the first one is just to rectify the inclination of the incisors and relieve crowding of the teeth. The canine and molar relationships would retain class II on the right side. Also, the denture midline would not be corrected either

(ii) Option 2: the second one is to regain the space for dental prosthesis of undersized lateral incisors, to correct the canine and molar relationship, and to adjust maxillary denture midline. The maxillary molars would be distalized by miniscrew implant anchorage to relieve the crowding

After full communication, he rejected the second option and emphasized that his chief concern was to correct retroclined upper incisors. He wanted to maintain the occlusion of the posterior element. According to this chief complaint, we reached a consensus and chose the first option. However, root torque control during tooth treatment is a tricky task for

many orthodontists to accomplish. In this case, if space created by molar distalization is not enough for relieving crowding and controlling the movement of roots of upper incisors, the upper incisors will inevitably be flared at the initial alignment stage which will result in a worsening of the alveolar bone defect. To avoid this problem, we fabricated the MNA, which will be described below in detail.

5. Treatment Progress

The treatment was commenced with the placement of the MNA. The appliance consisting of two connecting palatal archwires made of 1.2 mm stainless steel wire, palatal button made of acrylic resin, and two additional hooks made of 0.7 mm stainless steel wire was cemented on both upper first molars to keep the crown of the upper incisors in position (Figure 4). To effectively control the movement of upper incisors, two metal buttons were placed gingivally on the lingual surface of upper incisors and were activated by stainless steel ligature tying to the hooks on MNA.

Self-ligating brackets (Damon Q, 0.022 × 0.025, High Torque, ORMCO) were bonded in the upper arch with a 0.013-inch CuNiTi wire engaged. Additionally, the brackets were placed 0.5 mm close to the incisal edge of upper incisors for the intrusion. Meanwhile, glass ionomer cement was

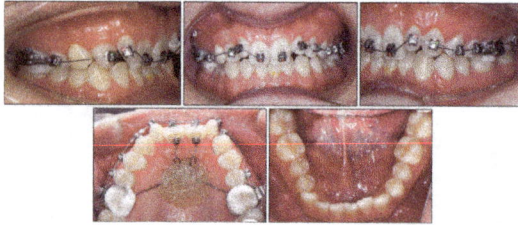

FIGURE 5: Self-ligating brackets (High Torque) were bonded in the maxillary arch.

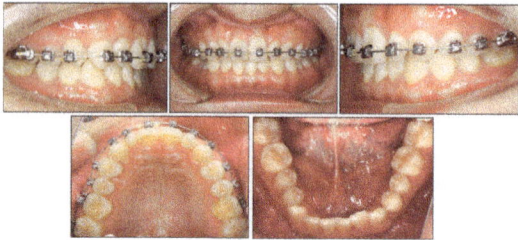

FIGURE 6: Four months after initial bonding. The MNA and occlusal stop were removed, and the upper arch form was changed from square to ovoid.

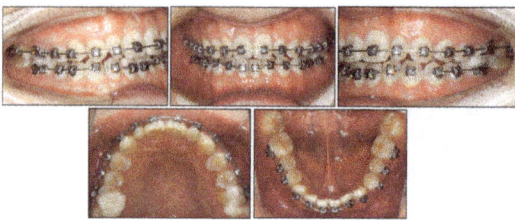

FIGURE 7: Initial bonding on the lower arch.

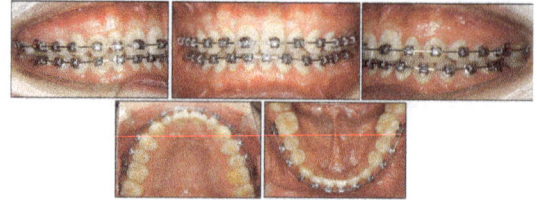

FIGURE 8: Eighteen months after initial bonding. 0.018×-0.025-inch nickel-titanium archwire in the maxillary arch and 0.017×0.025-inch stainless steel archwire in the mandibular arch were applied.

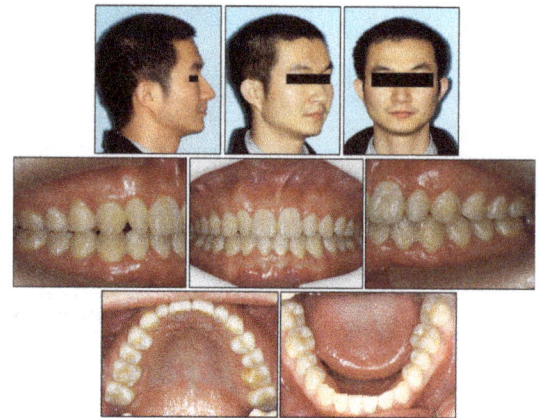

FIGURE 9: Posttreatment facial and intraoral photographs.

relationship, and the functional class II canine and molar relationship on the right side was achieved. After 22 months, the appliance was removed, the upper and lower Hawley retainers were placed with a protocol of wearing full time for the first six months.

6. Treatment Results

Patient cooperation throughout the treatment was excellent. The posttreatment records indicated that the treatment objectives were achieved. The facial photographs demonstrated significant improvements in his soft tissue profile with increased anterior lower facial height. He was very happy with the outcome (Figure 9).

Intraorally, the retroclination of upper and lower incisors was corrected. Optimal overjet (4 mm) and overbite (2.0 mm), a class I canine and molar relationships on the left side, and a class II canine and molar relationship on the right side were reached (Figures 9 and 10). Remarkably, the torque of the upper incisors was in good control as expected (U1-SN, 102.4°). Root control and absolute intrusion of the maxillary incisors were achieved at the initial stage. The lingual movement of root of upper incisors was attained easily by using a high-torque version of self-ligating brackets. Meanwhile, the crown was avoiding extra labial tipping all through the treatment (Figure 11 and Table 1). Through good oral health education, the patient became more conscious of oral hygiene after the treatment. Clinical indicators including PD (2 mm), GI (1), and BOP positive percentage

cemented on the occlusal surface of the upper first molars as an occlusal stop to eliminate occlusal inference (Figure 5). The initial aligning and leveling stage took place over the first 3 months while the roots of upper incisor were moving lingually.

At month 4, the upper arch form was changed from square to ovoid. The MNA and occlusal stop were removed. After the removal, the cephalometric radiograph was retaken for observing the roots of upper incisors. As was shown in Figure 6, in the upper arch, the movement of the crown of upper incisors was under control as well as the root retraction without the exaggerated dehiscence on the buccal root surface of upper incisor.

For further alignment and leveling, a 0.014×0.025-inch CuNiTi archwire was changed by a 0.017×0.025-inch NiTi archwire. At month 12, the deep bite was almost corrected. At this point, the lower arch was bonded and leveled (Figure 7). To achieve more favorable torque expression in the upper teeth, 0.019×0.025-inch stainless steel archwires were engaged in the end (Figure 8). The near end stage of treatment was to adjust midline and occlusal relationship for better intercuspation. The patient was instructed to wear class II elastics (5/16, 3.5 orz) full time for three months. In the end, the teeth were well aligned with the good intercuspal

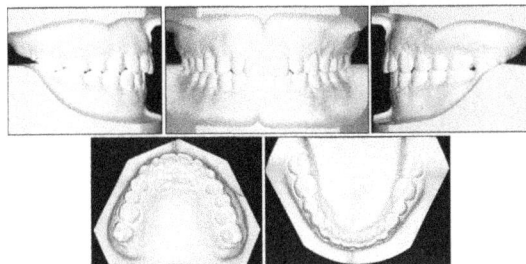

FIGURE 10: Posttreatment dental casts.

(0%) show a healthy periodontal state after treatment. Therefore, the absolute intrusion of the maxillary incisors did not worsen the periodontal problems but enhance the bony support for teeth.

The panoramic radiograph showed no significant bone loss or root resorption, and all tooth roots were parallel to each other (Figure 11). Cephalometric superimposition registered on the SN line showed the intrusion of the maxillary incisors by 2 mm with lingual root movement by 25.6 degrees and the increased mandibular plane angle (FMA, 25.9°) (Figure 12 and Table 1). As a result, the anterior lower facial height was increased to 2 mm. According to CBCT image, we had found excitedly the original dehiscence on cervical root surface of upper incisor restored on the labial surface instead of getting worse (Figure 11). There was a thin layer of bone covering on the cervical root surface of upper incisor visibly.

After 22 months of treatment, the patient was satisfied with the outcome. However, the patient studied abroad later and out of contact. We lost follow-up unfortunately.

7. Discussion

As to CII/2 malocclusion, the objectives of treatment mainly focus on correction of anterior deepbite, correction of upper incisor inclination, and correction of class II molar relationships [13–16]. Clinically, correction of deep overbite can be achieved by molar extrusion, incisor intrusion, or a combination of these two types of tooth movement. Extrusion of posterior teeth is stable in growing patients when the growth potential of mandibular condylar remains. In adult patients, posterior teeth extrusion is probably counteracted by the posterior occlusion, especially in the hypodivergent skeletal pattern.

For this specific patient, to some extent, deep overbite could be corrected by intruding the maxillary and mandible incisors. Nevertheless, with a dehiscence defect existed in maxillary anterior teeth, a careful consideration of avoiding further dehiscence of the alveolar bone should be addressed. According to Carranza [17], dehiscences were defined as bony defects in which the denuded areas involve the alveolar bone margin. Previous studies used various criteria for the definition of dehiscences, including any defect greater than 1 mm near the cementoenamel junction (CEJ) [18], 4 mm apical to the interproximal bone crest [19–21], and exposure of half of the root [22]. The presence of these buccal alveolar bone defects weakened the bony support for teeth. Inadequate bone support during orthodontic tooth

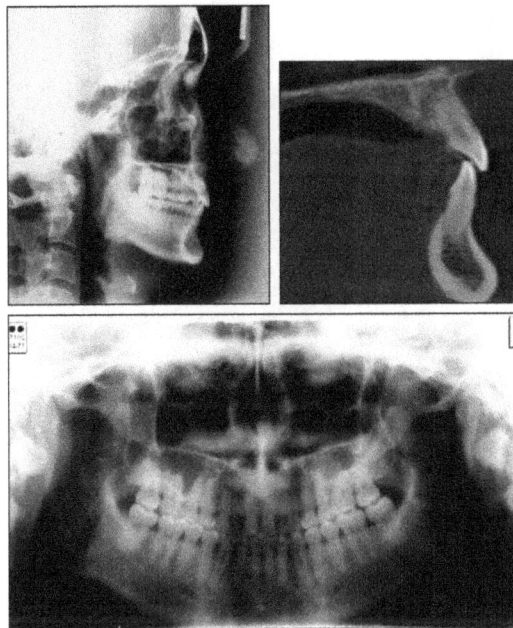

FIGURE 11: Posttreatment cephalograph, panoramic radiograph, and posttreatment image of maxillary left central incisor from CBCT.

movement may have deleterious effects on teeth and the periodontium [23]. Additionally, rapid movement of these teeth may also reduce the amount of radicular bone, enlarge the alveolar defect, and increase the risk of gingival recession. Studies have shown greater prevalence of alveolar defects on the buccal surface than on the lingual surface [1, 21]. This may be attributed to narrow bone at the buccal surface, where the amount of marrow bone is less dense than that in the lingual region.

Currently, periodontally accelerated osteogenic orthodontics (PAOO) is one of the most classic techniques for the alveolar bone defect. This approach includes buccal and lingual full-thickness flaps, selective partial decortication of the cortical plates, concomitant bone grafting or augmentation, and primary flap closure [24]. The aim of the surgery is focused on covering bony dehiscences and reshaping alveolar bone, thus provides additional support for the roots of the teeth and diminishes risk of periodontal recession. However, for this patient, PAOO is not a smart choice. Patients with characteristic CII/2 malocclusion always show a prognathic maxilla, retroclined maxillary central incisors, a retrusive mandible, and a deep curve of Spee [6]. Abovementioned PAOO would augment the thickness of alveolar bone and make A point move forward, which would lead to further increase of the prominence of upper lip and an adverse influence on the soft-tissue profile. Therefore, in such cases, a noninvasive and cost-effective method of treatment is needed. Through the CBCT, dehiscence was found on the facial root surface of upper incisor. To avoid enlarged alveolar defect, labial tipping should be under precise control. For this reason, we fabricated the MNA. The two metal buttons bonded gingivally on the lingual surface functioned as the pivot. The labio-lingual inclination of the upper central

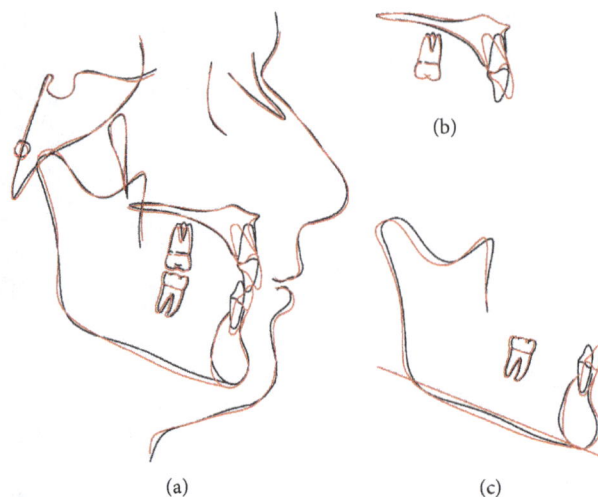

FIGURE 12: Cephalometric superimpositions showed marked differences between pretreatment (black) and posttreatment (red): (a) SN plane; (b) maxillary plane; (c) mandibular plane.

incisors would move around the pivot which attached to hooks on the MNA. After 0.013-inch CuNiTi archwire was fully engaged into the bracket slots of the malpositioned teeth, the gentle force delivered by the archwire progressively aligned the maxillary teeth. During the initial alignment stage, the crowns of maxillary incisors were held by the hooks and the roots moved lingually. By using the MNA, full control of the tipping of the upper incisors and absolute intrusion of the maxillary incisors were achieved. To avoid deteriorating alveolar bone defect, the gentle force and slow movement of teeth should be taken into account at the initial stage. At the end of treatment, we could find a thin layer of bone covering the cervical root surface of maxillary incisor followed by the successful lingual movement of roots of maxillary incisors.

As known, the interincisal angle has been considered as a factor related to long-term stability. Riedel [25] indicated that a large interincisal angle at the end of treatment would be associated with the relapse of deep overbite. Proper palatal root torque of the maxillary incisors plays an important role in maintaining a normal interincisal angle and establishing anterior occlusal stop [26]. In this case, we corrected the torque of the retroclined upper incisors (Figure 12 and Table 1), which was beneficial to maintain an optimal interincisal angle and overbite stability. The idea that bone traces tooth movement indicates whenever orthodontic tooth movement occurs, the bone around the alveolar socket would remodel to the same extent [27]. When the angle of upper incisors to SN plane changed from 76.8° to102.4°, the anterior alveolar bone underwent remodeling at the same time. The A point moved backward subsequently which caused SNA angle changed from 84.2° to 81.7° (Table 1).

Although, there are some other clinical treatment approaches reported for controlling root torque, such as auxiliary arch, rectangular loops, and reverse-curve archwire. However, the MNA fabricated in this case shows some merits. It could achieve root control and absolute intrusion of the maxillary incisors at the initial stage. Combined with a high-torque version of self-ligating brackets, the lingual

movement of root of upper incisors could be attained easily. Remarkably, it is noninvasive, cost-effective, and easy to handle without repeated adjustment.

The patient in this case chose to maintain the dental midline and the occlusion of the posterior element and rejected to restore his undersized lateral incisors. Given the reason that satisfaction with the outcome depends on the expectations of patients, their point view of the assessment of final aesthetics is decisive. Therefore, acceptable overjet and a class II canine and molar relationship on the right side were achieved after treatment. The posttreatment occlusion was improved both functionally and aesthetically. The outcome of treatment was favorable. Further follow-up on the stability of the MNA would be scheduled.

8. Conclusions

The clinical management for orthodontic patients with alveolar defects as dehiscence and fenestration remains a tricky task for orthodontists to accomplish, especially in adult class II division 2 malocclusion (CII/2) patients with deep overbite and dehiscence on the facial root surface of retroclined upper incisors. The MNA presented in this case showed a favorable potential in achieving satisfying results during active orthodontic treatment.

Disclosure

This work has been presented at 2018 American Association of Orthodontists Annual Session as an E-poster.

Authors' Contributions

Zhujun Li and Zhengxi Chen contributed equally to this work.

Acknowledgments

This study was supported by grants from National Key R&D Program of China (2017YFC0840100, 2017YFC0840110).

References

[1] K. Evangelista, K. . F. Vasconcelos, A. Bumann, E. Hirsch, M. Nitka, and M. A. G. Silva, "Dehiscence and fenestration in patients with class I and class II division 1 malocclusion assessed with cone-beam computed tomography," *American Journal of Orthodontics and Dentofacial Orthopedics*, vol. 138, no. 2, pp. 133.e1–133.e7, 2010.

[2] R. A. W. Fuhrmann, "Three-dimensional evaluation of periodontalremodeling during orthodontic treatment," *Seminars in Orthodontics*, vol. 8, no. 1, pp. 23–28, 2002.

[3] R. Mengel, M. Candir, K. Shiratori, and L. Flores-de-Jacoby, "Digital volume tomography in the diagnosis of periodontal defects: an in vitro study on native pig and human mandibles," *Journal of Periodontology*, vol. 76, no. 5, pp. 665–673, 2005.

[4] M. A. G. Silva, U. Wolf, F. Heinicke, A. Bumann, H. Visser, and E. Hirsch, "Cone-beam computed tomography for routine orthodontic treatment planning: a radiation dose evaluation," *American Journal of Orthodontics & Dentofacial Orthopedics*, vol. 133, no. 5, pp. 640.e1–640.e5, 2008.

[5] R. Fuhrmann, "Three-dimensional interpretation of labiolingual bone width of the lower incisors," *Journal of Orofacial Orthopedics*, vol. 57, no. 3, pp. 168–185, 1996.

[6] S. Ruf and H. Pancherz, "Class II division 2 malocclusion: genetics or environment? A case report of monozygotic twins," *The Angle Orthodontist*, vol. 69, no. 4, pp. 321–324, 1999.

[7] H. G. Coskuner and S. Ciger, "Three-dimensional assessment of the temporomandibular joint and mandibular dimensions after early correction of the maxillary arch form in patients with class II division 1 or division 2 malocclusion," *The Korean Journal of Orthodontics*, vol. 45, no. 3, pp. 121–129, 2015.

[8] N. C. Bock and S. Ruf, "Class II division 2 treatment does skeletal maturity influence success and stability?," *Journal of Orofacial Orthopedics*, vol. 74, no. 3, pp. 187–204, 2013.

[9] N. Bock and S. Ruf, "Post-treatment occlusal changes in class II division 2 subjects treated with the Herbst appliance," *European Journal of Orthodontics*, vol. 30, no. 6, pp. 606–613, 2008.

[10] A. Yagci, İ. Veli, T. Uysal, F. I. Ucar, T. Ozer, and S. Enhos, "Dehiscence and fenestration in skeletal class I, II, and III malocclusions assessed with cone-beam computed tomography," *The Angle Orthodontist*, vol. 82, no. 1, pp. 67–74, 2012.

[11] C. J. Hwang and J. L. Moon, "The limitation of alveolar bone remodeling during retraction of the upper anterior teeth," *The Korean Journal of Orthodontics*, vol. 31, no. 1, pp. 97–105, 2001.

[12] J. D. Decker and C. Chen, "Adaptive response of the human dental alveolar process: correction of a class I protrusive and mutilated dentition, with 32-year follow-up," *American Journal of Orthodontics & Dentofacial Orthopedics*, vol. 135, no. 4, pp. S113–S122, 2009.

[13] N. C. Bock, C. Santo, and H. Pancherz, "Facial profile and lip position changes in adult class II, division 2 subjects treated with the Herbst-multibracket appliance. A radiographic cephalometric pilot study," *Journal of Orofacial Orthopedics*, vol. 70, no. 1, pp. 51–62, 2009.

[14] H. Devreese, G. de Pauw, G. van Maele, A. Kuijpers-Jagtman, and L. Dermaut, "Stability of upper incisor inclination changes in class II division 2 patients," *European Journal of Orthodontics*, vol. 29, no. 3, pp. 314–320, 2007.

[15] T. W. Kim and R. M. Little, "Postretention assessment of deep overbite correction in class II division 2 malocclusion," *The Angle Orthodontist*, vol. 69, no. 2, pp. 175–186, 1999.

[16] J. Kinzel, P. Aberschek, I. Mischak, and H. Droschl, "Study of the extent of torque, protrusion and intrusion of the incisors in the context of class II, division 2 treatment in adults," *Journal of Orofacial Orthopedics*, vol. 63, no. 4, pp. 283–299, 2002.

[17] F. A. Carranza and G. W. Bernard, "The tooth-supporting structures," in *Carranza's Clinical Periodontology*, M. G. Newman, H. H. Takei, and F. A. Carranza, Eds., pp. 36–57, W.B. Saunders, Philadelphia, PA, USA, 9 edition, 2002.

[18] K. Jorgić-Srdjak, D. Plancak, A. Bosnjak, and Z. Azinović, "Incidence and distribution of dehiscences and fenestrations on human skulls," *Collegium Antropologicum*, vol. 22, pp. 111–116, 1998.

[19] R. M. Davies, M. C. Downer, P. S. Hull, and M. A. Lennon, "Alveolar defects in human skulls," *Journal of Clinical Periodontology*, vol. 1, no. 2, pp. 107–111, 1974.

[20] A. Edel, "Alveolar bone fenestrations and dehiscences in dry Bedouin jaws," *Journal of Clinical Periodontology*, vol. 8, no. 6, pp. 491–499, 1981.

[21] R. D. Rupprecht, G. M. Horning, B. K. Nicoll, and M. E. Cohen, "Prevalence of dehiscences and fenestrations in modern American skulls," *Journal of Periodontology*, vol. 72, no. 6, pp. 722–729, 2001.

[22] D. C. Larato, "Alveolar plate fenestrations and dehiscences of the human skull," *Oral Surgery, Oral Medicine, and Oral Pathology*, vol. 29, no. 6, pp. 816–819, 1970.

[23] J. L. Wennstrom, B. L. Stokland, S. Nyman, and B. Thilander, "Periodontal tissue response to orthodontic movement of teeth with infrabony pockets," *American Journal of Orthodontics and Dentofacial Orthopedics*, vol. 103, no. 4, pp. 313–319, 1993.

[24] W. M. Wilcko, T. Wilcko, J. E. Bouquot, and D. J. Ferguson, "Rapid orthodontics with alveolar reshaping: two case reports of decrowding," *The International Journal of Periodontics & Restorative Dentistry*, vol. 21, pp. 9–19, 2001.

[25] R. A. Riedel, "A review of the retention problem," *The Angle Orthodontist*, vol. 30, pp. 179–199, 1960.

[26] L. R. Dermaut and G. De Pauw, "Biomechanical aspects of Class II mechanics with special emphasis in deep bite correction as part of the treatment goal," in *Biomechanics in Clinical Orthodontics*, R. Nanda, Ed., pp. 86–98, W.B. Saunders, Philadelphia, PA, USA, 1997.

[27] K. Reitan, "Effects of force magnitude and direction of tooth movement on different alveolar bone types," *The Angle Orthodontist*, vol. 34, no. 4, pp. 244–255, 1964.

36

A New Intraoral Appliance for Trismus in Oral Submucous Fibrosis

Nallan C. S. K. Chaitanya ⑩,[1] **C. M. S. Krishna Prasad,**[2] **Reshma Priyanka Danam,**[1] **Madireddy Nithika,**[1] **Chintada Suvarna,**[1] **Jampala Nancypriyanka,**[1] **and Rajkumar Badam**[2]

[1]*Department of Oral Medicine and Radiology, Panineeya Institute of Dental Sciences, Hyderabad, India*
[2]*Department of Orthodontics and Dentofacial Orthopedics, Panineeya Institute of Dental Sciences, Hyderabad, India*

Correspondence should be addressed to Nallan C. S. K. Chaitanya; nallanchaitanya@gmail.com

Academic Editor: Tommaso Lombardi

Trismus is the most common sequelae of various pathological processes leading to compromised nutritional state in addition to physical and psychological disabilities. Therapeutic interventions are available to relieve trismus, which range from oral usage of pharmacological agents to intralesional steroid therapy. Intraoral appliance therapy can be employed as an alternative or adjuvant treatment for radiotherapy-induced fibrosis and autoimmune disorders such as scleroderma, psychogenic trismus, and oral submucous fibrosis, decreasing the adverse effects associated with other pharmacological interventions. A novel intraoral appliance—"Nallan C-H"—has been developed and tried for trismus producing better results. A report on three such cases having trismus due to a premalignancy has been presented. It is hypothesized that the same appliance can be used for treating inoperable trismus in palliative care setting additionally or as an adjuvant to pharmacological approach.

1. Introduction

Trismus refers to the condition where an individual is unable to open the mouth, occurs due to various causes ranging from simple, nonprogressive to potentially life-threatening [1]. It is often considered as a common complication of dental treatment. It has further implications on both mastication and speech [2]. Studies also had shown that trismus is associated with a significant impact on health-related quality of life (HRQOL) [3]. Normal mouth opening in individuals ranges from 40 to 60 mm; in patients with trismus, its restriction varies from a few millimetres (mm) to even several centimetres (cm). For its successful treatment, recognition of its cause followed by initiation of effective management is vital or it may lead to permanent functional impairment [1]. Complications due to radiotherapy include osteoradionecrosis which results in pain, trismus, suppuration, and wound [2]. Most commonly encountered noninfectious causes of trismus are oral submucous fibrosis and radiation-induced fibrosis.

Oral submucous fibrosis (OSMF) refers to chronic, premalignant condition of the oral mucosa. It is prevalent in India affecting 0.2% to 0.5% of the general population with gender variation of 0.2–2.3% in males and 1.2–4.57% in females. Age distribution of patients with OSMF is wide, ranging between 20 and 40 years. The initial presentation of OSMF is inflammation, followed by hypovascularity and fibrosis. Moderate stage of OSMF (group II and group III by Khanna et al.) is characterised by irreversible fibrosis which is progressive, invariably leading to trismus with variable mouth opening. Trismus in oral submucous fibrosis is due to fibrosis of the lamina propria resulting in loss of elasticity and stiffness. It is different in other conditions such as space infections, muscle spasm due to tetanus, maxillomandibular factures in which collagen fibres are unaffected, and no loss of elasticity. OSMF-related trismus has further

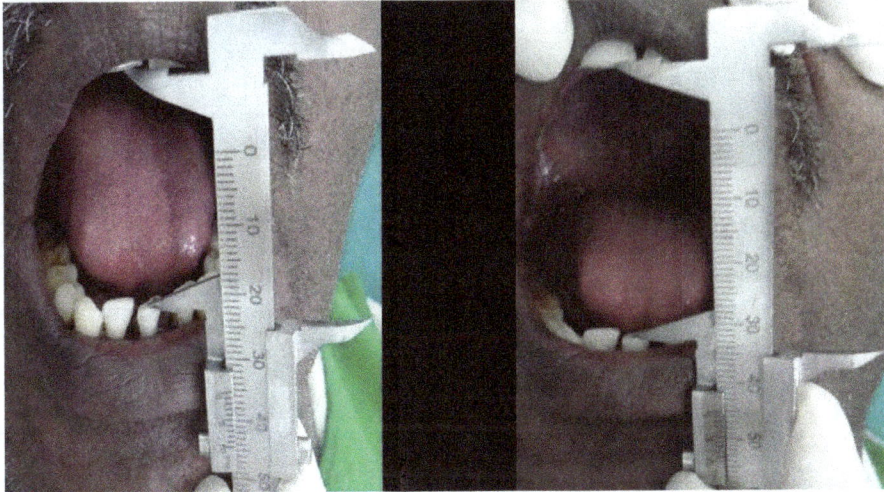

FIGURE 1: Pre and post appliance therapy.

bearing on oral hygiene, speech, mastication, and possibly swallowing. Moreover, the risk for its malignant transformation is found to be varied from 7% to 30% [4].

Along with other treatment modalities such as intralesional corticosteroids with and without combination of placentrex, surgical release of the fibrous bands is another treatment modality for this condition. Relapse is the common complication during and after treatment, and the compliance with treatment is a major detrimental factor for successful outcome. Alternative options in treating are pentoxifylline 400 mg thrice daily medication, vitamin A supplements, heat short-wave diathermy, antioxidants, immunised milk, turmeric, and aloe vera oral applications. All of these modalities have limitations and relapse [5].

An intraoral appliance which would not be cumbersome and bulkier in oral cavity and also comfortable for the patient to wear would be beneficial. The appliance should not demonstrate functional changes in the teeth as well as in the occlusion. It should cause desirable mouth opening with minimal side effects. This case series focuses on the development and fabrication of a novel intraoral appliance called "Nallan C-H appliance" for the improvement of mouth opening in patients with trismus. It is noninvasive, economical, and had fair compliance with the patients.

2. Case Reports

2.1. Case 1. A male patient, aged 39 years, presented to a private clinic with a chief complaint of difficulty in mouth opening since one and half years. The patient had a habit of chewing *gutka* for the past eight years. It was observed that there is noticeable decline in mouth opening of 17 mm (intercanine distance) and tongue protrusion of 10 mm. On intraoral examination, generalized blanching of the oral mucosa with grayish black pigmentation was seen. And also, multiple vertical palpable fibrous bands with loss of elasticity and leathery in texture were noticed. OSMF was diagnosed, and the patient was treated with conventional intralesional steroid injections. Since the patient has been under similar

treatment for over a period of time with no recognisable change or relief, he requested for an alternative therapy. Intraoral appliance therapy was considered, and prior consent was obtained from the patient. The patient was duly provided with necessary precautions regarding the usage of appliance and weekly follow-up without discontinuing the treatment. The treatment was carried out for a total period of 8 weeks and a follow-up of two months after completion of the therapy (Figure 1).

2.2. Case 2. A female patient, aged 56 years, presented to the private clinic with chief complaint of difficulty in mouth opening since one month. During her first visit, i.e., approximately a year back, she reported about the treatment that she received for trismus (due to OSMF) using intralesional injections. At that time, the patient had marginal relief from the symptoms. Again, she started developing trismus since one month and also had burning sensation in the oral cavity. Patient had restricted mouth opening of 30 mm (canine-canine distance) and tongue protrusion of 12 mm with all signs of OSMF (group 2 by Khanna et al.) in the oral cavity. As she was not able to tolerate any more pain from intralesional steroid injections, she was advised intraoral appliance therapy for 8 weeks. She was also instructed for weekly follow-ups with precautions during appliance position in the oral cavity.

2.3. Case 3. A male patient, aged 40 years, with a history of chewing betel quid for the past 15 years, presented to the private clinic with reduction in mouth opening since one year. Patient had a restricted mouth opening of 35 mm (canine-canine distance) and tongue protrusion of 12 mm with all signs of OSMF (group 2 by Khanna et al.) in the oral cavity. The patient was then started with intralesional corticosteroids, which showed improved mouth opening till 42 mm (canine-canine distance), and then this treatment modality was discontinued due to pain arising from repeated punctures. The patient then requested for alternative therapy. He was advised appliance therapy and was instructed

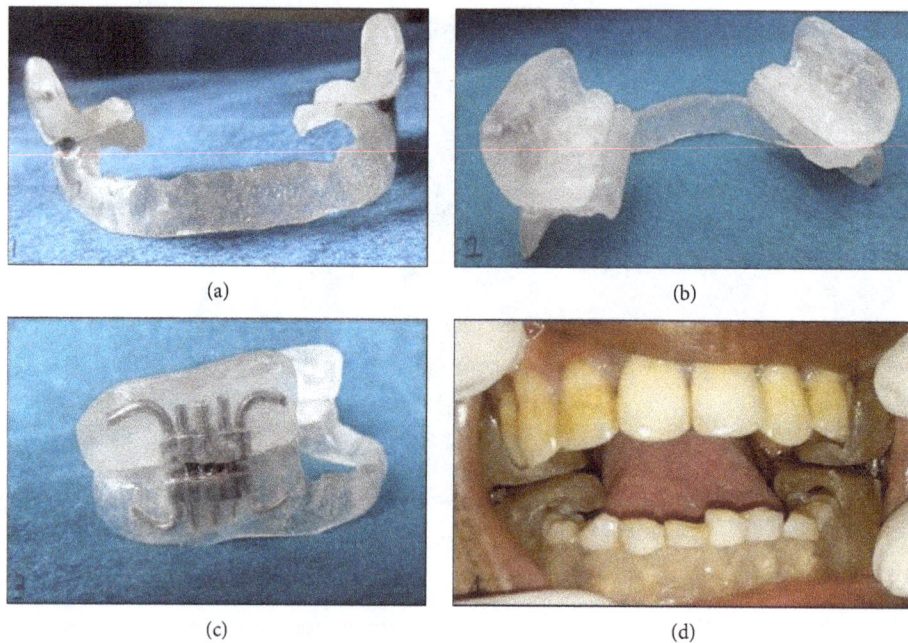

FIGURE 2: (a) Frontal view of the appliance with labial extension in the lower arch. (b) Posterior view of the appliance with occlusal plates and buccal extensions in both upper and lower arches. (c) Lateral view of the appliance with hyrax screws placed within the acrylic plates. (d) Intraoral placement with activated appliance and separation in progress.

for weekly follow-ups for 8 weeks with precautions in positioning and usage of the appliance in the oral cavity.

3. Clinical Procedure and Fabrication of the Appliance

For all patients, maximum mouth opening was recorded using appropriate measuring device at baseline prior to the initiation of the appliance therapy. Necessary precautions were taken during the fabrication of the appliance such as the following:

(1) The appliance should not impinge gingival margins

(2) It should be easy to manipulate by the patient

(3) Should be comfortable to use and also rigid enough to resist masticatory forces

Alginate impression was taken for both upper and lower arches with stock metal trays. Impression was poured using dental stone. The obtained casts were then articulated with an apex articulator. Fabrication of appliance was done by using self-cure acrylic resin and sprinkle on technique covering the sulcus area in the anterior region, which broadens posteriorly to cover the buccal area and occlusal surface of the lower arch. On the upper arch, only the molar area covered the teeth both occlusally and buccally. Mounting of cast in the occlusion was done in a hinge articulator so that occlusal relation was maintained. The wax was then adapted on the buccal surface of the lower arch to keep the distance of 2 mm from the gingiva, so that it did not impinge the soft tissues. Hyrax screws of 12 mm gauge were adapted

bilaterally on the buccal aspects of the molars on the wax. Precaution was taken to avoid blocking the activation hole of the screws. Once the acrylic had begun to set, the appliance was removed cleaned, trimmed, and polished. A lower labial extension was given for the appliance in order to prevent accidental breakage and subsequent aspiration of the appliance (Figure 2).

The appliance was then tried in the patient's mouth and adjusted according to his/her convenience. Care was taken to avoid excess pressure. The patients were educated regarding proper insertion, removal, and maintenance of the appliance and oral care. Moreover, they were encouraged to wear the appliance 12 hours overnight for 8 weeks and followed up every week to check any improvement. Patients were also encouraged to perform isometric mouth exercises daily according to their comfort. For every visit, the mouth opening was measured and the screw was released 1 mm on each side to improve mouth opening. A follow-up of 2 months was performed on each patient (Table 1).

4. Treatment Evaluation and Follow-Up

It was observed that there was significant increase in mouth opening in all three patients ranging from 2 to 8 mm. None of the patients reported difficulty in the placement of appliance in the oral cavity during the treatment phase. No significant decrease in mouth opening was observed during post appliance follow-up of 2 months. However, there was a decrease of 2 mm in the third patient and 0.5 mm in the first patient.

TABLE 1: Treatment evaluation at various stages for all 3 patients.

(a)

Phase 1 Cases	(At diagnosis) Mouth opening (mm)
Case 1	17
Case 2	30
Case 3	35

(b)

Phase 2 Cases	(After complete treatment) Mouth opening (mm)
Case 1	22.5
Case 2	32
Case 3	45

(c)

Phase 3 Cases	(Follow-up after 2 months) Mouth opening (mm)
Case 1	22
Case 2	32
Case 3	42

5. Discussion

Trismus is defined as a prolonged tonic spasm of the muscles, which results in restricted mouth opening. OSMF is a potentially malignant, chronic, progressive disorder seen mostly in people from Asia and is found to affect most of the parts of the oral cavity that includes the lips, tongue, palate, pharynx, and even the upper third of the oesophagus. In later stages, further stiffening occurs due to myofibrosis of the subepithelial and submucosal tissues, thereby resulting in limitations in the mouth opening and tongue protrusion causing difficulty in eating, swallowing, and also phonation-related issues [6]. Various treatment modalities such as physical oral therapy, intralesional corticosteroids, ultrasound therapy, and surgical modalities were tried till date [4].

In the present case series, a newer treatment procedure is tried on patients suffering from OSMF. An appliance that can be easily fabricated was designed and used in patients with trismus due to any noninfectious pathology. For patients who are not comfortable or given consent for treatment with intralesional steroids, this appliance therapy could be an alternative treatment modality. Moreover, cost and the adverse effects are involved in this treatment when compared with steroid therapy. Yadav et al. believed that protecting surgically reconstructed defects using flaps is vital, and the authors fabricated an appliance in order to avoid trauma to the flap in the postoperative period [6]. It is further believed that physiotherapeutic effect is a probable mechanism behind appliance therapy, which causes remodelling of the tissues for improving mouth opening [7].

From design, the appliance works by causing mechanical force which then induces the stretching of the elevator and depressor muscles. Based on the design, these appliances are classified into externally and internally activated types. Externally activated appliances exert force by stretching the elevator muscles and depressing the mandible whereas internally activated appliances employ the force on the depressor muscles to stretch the elevator muscles. They impart forces which are continuous or intermittent, elastic or nonelastic, and light or heavy. The force generated by the elevator muscles is greater than that by the depressor muscles. The amount of force delivered depends on the strength, frequency, duration of stretching, and motivation of the patient [8].

The activation cycle is unique to the appliance. The key which is provided for opening up the hyrax screws during rapid palatal expansion is used for activation purposes in relieving the trismus. Each full turn is equal to approximately 0.2 mm and total number of 4 full turns is given which account to 0.8 mm per week. The patient is followed up every week for 8 weeks. The approximate mouth opening hypothesized ranges from 5 mm to 1.5 cm.

In the present case series, the appliance emits intermittent and bilateral forces, which help to depress the mandible and make the maxillary and mandibular teeth apart thereby relieving the trismus. Physical therapy improves the range of motion of temporomandibular joint, reduces pain, prevents hypomobility, avoids fibrosis formation, strengthens the musculature, and improves flexibility, tissue elasticity, and blood circulation.

The appliance can be fabricated in patients who are completely edentulous and also in those partially edentulous patients. As the appliance is passive over the teeth and does not cause functional tooth movements, it can be comfortably worn in patients with missing dentition. As the occlusion is undisturbed, there is elimination of alteration in the occlusion sequence. Caution has to be maintained when there are periodontal compromised teeth. Excessive vertical forces may further breakdown the periodontium. Periodontal assessment has to be carried out before the appliance fabrication. Teeth with excessive mobility and poor prognosis should be managed prior to appliance insertion. Mild-to-moderate periodontitis is not a contraindication for appliance fabrication.

Patil et al. from their study concluded that the use of mouth exercising device appears to be effective for the separation of collagen fibers and increased the subcutaneous matrix area leading to improved blood circulation [9]. Oswal et al. fabricated an oral screen prosthesis to stabilize the secured flaps and to prevent it from being bitten into occlusion, and the same can also be used as an oral stent to prevent relapse [10]. Similarly, Li et al. fabricated a EZBite open mouth device and conducted a 12-week structured open mouth training program and stated a marked improvement in mouth opening [11].

Till date, there are two jaw-exercising devices used in palliative care. "TheraBite" is a mechanical device with lever system which assists mouth opening by squeezing the handle of the device and is able to control the extent of the stretch to the tissues. Another appliance is "Dynasplint trismus system" which is used with a low-torque and prolonged duration stretch designed to lengthen connective tissue [12, 13]. Both of these appliances are used effectively to relieve trismus due to various causes. TheraBite is a lever system which is patient dependent, and the maximum opening claimed is almost 41 mm. Dynasplint trismus system is bulkier compared to the presently described appliance. The present appliance is not visible outside the oral cavity unlike the two above-described systems. The mandibular range of motion may not be achieved with the present model, and modifications may be required to assess the same in further fabrication.

6. Biocompatibility of the Appliance

The appliance is made up of acrylic resin material which is routinely used in the fabrication of partial or complete removable dentures and hyrax screw which may be used for palatal expansion in orthodontic treatment. The components have been proven to be biocompatible in the patients. The labial extension of the appliance is a safety measure which enables the appliance to stay fit in the oral cavity without breakage and accidental slip into the oral mucosa and esophagus.

7. Limitations and Adverse Effects

The adverse effects with present appliance were as follows:

(1) Difficulty to insert intraorally during the initial phases of treatment

(2) Excessive salivation

(3) Reduced strength of appliance after weeks of usage may be due to fabrication errors

8. Conclusion and Future Recommendations

The present appliance can also be successfully intervened in trismus arising from any of the abovementioned causes without much adverse effects. Long-term studies are required to evaluate the effectiveness of the appliance over a large group of population and its compliance among the patients. Follow-up at regular intervals may be required for effective management of the patients with trismus and relapse.

Acknowledgments

We acknowledge the staff of the Department of Oral Medicine and Radiology, Panineeya Institute of Dental Sciences, and Dr. Shivaram, senior lecturer, Department of Orthodontics and Dentofacial Orthopaedics, for their support in each step of this case study.

References

[1] M. Marien Jr, "Trismus: causes, differential diagnosis, and treatment," *General Dentistry*, vol. 45, no. 4, pp. 350–355, 1997.

[2] P. J. Dhanrajani and O. Jonaidel, "Trismus: aetiology, differential diagnosis and treatment," *Dental Update*, vol. 29, no. 2, pp. 88–94, 2002.

[3] J. Johnson, M. Johansson, A. Ryden, E. Houltz, and C. Finizia, "Impact of trismus on health-related quality of life and mental health," *Head & Neck*, vol. 37, no. 11, pp. 1672–1679, 2015.

[4] U. Wollina, S. B. Verma, F. M. Ali, and K. Patil, "Oral submucous fibrosis: an update," *Clinical, Cosmetic and Investigational Dermatology*, vol. 8, pp. 193–204, 2015.

[5] U. Dayanarayana, N. Doggalli, K. Patil, J. Shankar, K. Mahesh, and Sanjay, "Non surgical approaches in treatment of OSF," *IOSR Journal of Dental and Medical Sciences*, vol. 13, no. 11, pp. 63–69, 2014.

[6] A. O. Yadav, B. H. Vanza, R. M. Borle, and K. A. Joglekar, "Custom made protective appliance for oral submucous fibrosis," *Journal of Maxillofacial & Oral Surgery*, vol. 12, no. 4, pp. 472–474, 2013.

[7] S. Cox and H. Zoellner, "Physiotherapeutic treatment improves oral opening in oral submucous fibrosis," *Journal of Oral Pathology & Medicine*, vol. 38, no. 2, pp. 220–226, 2009.

[8] V. Mehrotra, K. Garg, Z. Sajid, and P. Sharma, "The saviors: appliances used for the treatment of trismus," *International Journal of Preventive & Clinical Dental Research*, vol. 1, no. 3, pp. 62–67, 2014.

[9] P. Patil, V. Hazarey, R. Chaudhari, and S. Nimbalkar-Patil, "Clinical efficacy of a mouth-exercising device adjunct to local ointment intra-lesional injections and surgical treatment for oral submucous fibrosis: a randomized controlled trial," *Asian Pacific Journal of Cancer Prevention*, vol. 17, no. 3, pp. 1255–1259, 2016.

[10] C. Oswal, P. Gandhi, and A. Sabane, "Prosthodontic management of surgically treated oral sub mucous fibrosis using the oral screen prosthesis," *IOSR Journal of Dental and Medical Sciences*, vol. 10, no. 4, pp. 33–36, 2013.

[11] Y.-H. Li, C. C. Liu, T. E. Chiang, and Y. W. Chen, "EZBite open-mouth device: a new treatment option for oral submucous fibrosis-related trismus," *Journal of Dental Sciences*, vol. 13, no. 1, pp. 80-81, 2018.

[12] J. I. Kamstra, J. L. N. Roodenburg, C. H. G. Beurskens, H. Reintsema, and P. U. Dijkstra, "TheraBite exercises to treat trismus secondary to head and neck cancer," *Supportive Care in Cancer*, vol. 21, no. 4, pp. 951–957, 2013.

[13] J. I. Kamstra, H. Reintsema, J. L. N. Roodenburg, and P. U. Dijkstra, "Dynasplint trismus system exercises for trismus secondary to head and neck cancer: a prospective explorative study," *Supportive Care in Cancer*, vol. 24, no. 8, pp. 3315–3323, 2016.

Permissions

The contributors of this book come from diverse backgrounds, making this book a truly international effort. This book will bring forth new frontiers with its revolutionizing research information and detailed analysis of the nascent developments around the world.

We would like to thank all the contributing authors for lending their expertise to make the book truly unique. They have played a crucial role in the development of this book. Without their invaluable contributions this book wouldn't have been possible. They have made vital efforts to compile up to date information on the varied aspects of this subject to make this book a valuable addition to the collection of many professionals and students.

This book was conceptualized with the vision of imparting up-to-date information and advanced data in this field. To ensure the same, a matchless editorial board was set up. Every individual on the board went through rigorous rounds of assessment to prove their worth. After which they invested a large part of their time researching and compiling the most relevant data for our readers.

The editorial board has been involved in producing this book since its inception. They have spent rigorous hours researching and exploring the diverse topics which have resulted in the successful publishing of this book. They have passed on their knowledge of decades through this book. To expedite this challenging task, the publisher supported the team at every step. A small team of assistant editors was also appointed to further simplify the editing procedure and attain best results for the readers.

Apart from the editorial board, the designing team has also invested a significant amount of their time in understanding the subject and creating the most relevant covers. They scrutinized every image to scout for the most suitable representation of the subject and create an appropriate cover for the book.

The publishing team has been an ardent support to the editorial, designing and production team. Their endless efforts to recruit the best for this project, has resulted in the accomplishment of this book. They are a veteran in the field of academics and their pool of knowledge is as vast as their experience in printing. Their expertise and guidance has proved useful at every step. Their uncompromising quality standards have made this book an exceptional effort. Their encouragement from time to time has been an inspiration for everyone.

The publisher and the editorial board hope that this book will prove to be a valuable piece of knowledge for researchers, students, practitioners and scholars across the globe.

List of Contributors

P. Santander and S. Batschkus
Department of Orthodontics, University Medical Center, Göttingen, Germany

E. M. C. Schwaibold
Institute of Human Genetics, University Medical Center, Göttingen, Germany

F. Bremmer
Institute of Pathology, University Medical Center, Göttingen, Germany

P. Kauffmann
Department of Maxillofacial Surgery, University Medical Center, Göttingen, Germany

Priyanka Agarwal, Rashmi Nayak and Ghayathri Elangovan
Department of Pedodontics and Preventive Dentistry, Manipal College of Dental Sciences, Manipal 576104, Karnataka, India

Gregor-Georg Zafiropoulos
College of Dental Medicine, University of Sharjah, Sharjah, UAE

Andreas Parashis
College of Dentistry, Ohio State University, Columbus, OH, USA

Taha Abdullah and Evangelos Sotiropoulos
College of Dental Medicine, Mohammed Bin Rashid University of Medicine and Health Sciences, Dubai, UAE

Gordon John
School of Dentistry, University of Duesseldorf, Duesseldorf, Germany

**Dhana Lakshmi Jeyasivanesan, Shameena Pazhaningal Mohamed
and Deepak Pandiar**
Department of Oral Pathology and Microbiology, Government Dental College, Kozhikode, India

Yoselíin Méndez-Salado, Paola De Ávila-Rojas, Amaury Pozos-Guillén, Raúl Márquez-Preciado, Miguel Ángel Noyola-Frías, Socorro Ruiz-Rodríguez and Arturo Garrocho-Rangel
Pediatric Dentistry Postgraduate Program, Faculty of Dentistry, San Luis Potosi University, San Luis Potosi, SLP, Mexico

Farzad Piroozmand
Department of Orthodontics, School of Dentistry, Tehran University of Medical Sciences, International Campus, Tehran, Iran

Hossein Hessari and Pegah Khazaei
Research Center for Caries Prevention, Dentistry Research Institute, Tehran University of Medical Sciences, Tehran, Iran

Mohsen Shirazi
Department of Orthodontics, School of Dentistry, Tehran University of Medical Sciences, Tehran, Iran

Ravi Kumar Mahto, Dashrath Kafle and Aradhana Agarwal
Department of Orthodontics, Dhulikhel Hospital, Kathmandu University School of Medical Sciences,Dhulikhel, Nepal

Shantanu Dixit
Department of Oral Medicine and Radiology, Dhulikhel Hospital, Kathmandu University School of Medical Sciences,Dhulikhel, Nepal

Michael Bornstein
Oral and Maxillofacial Radiology, Applied Oral Sciences, Faculty of Dentistry, University of Hong Kong,Pokfulam, Hong Kong

Sanad Dulal
Department of Oral and Maxillofacial Surgery, Dhulikhel Hospital, Kathmandu University School of Medical Sciences,Dhulikhel, Nepal

Norberto Sugaya and Dante Migliari
Division of Oral Medicine Clinic, Department of Stomatology, School of Dentistry, University of Sao Paulo, Sao Paulo, SP, Brazil

Nikolaos Soldatos, Michelle Michaiel, Ali Sajadi, Nikola Angelov and Robin Weltman
Department of Periodontics and Dental Hygiene, School of Dentistry, University of Texas Health Science Center at Houston,Houston, TX, USA

Georgios E. Romanos
Department of Periodontology, School of Dental Medicine, Stony Brook University, Stony Brook, NY, USA

Georgios E. Romanos
Department of Oral Surgery and Implant Dentistry, Johann Wolfgang Goethe University of Frankfurt, Frankfurt, Germany

Peter Fairbairn
Department of Periodontology and Implant Dentistry, School of Dentistry, University of Detroit Mercy, 2700 Martin Luther King Jr. Boulevard, Detroit, MI 48208, USA

Minas Leventis
Department of Oral and Maxillofacial Surgery, Dental School, National and Kapodistrian University of Athens, 2,ivon Street,Goudi, Athens 115 27, Greece

Chas Mangham
Manchester Molecular Pathology Innovation Centre,,e University of Manchester, Nelson Street, Manchester M13 9NQ, UK

Robert Horowitz
Departments of Periodontics, Implant Dentistry, and Oral Surgery, New York University College of Dentistry, 345 E. 24th Street,New York, NY 10010, USA

Geórgia Silva and Ana Cristina Normandes
School Superior of Amazonia (ESAMAZ), Bel´em, PA, Brazil

Edson Barros Júnior
College São Leopoldo Mandic (SLMANDIC), Bel´em, PA, Brazil

Joyce Gatti, Kalena Maranhão, Ana Cássia Reis, Fernanda Jasse´, Lucas Moura and Thaís Barros
School of Dentistry, School Superior of Amazonia (ESAMAZ), Belém, PA, Brazil

Arturo Garrocho-Rangel, Andrea Gómez-González, Adriana Torre-Delgadillo, Socorro Ruiz-Rodríguez and Amaury Pozos-Guillén
Pediatric Dentistry Postgraduate Program, Faculty of Dentistry, San Luis Potosi University, San Luis Potosi, SLP, Mexico

Zaki Hakami
Department of Preventive Dental Sciences, Division of Orthodontics, College of Dentistry, Jazan University, Jazan, Saudi Arabia

Po Jung Chen and Ahmad Ahmida
Division of Orthodontics, School of Dental Medicine, University of Connecticut, Farmington, CT, USA

Nandakumar Janakiraman
Georgia School of Orthodontics, Atlanta, GA, USA

Flavio Uribe
Division of Orthodontics, Department of Craniofacial Sciences, School of Dental Medicine, University of Connecticut,Farmington, CT, USA

Luca Francetti, Silvio Taschieri, Nicolò Cavalli and Stefano Corbella
Department of Biomedical, Surgical and Dental Sciences, Universit`a degli Studi di Milano, Milan, Italy
IRCCS Istituto Ortopedico Galeazzi, Milan, Italy

Vincenzo Luca Zizzari
Private Practice, Via Benedetto Croce, 85/D, Foggia 71122, Italy
Department of Medical, Oral and Biotechnological Sciences, University "G. d'Annunzio", Chieti-Pescara, Italy

Gianmarco Tacconelli
Department of Medical, Oral and Biotechnological Sciences, University "G. d'Annunzio", Chieti-Pescara, Italy

Dhanalaxmi Karre and Silla Swarna Swathi
Department of Pedodontics, Sri Sai College of Dental Surgery, Vikarabad, India

Mahesh Kumar duddu
Department of Pedodontics, G Pulla Reddy Dental College, Kurnool, India

Abdul Habeeb Bin Mohsin
Department of Prosthodontics, Sri Sai College of Dental Surgery, Vikarabad, India

Bhogavaram Bharadwaj
Department of Oral and Maxillofacial Surgery, Sri Sai College of Dental Surgery, Vikarabad, India

Sheraz Barshaik
Department of Oral and Maxillofacial Surgery, MNR Dental College and Hospital, Sangareddy, India

A. M. Espinoza-Coronado, J. H.Olvera-Delgado, J. O. García-Cortes and J. F. Reyes-Macías
Advanced Education in General Dentistry, Master Degree Program at San Luis Potosi University, Faculty of Dentistry of San Luis Potosi, Universidad Aut´onoma de San Luis Potosí, San Luis Potosi, SLP, Mexico

J. P. Loyola-Rodríguez
Escuela Superior de Odontolog´ıa y Doctorado en Ciencias Biom´edicas, Universidad Aut´onoma de Guerrero, Acapulco, GRO, Mexico

O. Marouane, N. Douki and F. Chtioui
Restorative Dentistry, Dental Surgery Department, Sahloul University Hospital, Sousse, Tunisia

Hind Alquthami
Department of Dentistry, Division of Endodontics, Prince Sultan Military Medical City, P.O. Box 7897, Riyadh 11159, Saudi Arabia

Abdulaziz M. Almalik
Department of Dentistry, Division of Periodontics, Prince Sultan Military Medical City, Riyadh, Saudi Arabia

Faisal F. Alzahrani
Department of Dentistry, Division of Orthodontics, Prince Sultan Military Medical City, Riyadh, Saudi Arabia

Lana Badawi
Department of Dentistry, Division of Endodontics, Prince Sultan Military Medical City, Riyadh, Saudi Arabia

Rafael de Lima Franceschi and Luciano Drechsel
Brasilian Association of Dental Surgeons, Curitiba, PR, Brazil
Dental Institute of the Americas, Balneário Camboriú, SC, Brazil
São Leopoldo Mandic University, Curitiba, PR, Brazil

Luciano Drechsel
Brazilian Dental Association (ABO), Ponta Grossa, PR, Brazil

Guenther Schuldt Filho
Federal University of Santa Catarina, Florianópolis, SC, Brazil

Bianca Tozi Portaluppe Bergantin, Daniela Rios and Heitor Marques Honório
Department of Pediatric Dentistry, Orthodontics and Public Health, Bauru School of Dentistry, University of São Paulo, Bauru,SP, Brazil

Daniela Silva Barroso Oliveira
Department of Clinic and Surgery, Federal University of Alfenas, Rua Gabriel Monteiro da Silva, 700, 37130000 Alfenas, MG, Brazil

Edmêr Silvestre Pereira Júnior and João Adolfo Costa Hanemann
Department of Clinic and Surgery, Pediatric Dentistry, Federal University of Alfenas, Rua Gabriel Monteiro da Silva, 700, 37130000 Alfenas, MG, Brazil

Marina Consuelo Vitale, Maria Francesca Sfondrini, Lorenzo Carbone, Paola Gandini and Andrea Scribante
Unit of Orthodontics and Paediatric Dentistry, Section of Dentistry, Department of Clinical, Surgical,Diagnostic and Paediatric Sciences, University of Pavia, Pavia, Italy

Giorgio Alberto Croci and Marco Paulli
Unit of Anatomic Pathology, Department of Molecular Medicine, University of Pavia and Fondazione IRCCS Policlinico San Matteo, Pavia, Italy

Gianluca Tenore, Ahmed Mohsen, Giorgio Pompa, Edoardo Brauner, Andrea Cassoni, Valentino Valentini, Antonella Polimeni and Umberto Romeo
Department of Oral and Maxillofacial Sciences, "Sapienza" University of Rome, Rome, Italy

Hayati Murat Akgül, Fatma Çağlayan and Gözde Derindağ
Department of Oral and Maxillofacial Radiology, Faculty of Dentistry, Ataturk University, Erzurum, Turkey

Sevcihan Günen Yılmaz
Department of Oral and Maxillofacial Radiology, Faculty of Dentistry, Akdeniz University, Antalya, Turkey

I. Kanimozhi
Government Medical College, Tuticorin, Tamil Nadu, India

Mahesh Ramakrishnan and Dhanalakshmi Ravikumar
Department of Pedodontics and Preventive Dentistry, Saveetha Dental College, Chennai, Tamil Nadu, India

Ningthoujam Sharna
Private Pratice, Imphal, Manipur, India

Aminah M. El Mourad
Department of Restorative Dental Sciences, King Saud University, Riyadh, Saudi Arabia

Vasileios I. Theofilou, Alexandra Sklavounou and Evanthia Chrysomali
Department of Oral Medicine and Pathology, School of Dentistry, National and Kapodistrian University of Athens, Athens, Greece

Prokopios P. Argyris
Department of Diagnostic and Biological Sciences, School of Dentistry, University of Minnesota, Minneapolis, MN, USA

Amanda Phoon Nguyen, Norman Firth and Omar Kujan
UWA Dental School, University of Western Australia, Nedlands, WA 6009, Australia

Sophie Mougos
Private Practice, OMFSurgery, Cambridge Street, Wembley, WA, Australia

G. Esteve-Pardo and L. Esteve-Colomina
Private Practice at Clínica Dental Esteve SL, Group Aula Dental Avanzada, Alicante, Spain

Sankalp Mittal
Department of Oral and Maxillofacial Surgery, Government Dental College (RUHS-CODS), Jaipur, India

Manoj Agarwal
Department of Conservative, Government Dental College (RUHS-CODS), Jaipur, India

Debopriya Chatterjee
Department of Periodontics, Government Dental College (RUHS-CODS), Jaipur, India

Manveen Kaur Jawanda and Chitra Anandani
Department of Oral Pathology, Luxmi Bai Institute of Dental Sciences, Patiala, Punjab, India

R. V. Subramanyam
Department of OMFS and Diagnostic Sciences, College of Dentistry, King Faisal University, Al-Ahasa 31982, Saudi Arabia

Harshaminder Grewal
Department of Oral Pathology, Desh Bhagat Dental College, Mandi Gobindgarh, Punjab, India

Ravi Narula
Department of Oral and Maxillofacial Surgery, Guru Nanak Dev Dental College, Sunam, Punjab, India

Tsz Leung Wong and Michael George Botelho
Prosthodontics, Faculty of Dentistry, The University of Hong Kong, Sai Ying Pun, Hong Kong

Houda Dogui, Feriel Abdelmalek, Adel Amor and Nabiha Douki
Department of Dental Medicine, Hospital Sahloul, Sousse, Faculty of Dental Medicine, Monastir, Tunisia
Laboratory of Research in Oral Health and Maxillo Facial Rehabilitation (LR12ES11), University of Monastir, Monastir, Tunisia
Faculty of Dental Medicine, University of Monastir, Monastir, Tunisia

Hisashi Ozaki
Department of Dentistry, Oral and Maxillofacial Surgery, Yamagata Prefectural Central Hospital, Yamagata, Japan
Department of Dentistry, Oral and Maxillofacial-Plastic and Reconstructive Surgery, Faculty of Medicine, Yamagata University, Yamagata, Japan

Yukie Yoshida, Hideyuki Yamanouchi and Mitsuyoshi Iino
Department of Dentistry, Oral and Maxillofacial-Plastic and Reconstructive Surgery, Faculty of Medicine, Yamagata University,Yamagata, Japan

Hiromasa Sakurai
Department of Dentistry, Oral and Maxillofacial Surgery, Nihonkai General Hospital, Yamagata Prefectural and Sakata Municipal Hospital Organization, Sakata, Japan

Zhujun Li, Zhengxi Chen and Zhenqi Chen
Department of Orthodontics, Shanghai Ninth People's Hospital, School of Stomatology, Shanghai Key Laboratory of Stomatology,Shanghai Jiao Tong University, Shanghai, China

Jian Sun
Department of Stomatology, Shanghai East Hospital, Tongji University School of Medicine, Shanghai, China

Li'an Yang
Department of Stomatology, Xin Hua Hospital Affiliated to Shanghai Jiao Tong University School of Medicine,Shanghai Jiao Tong University, Shanghai, China

Nallan C. S. K. Chaitanya, Reshma Priyanka Danam, Madireddy Nithika, Chintada Suvarna and Jampala Nancypriyanka
Department of Oral Medicine and Radiology, Panineeya Institute of Dental Sciences, Hyderabad, India

C. M. S. Krishna Prasad and Rajkumar Badam
Department of Orthodontics and Dentofacial Orthopedics, Panineeya Institute of Dental Sciences, Hyderabad, India

Index